Developmental Hand Dysfunction

Theory, Assessment, and Treatment
(Second Edition)

Rhoda P. Erhardt, M.S., OTR, FAOTA

Illustrations by Gary Baune

Therapy Skill Builders® 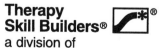®
a division of
The Psychological Corporation

555 Academic Court
San Antonio, Texas 78204-2498
1-800-228-0752

Reproducing Pages from This Book

As described below, some of the pages in this book may be reproduced for instructional or administrative use (not for resale). To protect your book, make a photocopy of each reproducible page. Then use that copy as a master for photocopying.

 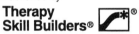

The first edition of this book was dedicated to

My children, Edward, Elizabeth, Jane, and Sally, who taught me how to love other children.

This second edition is dedicated to

Gloria Dosland, 1930-1991, the first of many parents who have had a profound influence on my professional philosophies and attitudes toward children with disabilities and their families. Her fierce determination to help her daughter Joanne reach her full potential was the original inspiration for my work in the area of cerebral palsy.

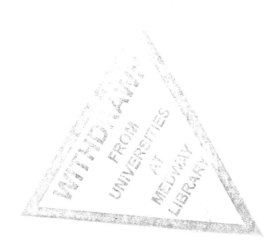

About the Author

Rhoda Priest Erhardt, M.S., OTR, FAOTA, received her bachelor of science degree in occupational therapy from the University of Illinois, and her master's degree in child development and family relations from North Dakota State University. She was trained in pediatric Neuro-Developmental Treatment (NDT) in London, England.

The former director of the Easter Seal Mobile Therapy Unit in Fargo, North Dakota, Mrs. Erhardt is currently in private practice in the Minneapolis/St. Paul area, providing evaluation and consultation services to a variety of health agencies, educational systems, and national corporations, as well as presenting workshops throughout the world. She has served on the editorial board of the *American Journal of Occupational Therapy* and the Board of Occupational Therapy Practice of the state of North Dakota, and was enrolled in the AOTA Roster of Fellows in 1983.

Mrs. Erhardt's publications include books, chapters, journal articles, assessments, and videotapes on topics such as prehension, vision, eye-hand coordination, and feeding problems in children with cerebral palsy as well as perceptual problems in children with learning disabilities. Her videotape on normal hand development received an award from the American Academy for Cerebral Palsy and Developmental Medicine.

Contents

Preface and Acknowledgments to the First Edition

How does a book get written? I don't think anyone suddenly decides one day to write a book. A more likely thought, one I have had many times, is "I wish I could write a book."

After graduating from the University of Illinois in 1953 and serving for two years in the Women's Medical Specialist Corps of the U.S. Army, I relinquished my profession to become a full-time housewife and mother. During that ten-year hiatus, reading became a primary source of mental stimulation. I remember wishing fervently that I could write a novel, but I was very well aware that I lacked the ability and the energy. I satisfied my creative writing urge as best I could with yearly Christmas letters, which were sometimes described as similar to the writings of Erma Bombeck.

Shortly after resuming my career in 1967, my interests and skills began to focus, first on the field of pediatrics, then developmental disabilities (especially cerebral palsy), and finally on prehension. Because I had been out of the field for so many years, I needed to resume intensive professional reading, attend workshops, and finally, from 1972 to 1974, pursue graduate study, while simultaneously applying this new information to clinical experiences. The publication of two journal articles (1970 and 1974) was an impetus to continue writing.

Probably the most significant influence on my theoretical thinking, as well as on that of therapists, physicians, and teachers all over the world, was the work done in the field of cerebral palsy by Dr. Karel Bobath and his wife, Berta Bobath, who originated Neuro-Developmental Treatment. The opportunity to travel to London, England, and attend the Bobaths' NDT training course in 1977 was made possible by Dr. D. Ross Halliday, president of the North Dakota Medical Association, and Wilbur Ashworth, director of the Easter Seal Society of North Dakota.

By the spring of 1981, with the help and expert research skills of Dr. Patricia Beatty, department of psychology, and Dr. Doris Hertsgaard, department of mathematical science, North Dakota State University, an interrater reliability study of the Erhardt Developmental Prehension Assessment was completed and reported in another published article. An integral component of that study was a series of videotapes meticulously produced by David Roberts, chief of medical photography, Biomedical Media, University of North Dakota School of Medicine.

Another videotaped project, *Normal Hand Development: Birth to 15 Months,* begun in the summer of 1980, was completed in the fall of 1981 after approximately 40 hours of filming time and 200 hours of editing. Dan Pullen, studio director of the TV Production Center, Moorhead State University, contributed his high professional standards and rare sense of humor to this study, which was sponsored by the special education department, with the assistance of Dr. Norman Buktenica, chairperson of the education department. The videotape was delightfully narrated by Marjorie Sanders, educational consultant, who not only spent many hours editing this manuscript, but was also an inspiring mentor for many years.

Ongoing professional support was also received from many Fargo physicians, especially Dr. Joseph Cullen, Dr. D. Ross Halliday, and Dr. Marvin Kolb, who all consented to review and edit the manuscript from the physician's viewpoint and to collaborate in writing the foreword.

The actual writing of the book took exactly one year, after at least 12 years of preparation. During that time the mass of ideas whirling around in various states of confusion in my head was directly proportional to the size of my collection of reference materials, card files, and voluminous notes. The final synthesis of these ideas and information seemed to occur miraculously when my stepsister, Wendy, and her husband, Jere, provided an ideal supportive living environment during the three-week NDT Baby Course in New York in the summer of 1981. My brother, Ben, added his personal encouragement at that time, also.

The writing began. Now the help from many sources became even more practical. Vern Hunter, architect with Hunter and Grobe, Architects/Planners, gave generously of his time, granting interviews, suggesting valuable references, editing certain sections of the manuscript, and posing as the model to illustrate normal adult patterns. Sheldon Green, editor of *Horizons* magazine, provided vivid photographs of impressive quality. Colburn Hvidston III, president of the National Press Photographers Association and photo chief of *The Forum,* secured permission for our use of photos from feature articles previously published in that newspaper. Gary Baune, whose previous art work has been described by the *New England Journal of Medicine* as "artistically valid" and "providing memorable images," produced an incredible quantity of exciting, accurate, and charming illustrations. Dr. Anne Brunton, chairperson of the sociology and anthropology department, Moorhead State University, and Dr. Bill Brunton, chairperson of the department of sociology-anthropology, North Dakota State University, were among countless other colleagues who recommended references in less familiar fields such as anthropology, education, and psychology.

When the book was finished, almost one year to the day from when it was begun, it seemed as though it had written itself. Through discussions with the parents of the three children whose case studies are presented, I came to realize that the book's content was derived directly from the children themselves. They have taught us what we need to know. I am deeply grateful to Gloria and Joanne Dosland; Sallie, John, and Patrick Mooneyham; and Carmon, Mike, and Kristy Cymbal. They have amazed me with their determination, patience, and creativity. But most of all, I value their friendship.

The following therapists participated in the 1979 interrater reliability study and the 1981 information field testing of the Erhardt Developmental Prehension Assessment (EDPA). Their help is very much appreciated.

> Judy Bartels
> Katherine Bellin
> Regina Bergantine
> Gloria Frolek Clark
> Jeannine Colburn
> Janet Engbring
> Nancy Fridley
> Karen Johnson
> Mary Jo Krahn
> Lori Kubat
> Sherry Loen-Brakke
> Mary Lou Lorenz
> Linda Malloy
> Joanne Mauch
> Anne Moore
> Janet Smith Olson
> Diane Rath
> Sheila Allen Robley
> Barbara Schnobrick
> Martha Talmadge
> Sally Wieland
> Mary Lou Wittman
> Nancy Koering Wolff

The ten babies whose parents graciously allowed them to be videotaped for the study *Normal Hand Development: Birth to 15 Months* were:

> David, son of Virginia and Tom Elliott
> Cathy, daughter of Sharon and Gary Fettes
> Shannon, daughter of Char and Charles Krieg
> Randy, son of Denice and Terry McLeod
> Tim, son of Sharon and John Michlitsch
> Ryan, son of Sallie and John Mooneyham
> Joshua, son of Susan and Craig Nelson
> Mikkel, son of Jana and Tom Rockne
> Erin, daughter of Mary Ann and Curt Smith
> Erica, daughter of Georgene and Mike Stone

Developmental Hand Dysfunction

Preface and Acknowledgments to the Second Edition

After publication of the first edition of this book in 1982, I continued my involvement with the families of the three children whose case studies were presented. My role as Kristy's occupational therapist changed from direct service provider to evaluator and consultant to her school staff (occupational therapist, physical therapist, speech therapist, teachers, paraprofessionals) and home caregivers (family, home health aides, respite care providers). Patrick's family had been transferred to three different states, but my lecture travel schedule allowed me to visit him every few years for consultation to his family and current therapists. When Joanne's family moved out of town, I provided intermittent evaluation and consultation under contract with her school district until she moved into an adult foster care home out of state.

Early in 1992, I realized that ten years had passed, and "my" children were transitioning into adulthood. They were changing, and so was the world in which they were living. They and their families had different priorities, and new federal legislation for persons with disabilities promised opportunities for increased independence through technology, funding for caregivers, and supportive employment programs. At the same time, changes were occurring in my profession of occupational therapy and in the multidisciplinary area of cerebral palsy. Frames of reference were moving from developmental to more functional approaches, with emphasis on occupational performance. Newer terminology was replacing language that had developed negative connotations (for example, "atypical" rather than "abnormal"). Neuro-Developmental Treatment (NDT) theory was in the process of incorporating the new theories of motor control and motor learning. It was apparent that a second edition of *Developmental Hand Dysfunction* was needed to update the theoretical material and show its application to current treatment models.

My conversations with the parents reflected their concerns about these changes and the new decisions to be made that would affect their children, siblings, and themselves during these transitions to adulthood. The Individual Education Plans (IEP), Individual Transition Plans (ITP), and Individual Service Plans (ISP) being written for these teenagers and adults placed heavy emphasis on functional environmental domains: domestic, vocational, leisure, and community. It was an ideal time to re-evaluate their hand function and make specific recommendations for intervention which would address their concerns for the future. I had been in the process of revising the language of the Erhardt Developmental Prehension Assessment (EDPA), using extensive feedback from colleagues and workshop participants, as well as my own experience with the assessment during the last ten years. The newly revised EDPA was ready to be used for the three case studies, and I was fortunately able to connect once more with each of them.

All three evaluations were videotaped, scored, and interpreted, with input from families and certain team members, who also assisted in planning the treatment programs and participated in the photo illustrations. Appreciation for their creativity and patience is extended to:

Joanne Dosland, her father Peter, sisters Valerie, Catherine, and Jacki Williams, niece and nephew Leigh and Christopher Hale, adult foster care supervisor Kristi Middleton, and job coach Barb Thoren,

Patrick Mooneyham, his parents Sallie and John, his brother Ryan, his personal trainer Darrel Hutchinson, and his physical therapists Kirsten Ness and Susan Ducote, and

Kristy Cymbal, her parents Carmon and Mike, her sister Tracy, her occupational therapist Val Schock, and her caregiver Becky Kleinknecht.

Special thanks is extended to Godfather's Pizza, Inc., Joanne's place of employment.

Foreword to the First Edition

The management and treatment of children who are physically impaired has been an ongoing concern and challenge not only to pediatricians, orthopedists, and neurologists, but also to therapists, teachers, and parents. New and more effective solutions to puzzling problems frequently result from the recognition and application of changing theoretical principles. The area of prehension, in particular, has deserved more attention because of the importance of hand use for intellectual growth and independence in self-help skills.

This book, a result of the author's many years of study, clinical experience, advanced training, research, and teaching, comprehensively reviews the work of other professionals from a variety of fields and clearly illustrates how this cumulative scientific knowledge can be creatively integrated and interpreted for practical use in therapy, education, and daily living activities.

Significant improvement in many handicapped children has already been demonstrated as the development of innovative theories leads to exploration of new methods and modalities. It is anticipated that through dissemination and reception of the information in this book, advances will continue to be made in the remediation of upper extremity dysfunction.

Joseph M. Cullen, M.D.
Pediatric Neurologist, The Neuropsychiatric Institute, Fargo, North Dakota

Assistant Clinical Professor of Neurology, University of North Dakota School of Medicine

D. Ross Halliday, M.D.
President, North Dakota Medical Association

Associate Clinical Professor of Orthopedic Surgery, University of North Dakota School of Medicine

Marvin O. Kolb, M.D.
Chairman, Department of Pediatrics, Fargo Clinic, Fargo, North Dakota

Assistant Clinical Professor of Pediatrics, University of North Dakota School of Medicine

Foreword to the Second Edition

I have never known a child with handicaps who improved without the efforts of loving parents and dedicated therapists. The most caring of parents and the most involved therapists will be "handicapped" without the knowledge contained in Rhoda Erhardt's newest book, *Developmental Hand Dysfunction: Theory, Assessment, and Treatment (Second Edition)*.

This book is a result of the author's many years of experience, training, and research applied to a select group of children over a long period of time. Remediation of upper extremity dysfunction through the therapeutic modalities graphically demonstrated in the following pages will allow children's therapists to give their patients the best chances for success in school and in life.

Ron H. Miller, M.D.

Clinical Associate Professor of Pediatrics

University of North Dakota School of Medicine

Former Chair, Department of Pediatrics, Fargo Clinic

The Children . . .

Joanne
(photo courtesy of
Gloria Dosland)

Kristy
(photo courtesy of
Carmon and Mike Cymbal)

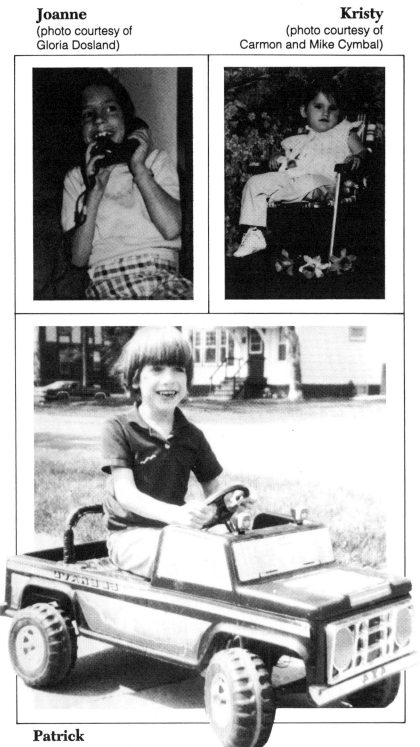

Patrick
(photo courtesy of
Sallie and John Mooneyham)

Transitions to Adulthood

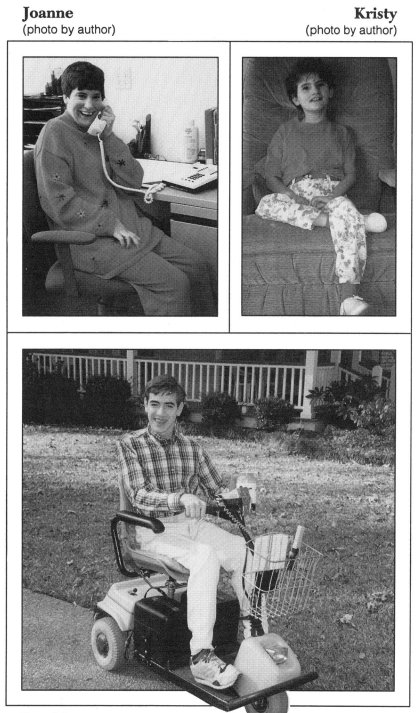

Joanne
(photo by author)

Kristy
(photo by author)

Patrick
(photo by author)

Introduction: The Children
Three Case Studies

The hand is a masterpiece. It can sense and act at the same time.
It acts as if it had the gift of vision . . . the hand adjusts itself to the hardest as
well as to the most sensitive work: with equal ease it has handled the stone knife
of the prehistoric hunter, the hammer of the blacksmith, the ax of the woodcutter,
the plow of the peasant, the sword of the medieval knight . . .
the brush of the artist, the pen of the writer. . . .
(paraphrased from Carrel 1935, 97-98)

Joanne

The first time I saw Joanne, she was 15 months old. She lay on the floor, soundless and almost motionless, barely aware of her mother or her twin sister, Valerie, who squatted beside her, offering an unnoticed toy (figure 1).

Despite being born six weeks prematurely and having a low birth weight (2 pounds, 9 ounces), Valerie had developed normally. She moved constantly around the room, crawling on hands and knees, climbing up on furniture, walking back and forth, always reaching, touching, grasping, and exploring.

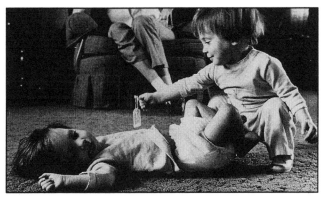

Figure 1. Joanne and her twin sister Valerie at 15 months: comparisons of arm and hand use (photo by Colburn Hvidston III, courtesy of *The Forum*)

Joanne, however, who had weighed 2 pounds, 8 ounces, had not breathed spontaneously and had suffered several episodes of apnea (cessation of breathing) during her first few days. She did not follow faces or objects with her eyes and did not turn her head consistently to sounds. Joanne had never rolled over, crawled, sat, or stood. Her hands remained closed, a symbol of Joanne herself, who, unlike Valerie, had not experienced the crucial first year of exploration and interaction with the world around her.

Importance of the Hand in Total Sensorimotor Development

Maria Montessori termed the hand "the instrument of intelligence" (Orem 1965). From the very beginning of life, the infant's hands are intricately involved in every aspect of total development: motor, social, language, and cognitive.

Even before birth, a total array of movements needed in later life is present and functional, according to Milani, who documented his findings on film with an ultrasound scanner (Milani-Comparetti 1980). Milani saw the fetus exploring the placenta as well as her own body with open hands, grasping and immediately releasing the umbilical cord, and sucking her thumb.

This first sensorimotor awareness of body image is expanded in the newborn, who strokes the mother's breast and gazes into her eyes during feeding, linking motor-social experience with the bonding process. Increasingly voluntary, repetitive, enjoyable movements such as arm waving are accompanied by spontaneous vocalizations, which elicit immediate verbal responses from the baby's mother. This first language, a dialogue of sounds between baby and caregiver, is enhanced by the interaction of motor and social stimuli.

Throughout the first year of life, the orderly progression of eye, head, shoulder, and trunk control enables the arm and hand to explore, manipulate, and control objects of various textures, shapes, sizes, and weights. This manual involvement with both animate and inanimate parts of the environment stimulates social development through motivation and imitation, language development through assignment of names and descriptive terms based on concrete experience, and cognitive development through organization and causal relationships.

But what happens to the total development of a child whose hands remain tightly closed during the first entire year of life?

Patrick

Even at the age of 4 years, Patrick used his left hand almost exclusively (figure 2). His right hand rarely helped to hold a toy, but it didn't lie limply in his lap, either. Patrick had a "flying hand," as his mother called it. No matter how often she reminded him, he could

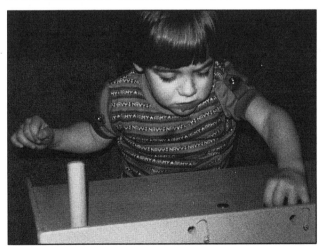

Figure 2. Position of Patrick's right arm during reaching with the left (photo by author)

not remember to keep his arm down and forward. Patrick could roll, sit unsteadily, and crawl, but he could neither stand nor walk. He understood almost everything that was said to him, but although he used a variety of sounds, he spoke only a few words clearly.

During the first few weeks of his life, he arched his neck and back so sharply that his shoulder blades almost touched in the back. It took many years before Patrick could clasp his hands together or transfer an object from one hand to the other. He tried to use his hands like other children, but all his effort only made his arms get tighter and his shoulders pull up higher, almost to his ears. He did not always look at what his hands were doing.

Abnormal Patterns Redefined as Developmentally Inappropriate

Milani refuted the traditional concept that the postures and movements of children with brain damage should simply be termed abnormal (Milani-Comparetti 1980). He observed that "fetal propulsion," for example, used for collaboration with uterine contractions during the labor process, resembles opisthotonia (hyperextended neck, back, arms, and legs, with internally rotated arms and fisted hands). He concluded that these patterns should be called regressive rather than abnormal, because they were seen in normal babies but developmentally earlier. He also traced the persistence of such patterns in the postnatal period to a prenatal or perinatal central nervous system insult.

Primitive reflexes, such as the Asymmetrical Tonic Neck (often described as the "fencing position"), are important in the normal baby's development to focus the eye on the hand for the first time (Fiorentino 1965). However, delayed integration, which interferes with progression from asymmetry to symmetry, results in the inability of the older child with brain damage to maintain visual fixation on an arm engaged in activities of flexion, such as spoon feeding. Instead, the child's head turns automatically toward the extended arm on the face side of the head as the arm on the skull side flexes.

The excess effort required to perform highly skilled hand movements that are above a child's present developmental level usually causes stress and reversion to earlier patterns such as asymmetrical neck extension, shoulder elevation, and scapular adduction, described by Haebig as blocks or fixes (Haebig 1980).

Developmental Hand Dysfunction

These patterns, which are normal in the very young infant, could be described as developmentally inappropriate rather than abnormal, a term which had developed a negative connotation.

Kristy

When Kristy was 2 years old, she spent most of her day on her back, contentedly watching people (figure 3). Attention from her family, especially her mother, excited her. She breathed faster, wiggled her fingers and toes, and smiled. When she was held, her hands would sometimes touch her mother's face or her own face, but Kristy did not seem to be aware that those hands belonged to her or that she could control them. She was hardly ever on her stomach because she couldn't lift her head to see anything, and she never reached for toys. Kristy could not roll over, sit up, or crawl. When she was held upright, her head needed to be supported and her arms were held rigidly backward, hands out of her view. Kristy rarely vocalized unless she was unhappy.

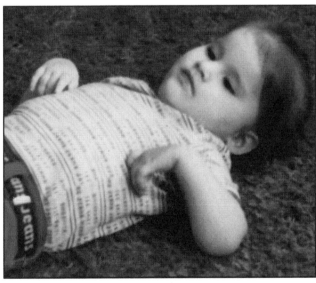

Figure 3. Upper extremity posture preventing Kristy's visual awareness of her hands (photo courtesy of Carmon and Mike Cymbal)

Cerebral Palsy and the Unique Child

Joanne, Patrick, and Kristy all have cerebral palsy and are developmentally delayed. Joanne's diagnosis is spastic quadriplegia. Patrick has athetoid quadriplegia with spasticity. Kristy, also quadriplegic, has hypotonia with spasticity. Each child has individual arm and hand patterns that are related to total body motor development as well as to latitudinal (cognitive, language, and social) growth. With or without handicaps, every child is a unique, complex integration of genetic and environmental influences, constantly changing, reacting, and, most of all, adapting to a world filled with objects and people. The child is an active participant.

This exciting process of development, although interrupted, delayed, and sometimes developmentally inappropriate, is illustrated by these three case studies. Theories are explored, evaluations administered, and intervention programs presented, all focused on prehension. To enhance the reader's learning process, comparisons of specific problems, individual learning styles, and treatment modifications are included. In addition, since the concept of development as a continuing process embraces the total life cycle, prehension patterns of adulthood are also considered.

The Architect

Perched on a stool at his drawing board, the architect quickly and skillfully sketches a perspective rendition of a new building. The pencil is held lightly in his fingers like a paintbrush (figure 4). As the drawing takes shape, he begins to define the lines carefully, now holding the pencil in a typical tripod grasp (figure 5). Precise lettering produces more changes in posture. His shoulders become more elevated, and as he rests his nondominant forearm on the board close to his chest, his hand closes tightly (figure 6). Rising, he moves to a flat table, where he places a large sheet of

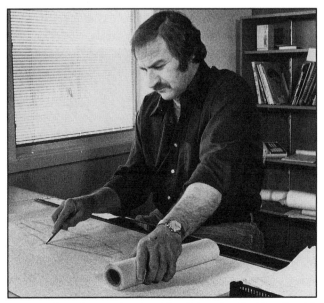

Figure 4. Pencil grasp for sketching (photo by Sheldon Green)

poster board. He begins to cut it with a knife, which he holds in his fist in a vertical power grip (figure 7).

In the space of a few minutes, a variety of hand grasps have been used. The essential activity, that of drawing or following a line on paper, is the same, but

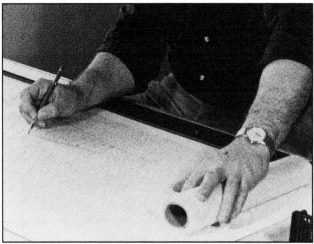
Figure 5. Typical tripod grasp (photo by Sheldon Green)

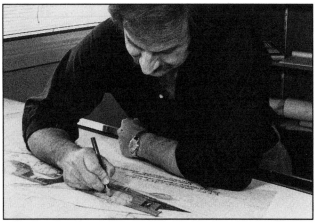
Figure 6. Postural stabilization for increased precision (photo by Sheldon Green)

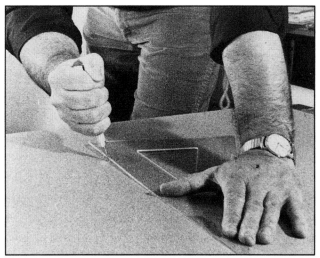
Figure 7. Power grip for knife use (photo by Sheldon Green)

the nature of the activity, the requirements of speed, precision, and strength, have obviously influenced the type of prehension of the tool and the position of the body (Napier 1956).

Many of the arm-hand postures and movements of adults with normal abilities are reminiscent of developing childhood patterns. Close observation and comparison of these patterns make the study of prehension more meaningful and relevant to the problems of developmentally delayed children, adolescents, and adults.

Bloom's Taxonomy: An Aid to the Study of Prehension

Bloom's taxonomy of educational objectives for the cognitive domain suggests that learning begins at the level of Knowledge, which can be described with verbs such as *list* and *define*. A study of prehension, then, may begin with a list of theories and definitions of terms. Level two, Comprehension, is concerned with *reviewing* and *discussing* those theories. Level three, Application, should *interpret* and *illustrate* the theories, using our case studies. Level four is termed Analysis, *comparing* and *differentiating* similarities and differences between normal and abnormal or atypical development.

By achieving these four levels, the reader is prepared for level five, Synthesis, *designing* and *constructing* a comprehensive, integrated, and practical theory of prehension, which serves as a framework for the evolving of a developmental prehension assessment. Level six, Evaluation, then proceeds with *measuring* and *scoring* of the assessment (Bloom 1956).

References

Bloom, B. 1956. Taxonomy of educational objectives. In *Handbook 1: The cognitive domain*. New York: David McKay.

Carrel, A. 1935. *Man the unknown*. New York: Harper.

Fiorentino, M. R. 1965. *Reflex testing methods for evaluating C.N.S. development*. Springfield, IL: Charles C. Thomas.

Haebig [Boehme], R. 1980 (October). Developmental kinesiology. Presented at Neuro-Developmental Treatment (NDT) Refresher Weekend. Chicago, Illinois.

Milani-Comparetti, A. 1980 (October). The prenatal development of movement: Implications for developmental diagnosis. Presented at Professional Development Programs. St. Paul, Minnesota.

Napier, J. R. 1956. The prehensile movements of the human hand. *Journal of Bone and Joint Surgery* 38B:902-13.

Orem, R. C. 1965. *Montessori handbook*. New York: G. P. Putnam's Sons.

PART ONE

Theoretical Rationale

Chapter One
Joanne

The Medical Orthopedic Approaches

Occupational therapists traditionally have been involved with the evaluation and treatment of hand dysfunction because of the human hand's close association with adaptive and independence skills. For undergraduate students, the acquisition of knowledge begins with basic anatomy: the normal hand is both compact and complex, containing 27 bones and 18 intrinsic muscles (Johnson 1973).

No portion of the body of equal volume contains as many end-organs of cutaneous and kinesthetic senses as the hand; no other part incorporates in as limited a section as many possibilities for varied action. First, the hand possesses great range of movement because of its suspension at the end of the arm. Its freedom of operation is due to the three arm joints (shoulder, elbow, and wrist) and to the rotary action of the radius on the ulna bone in the forearm.

The hand's manipulatory and exploratory qualifications are impressive because of its five long digits with 14 phalangeal segments, the sensitive fingertips, and the prehensile value of the thumb opposition to the other four digits. The reach, strength, flexibility, and speed of the fingers and adaptabilities of grasp to the size, shape, weight, position, and disposal of the object are infinite in variety (Halverson 1931).

A Quantitative View

At the University of Illinois in the early 1950s, occupational therapy students were introduced to the developmental theories of Dr. Arnold Gesell, who had studied thousands of infants at the Yale Child Development Center in New York, but the major orientation from the College of Medicine, which housed the Occupational Therapy Department, was almost purely orthopedic. Most of the other several dozen accredited occupational therapy schools throughout the country at that time produced a generation of graduates who, like their physical therapist and physician contemporaries, considered assessment and treatment goals quantitatively—that is, in terms of degrees of joint range of motion, the number grade of muscle strength, coordination (usually timed tests), and activities of daily living (how many skills could be accomplished).

This approach was usually effective for patients with conditions such as polio, arthritis, and peripheral nerve injuries, but it was less satisfactory when dealing with stroke or cerebral palsy. Strengthening what were thought to be weak muscles only increased spasticity, particularly in other parts of the body (associated reactions). Excess effort during dressing, feeding, or writing activities resulted in patterns termed abnormal that became reinforced with repetition. Stress appearing whenever speed was required produced similar effects. Patients were sacrificing quality of movement in order to learn new skills, but there seemed to be no alternative.

Traditional Treatment vs. Neuro-Developmental Treatment

The typical treatment of cerebral palsy between 1930 and 1950 was described in a well-known retrospective study at the Children's Hospital in Boston as a heterogeneous group of methods including passive stretching, muscle re-education, functional training for self-care, bracing, and surgery (Paine 1962). The data presented in that study indicated little difference in improvement between the treated and untreated group, reflecting the generally pessimistic prognosis for cerebral palsy that pervaded professionals' attitudes at that time. Therapists taught children to perform what were considered necessary skills in any possible manner, despite movements which were described as ingenious but considered abnormal.

During the 1950s, however, a number of neurodevelopmental models for therapy gained international acceptance among physical, occupational, and speech therapists. Treatment no longer concentrated on strengthening or relaxing individual motor groups but aimed at improving postural tone and achieving more normal movement patterns. The most popular neurodevelopmental model was devised by Dr. Karel Bobath, a neurologist, and his wife, Berta Bobath, a physiotherapist, who together established a center in London, England.

The Bobaths' theories were supported by laboratory observations of animals with specific neurologic lesions and by clinical observations of children with cerebral palsy, although very few controlled studies were published (Marquis 1979). Patients were sufficiently dissimilar that it was almost impossible to set up adequate paired study, even if the parents and physicians had felt able to withhold treatment from 50% for comparison (Paine 1962).

Although physicians were made aware of the newer methods of treatment, a paucity of supportive research prolonged the controversies and delayed acceptance. Even in the 1970s, many physicians still favored therapy that was common several decades earlier.

Joanne

Joanne began receiving occupational therapy in her home from the Easter Seal Mobile Therapy Unit based in Fargo, North Dakota, when she was 15 months old. The year was 1970. Before that time, her only medically prescribed therapy from a physiatrist (physical medicine specialist) consisted of range-of-motion exercises, which her mother had attempted to do at home on a daily basis. Joanne resisted by crying, stiffening, and becoming tighter.

We had been asked to train a large group of volunteers to relieve her mother, who had four other children and a foster child, and was discouraged because of the lack of progress for more than a year. We

followed the doctor's orders, supervising the volunteers in shifts of two, ranging almost all the joints in Joanne's body twice daily.

Shortly after Joanne's program was initiated, a two-day workshop in St. Louis provided my first exposure to Neuro-Developmental Treatment. As Mrs. Bobath handled an assortment of babies and children with various types of cerebral palsy, her clear, logical explanations of theory and treatment triggered vivid insights into Joanne's characteristic problems. Copious notes and workshop bibliographies formed the first theoretical foundation for the beginning of a nine-year treatment program. Joanne became a guinea pig. With her mother's consent, the "new treatment" began with twice-weekly home visits, incorporating neurodevelopmental concepts into total handling by all family members in methods of carrying, feeding, dressing, and playing (figure 1.1). An 8mm film documented developmental changes every few months. Detailed progress notes were duplicated for the physician as well as the family.

Joanne's fisted hands first opened at 18 months when she began reaching for toys in supine (on her back); then at 21 months, as she lifted her head, pushed up on her hands, and crawled in prone (on her stomach); and later, at 24 months, when, sitting alone, she reached out to catch herself to protect her head when falling.

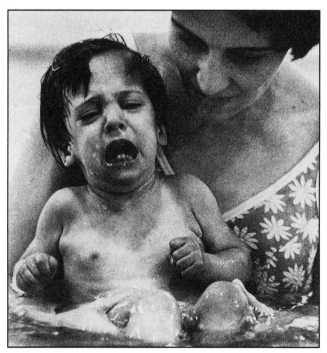

Figure 1.1. Therapeutic handling during play in the swimming pool (photo by Colburn Hvidston III, courtesy of *The Forum*)

Developmental Hand Dysfunction

As Joanne became actively involved in exploring her world with her new mobility, the importance of a systematic approach to her total developmental process became apparent. Further study of prehension within the framework of normal child development was needed to know how to stimulate learning, prevent atypical development, and coordinate the interrelationship of motor, social, language, and cognitive areas.

Child Development

The author's master's degree in child development and family relations became the vehicle for an integrated study of the prehension theories of Gesell, Piaget, and Halverson. That paper, later revised for publication in the *American Journal of Occupational Therapy* in 1974, demonstrated the relationship of those theories to clinical application, illustrated by a four-year case study of Joanne (Erhardt 1974).

Development was originally used as a biological term, meaning organic growth, but when it is applied to the behavioral sciences, it refers to an integration of constitutional and learned changes. Development is a process; change is a product. Development is based on both change and constancy. By its reliance on predictable change, it implies a variance from constancy (Maier 1969). Arnold Gesell, Jean Piaget, and Henry Halverson each examined the development of prehension in the human infant.

Gesell and the Developmental Pediatric Approaches

Gesell's studies were concerned with growth that produced changes in structure correlated with changes in function. He considered all maturing patterns to depend primarily on neuromotor readiness rather than environmental factors, and he attributed variances among children to fluctuations in mechanisms of self-regulation. He saw hand function developing like other motor behavior by expansion of the total reflex system; that is, first dependent on certain postural sets, then becoming independent, versatile, and smoothly synergized (Gesell and Amatruda 1969). Stages of motor development were classified as Pre-nascent, Nascent, Assimilative, Coordinating, and Synergic. Table 1 defines these stages and illustrates each with examples of prehension components, approach, grasp, and release.

Table 1. Stages of Motor Development

Stage	Definition	Approach	Grasp	Release
Pre-nascent	Complete absence of function	No reach before eye contact	No grasp until fisted hand is opened, then reflexive, not voluntary	No release by fisted hand
Nascent	Imperfect, sporadic, inadequate, dependent on certain postural sets	Insufficient arm extension to contact object consistently; in supine before prone or sitting	Precarious, inconsistent, not sustained	Involuntary release without awareness
Assimilative	Improved, functional, dependent on postural sets and accessory reinforcing attitudes	Underreaching or overreaching, but adjusting to succeed, with arm support	Sustained grasp with total flexion pattern (including wrist)	Assistive release (against a surface or simultaneous grasp of other hand)
Coordinating	Perfected, still linked to postural sets, but not dependent on accessory attitudes	Precise approach, one arm leading, other suppressed (first achieved in prone because other arm is weight bearing)	Grasp becomes specialized toward radial side, fingers rather than whole hand	Adept transfer, crude release above surface or into large container
Synergic	Versatile, individuated, independent from restricted postural sets	Approach and grasp become one skilled movement in sitting and standing, not just prone and supine	One finger can extend while others flex, thumb and index finger in fine pincer grasp	Precise release into small container

Some material in this table has been taken from Gesell and Amatruda (1969).

Joanne

At 1 year of age, Joanne's prehension level was clearly Pre-nascent. She did not reach for toys because the prerequisite visual regard was not present. No voluntary grasp or release was possible because her hands remained fisted.

Her first reaching (Nascent) was seen in supine, her most stable position (dependent on certain postural sets), but it was not consistently successful because of insufficient arm extension. Her first grasp was also Nascent, sporadic, not sustained, as was her release, which was involuntary and without awareness.

At the Assimilative stage, Joanne underreached or overreached but gradually learned to adjust and succeed in her approach. Grasp was characterized by total wrist and finger flexion, an accessory reinforcing attitude. Release also depended on an accessory reinforcing movement, simultaneous grasp of the other hand (the first crude transfer), or against a resistive surface, since true voluntary release was not possible.

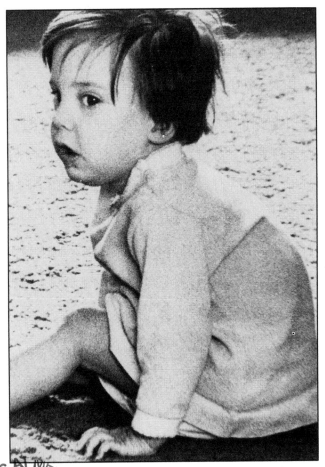

Figure 1.2. Both arms needed for support in sitting (photo by Colburn Hvidston III, courtesy of *The Forum*)

The Coordinating stage was evident when Joanne reached with one arm while weight bearing on the other arm in prone, which inhibited bilateral reaching. When first sitting alone, however, approach became Pre-nascent again, since both arms were needed for support (figure 1.2). Grasp at the Coordinating stage became specialized toward the radial or thumb side of the hand and fingers, instead of the whole hand being used as a paw (accessory attitudes). Her release of objects also became more independent of accessory attitudes, possible above a surface or into a large container.

The highest level, the Synergic stage, was not reached until Joanne's performance became versatile and skilled. Approach and grasp needed to be smoothly unified. The ability to extend the index finger and poke while keeping the other fingers flexed required a high level of digit individuation, preceding the ability to grasp a small pellet with thumb and finger. Release into a small container was not possible until a precise movement occurred at a precise time in a precise place.

Piaget and the Educational Psychological Approaches

Jean Piaget used detailed observations of his own three children to analyze the process of learning. He found that adaptation to the complex external environment depended on how innate neonate reflexes were modified by experience to evolve into intelligent behaviors. His concept of schema was that of an adaptive behavior proceeding from a simple reflex pattern, a sequence used repeatedly, continually applied to new objects, and interacting with other schemata (Piaget 1952). The grasping schema, for example, developed from reflexive grasp, was used repeatedly with a wide variety of objects, and interacted with the sucking and vision schemata.

Spirited disagreement exists in the literature, however, concerning the coordination of vision and reaching. Bower's claim that newborns can reach and grasp objects within the visual field is disputed by Gesell, Piaget, and others who feel that visually controlled prehension emerges at approximately 5 months (Gesell and Amatruda 1969; Piaget 1952; Bower 1979; Twitchell 1970; White, Castle, and Held 1964; Field 1977). It is doubtful that the newborn is capable of object vision because the optic nerve tracts and pathways are not myelinated at birth. Even during the first month, the structural development of the striate area is very slow (McGraw 1969).

Bower's attempts to discover to what extent manual skills are maturationally determined or developed through environmental interaction resulted in his conclusion that maturational processes use input from the environment but do not really need it (Bower 1979). He saw the environment operating as an accelerator or brake on a preprogrammed genetic process, but not as a switch, changing development from one path to another. Even the inhibitive or facilitative effect of the environment was perceived as only a slight loss or gain, a matter of a few weeks in time. Like several other researchers, Bower was convinced that all maturing behavior patterns depend primarily on intrinsic growth factors and neuromotor readiness rather than environmental influences (Gesell and Amatruda 1969; Illingworth 1970).

Piaget, however, considered environment to be extremely significant in that the varied experiences of individual children affected the rate—but not the order—of skill acquisitions. He stressed the invariant sequences of developmental stages, while admitting that ages varied considerably. He saw development not in a linear fashion, with one behavior pattern succeeding another (one stage disappearing as the next appeared), but as layers of a pyramid, new patterns added to the old, to complete, correct, or combine with them. Structures from earlier stages were incorporated into new stages with many intermediate transitional stages between. Disequilibrium was common during the initial period of learning for each new skill. Progression through each level depended on the state of equilibrium achieved at each level (Flavell 1963).

Like Gesell and Gibson, Piaget attributed variances among children to fluctuations in the mechanisms of self-regulation, which depend not on positive or negative reinforcement from external sources but on internal reinforcement, the reduction of uncertainty. The child's increasing ability to distinguish between appropriate and inappropriate application of the schema can be illustrated by the use of active touch, a method of searching for distinctive features and cognitive order (Gesell and Amatruda 1969; Piaget 1952; Gibson 1972).

Observations of babies exhibiting an indomitable urge to exercise emerging skills indicate that the fundamental need for repetition at an opportune time is essential for integration and perfection of new functions. Certain signals of readiness can be detected, and if opportunities for practice are provided, critical new learning can take place (McGraw 1969).

The first stage in the development of grasp (the newborn's hand closing when the palm is touched) was described by Piaget as pure reflex, with the impulsive, continuous movements of arms, hands, and fingers in the first weeks seen as a functional use of reflexes. The recognition, assimilation, and accommodation of hand to objects were designated as the first acquired adaptations and the primary circular reactions. Subsequent stages bring vision and the hand together (procedures for making interesting sights last and secondary circular reactions); coordinate vision, the hand, and outside objects (coordination of secondary schemata and their application to new situations); and culminate in a myriad of manipulative activities (tertiary circular reactions and the discovery of new means by active experimentation) (Flavell 1963). Table 2 defines these stages and illustrates each with examples of hand function.

Joanne

Joanne had remained at the reflexive grasp level for her entire first year. She had not passed through the transition stage of awareness during reflexive activities such as scratching, clutching, and grasping at her own body, her clothing, and her blankets, which usually lead to the beginning of tactile recognition and assimilation (primary circular reactions).

Because of the fisted hands and her general lack of mobility, Joanne had never rolled or crawled to explore the incredible variety of textures, shapes, and sizes of materials in the environment that the baby who is developing normally discovers and enjoys. A filmed case study shows Joanne touching grass for the first time at the age of 2¹/₂ years. She withdraws her arm suddenly in surprise at the unfamiliar sensation but tentatively reaches out again, grinning with delight.

The process of accommodation (the hand taking the form of new objects, thus learning new movements and positions) was extremely delayed, leaving Joanne with few hand patterns at her disposal.

Table 2. Stages of Development

Stage	Age	Definition of Hand Function
Reflexive grasp	0-1 month	Hand closes on any contact, without volition but with some awareness.
Primary circular reactions and first acquired adaptations	1-4 months	Hand movements controlled by reflexes, but also affected by the beginning of tactile recognition and assimilation (certain behaviors such as scratching become extended to everything: blanket, clothing, own face and body; recognition leads to repetition). Some accommodation also (the hand takes the form of the object, thus learning new movements and positions).
Secondary circular reactions and procedures for making interesting sights last	4-8 months	Hand schema interacts with other schemata (sucking, vision). Hand carries object to mouth, sucking on both. Vision influences hand movements, since the act of looking augments hand's activity, limiting its movement to the visual field. Reciprocal assimilation coordinates vision and prehension schemata: child observes moving hand, prolongs spectacle by keeping eyes on hand (assimilates vision to hand movement) and by keeping hand moving (assimilating movement to vision).
Coordination of secondary schemata and their application to new situations	8-12 months	Same schema is applied to other objects besides the hand. Hand and desired object are perceived in same visual field (neither sight of hand nor of object alone leads to grasping). Prehension is generalized and differentiated through repetition.
Tertiary circular reactions and the discovery of new means by active experimentation	12-18 months	Active experimental behavior of manipulating and combining objects. The hand grasps everything the eye sees; the eye looks at everything the hand grasps. Grasping possible without hand and object in same visual field simultaneously.

The material in this table is based on Flavell (1963).

Secondary circular reactions were also delayed, since Joanne's vision schema was incomplete. She did not fixate consistently on faces, visually inspect her own hands, or track moving objects. Like many other children with cerebral palsy, Joanne's hypertonus and retention of primitive patterns had kept her shoulders immobile, her arms flexed and somewhat asymmetrical, and her hands fisted, without the infinite variety of constant finger movements observed in normal babies.

The development of visual fixation, convergence, and tracking of new objects was hampered not only by Joanne's inability to bring her hands to midline but also by the concurrent incoordination of four pairs of ocular muscles. Thus, she did not experience reciprocal assimilation (prolonging the spectacle of her moving hand by keeping her eyes on her hand as well as keeping her hand moving).

In order to grasp an object, Joanne needed to perceive her hand and the desired object in the same visual field, since neither the sight of her hand nor the object alone would lead to voluntary prehension. The coordination of secondary schemata would not be possible until secondary circular reactions had

been achieved, because the one stage prepares for the next. Not until Joanne became actively manipulating, experimentally exploring, grasping everything she looked at, and looking at everything she grasped would she reach the stage of tertiary circular reactions, when prehension is possible without the hand and object necessarily being in the same visual field simultaneously.

Environmental influences interacting with maturational readiness were crucial factors in Joanne's developmental progress. Input from the environment did more than accelerate or brake her preprogrammed genetic process. Without appropriate stimulation, Joanne's development was blocked for more than a year. Providing the right amount and type of stimulation and methods of intervention was a challenge that required not only a comprehensive knowledge of normal child development and of the specific effects of motor damage to the central nervous system but, just as important, careful observations of Joanne's individual and distinctive learning style.

Although it appeared to be uneven, Joanne's rate of learning revealed a definite pattern. It was characterized by periods of rapid acquisition of clusters of new skills, followed by periods of plateaus, during which we suspected the skills were becoming integrated and automatic. Early performances were slow, awkward, and clumsy, almost always accompanied by increased spasticity. With repetition, each new skill eventually became more normalized as disequilibrium subsided, but only if the previous developmental skill had reached a reasonable state of equilibrium and if the new skill were developmentally appropriate; that is, in the next sequential order. If the new skill were at an inappropriately high level, either because of premature presentation by an eager therapist or parent, or even because of Joanne's motivation to imitate her twin sister, Valerie, the state of disequilibrium persisted. Repetition thus resulted in reinforcement and permanent incorporation of hypertonus and atypical movement into the newly learned pattern.

The real challenge, then, was to develop sensitive observational skills to detect Joanne's personal signals of readiness, both neuromotor and motivational, in order to capitalize on each critical learning period.

Halverson and the Anthropological and Psychological Approaches

Henry Halverson's analytic studies of prehension in babies recorded on film three principle behaviors: visual location of the object (regard), hand approach (backhand, circuitous, and direct), and grasp (ten different types ranging from primitive to mature) (Halverson 1931; see table 3).

From his review of the anthropological literature, Halverson concluded that the nervous system develops in an order favoring those sections that are of immediate concern to the infant's welfare. Thus, certain spinal reflexes, such as the Flexor Withdrawal (pulling the limb quickly away from danger), are functional before cerebellar functions of spatial orientation and general muscular coordination, which necessarily precede cortically mediated skills such as writing (Jackson 1932).

This neuroevolutionary concept of ascending development of brain center control was the foundation for some theorists' belief that ontogenetic development

Table 3. Types of Grasp

Type	Age	Definition
No contact	16 weeks	
Contact only	20 weeks	Hand touches but doesn't secure object.
Primitive squeeze	20 weeks	Hand thrusts beyond object, corrals it, squeezes it against other hand or body; not true grasp.
Squeeze grasp	24 weeks	Hand contacts object with palm laterally, fingers press object against heel of palm; no thumb involvement, unsuccessful, clumsy.
Hand grasp	28 weeks	Pronated hand brought down paw-like on object, fingers press it against palm; no thumb involvement, successful.
Palm grasp	28 weeks	Pronated hand set on object with fingers curled over the top and down on the far side, thumb opposes the fingers in pressing object against palm.
Superior palm grasp	32 weeks	Radial side of palm set on object, thumb opposing first two fingers only, pressing object against palm.
Inferior-forefinger grasp	36 weeks	Resembling superior-palm grasp, but digits pointing more medianward than downward; improved thumb opposition, without object against palm.
Forefinger grasp	52 weeks	Fingertips of first three or four fingers hold object with thumb opposed; only metacarpophalangeal joints flexed instead of all.
Superior-forefinger grasp	52 weeks	Similar to forefinger grasp but without hand needing a resting place for digits or leverage in lifting object.

The material in this table is based on Halverson (1931).

recapitulates phylogeny; that is, the normal infant passes through the same stages from which the species evolved (Swinyard 1967; Peiper 1963). Ayres, however, stated that although evolution of man as a vertebrate is reflected in every child's development, it is an oversimplification to say that each child repeats the species' evolutionary history. Innate adaptive behavioral patterns may be inherited, but individual maturation and expression depend on ontogenetic experience, as the environment demands constant interpretation of sensory stimuli and adaptive responses (Ayres 1973, 1974).

One of the earliest phylogenetic survival patterns of reflexive grasp is seen in the baby primate who needs to cling to the mother's fur as she runs from danger on all four limbs. Another reason for the predominant power of flexor muscles may be traced to the arboreal locomotion method of most primates (Connolly and Elliott 1972). In fact, the hands of certain species cannot be used flat as a means of support, because the ligaments retain a permanent, curved, hook-like shape adapted for brachiation (traveling from one tree branch to another by the arms) (Campbell 1966).

Halverson also related the development of specific movements to the phylogenetic order of appearance of muscular structures. For example, the trunk or axial muscles precede arm or appendicular muscles, and the gross muscles of the arms precede fine hand muscles. Thus, the trapezius and latissimus dorsi, with origins in the trunk, are the first muscles affecting the shoulder and arm to become activated. The newborn's shoulders are so elevated by the trapezius in prone, supine, and sitting positions that there appears to be no neck. The influence of the latissimus dorsi is seen in the adducted, internally rotated arms, part of the newborn's pattern of passive flexion. As the deltoid, teres major, supraspinatus, and infraspinatus become activated, the infant develops more abduction and external rotation. Elbow and wrist control develop with the triceps, biceps, and carpi ulnaris and radialis groups. Finally, extrinsic and intrinsic hand muscles are coordinated into patterns of prehension made possible by the child's gradual emancipation from postural attitudes (Halverson 1931).

Pencil Grasp

The development of pencil grasp in children from 1 to 6 years illustrates the principles of development from proximal to distal, global to differentiated, and axial to appendicular. Between the first and second years, the earliest grasp of a crayon or pencil has been described as palmar-supinate, with the wrist slightly supinated, the hand fisted, and shoulder motion predominating.

Stability in the shoulder and the beginning of elbow mobility is seen in the digital-pronate grasp, between ages 2 and 3, when the pencil is held by the fingers, wrist pronated. From age 3 onward, a tripod posture begins to emerge, static at first, with some wrist mobility, but with control largely based in the shoulder and elbow, and the arm moving as a unit. Although the pencil is held with the thumb and two fingers, approximation is proximal and rather crude.

Not until 4 years does a more dynamic tripod posture begin to be perfected, with shoulder, elbow, and wrist stabilization allowing the interphalangeal joints to perform very fine individuated movements. The flexed ring and little fingers provide stability, also, by resting on the surface, forming an arch. The tripod opposition of thumb and two fingers is precise and at the distal end of the pencil (Rosenbloom and Horton 1971).

Interestingly, stages of pencil grasp are remarkably similar to types of adult grasps described by various authors for classification purposes (Connolly and Elliott 1972; Napier 1956; Johnson and Cohen 1975; Skerik, Weiss, and Flatt 1971). The earliest palmar-supinate grasp approximates a power grip, followed by a modified power grip resembling the digital-pronate grasp. Certain variations of the tripod posture are often seen in older children and adults who may have fixated at an earlier level of prehension. The scissors grasp, for example, described by Gesell (object held by thumb and side of curled index finger) (Gesell and Amatruda 1969), is normally retained in adult life for specialized functions such as turning a key in a lock (lateral pinch), but it is first seen as a primitive, temporary grasp of the pellet.

Dominance

The establishment of definitive hand dominance appears to correlate with the developing mature dynamic tripod posture used by the 4- to 6-year-old. Normal 3-year-olds still show ambidexterity, alternating dominance from one hand to the other until 6 years (table 4). Completely integrated dominance does not always occur until 8 or 9 years. In fact, clear preference for one hand in the first 15 months of life indicates impairment in peripheral or central control of the other hand, because the normal child passes through stages of both unilateral and bilateral hand use, which prepare for using both hands separately and together (Gesell and Amatruda 1969).

Several studies relating lateral preferences and manual skills have concluded that bilateralization rather than unilateralization of function provides a more balanced repertoire of adaptive behaviors (Crinella, Beck, and Robinson 1971; Annett 1970). Situational variables that influence lateral preferences and that should be considered when assessing hand dominance in children include the shape, size, and placement of objects. Certain activities, such as drawing, cutting, and hammering, lend themselves to consistent preferential manipulation, while others, such as picking up and carrying objects, scrubbing, pulling a wagon, placing pegs, and stacking blocks, are of such a nature that the situation (convenience) often determines which hand will be used (Heinlein 1930).

Development of Sensation

Final perfection of the hand is evident not only in anatomy and motor control but in sensory perception. During evolution, innervation of the volar pads, particularly the terminal digital pads, increases in density, making them tactile sense organs of great importance. The tactile function of the hand almost completely replaces locomotor function in the human adult, but not in all other primates. Monkeys, apes, and man are the only animals with the ability to manipulate objects, turn them over, and examine form and texture. This ability to extract an object from the environment and examine it three-dimensionally from all sides is important, because it leads to analytic perception and eventually to conceptual thought (Campbell 1966).

Motor control of the hand must originate with sensory input, which is the source for movement behavior. The central nervous system receives information from a variety of receptors (skin, eyes, ears, nose,

Table 4. Development of Dominance

Age	Hand Use
3 months	Unilateral activation, no contact, usually nondominant hand
4 months	Bilateral approach and contact, as well as bidextrous (either hand)
5 months	Bilateral approach and grasp, one reaches, other joins, beginning transfer
6 months	Unilaterality, one hand dominant, two-stage transfer (momentarily bilateral)
7 months	Unilaterality, bidextrous (hands equal in skill), one-stage transfer, reaches for another object while first hand either drops or retains first object
8-9 months	Unilaterality, either hand predominating
10-11 months	Unilaterality, temporary dominance, alternating hands, other hand mirroring
12-13 months	Unilaterality, dominant hand actively manipulates, other hand passive
15 months	Unilaterality, dominant hand manipulates, other hand holds
18 months	Unilaterality and bilaterality, variability
2 years	Unilaterality, dominant hand
$2^1/_2$-$3^1/_2$ years	Bilaterality, simultaneous approach and manipulation or alternating hand use
4-6 years	Unilaterality, dominance gradually increasing, other hand passive

The material in this table is based on Gesell and Ames (1947).

tongue, bones, muscles, joints, and internal organs) through the afferent system. Organization of this information within the system, and the resulting output, or action on the environment through the efferent system, produces feedback that stimulates further interaction. Sensory modalities affecting tactile hand function include touch, pain, temperature, proprioception (joint position sense), and stereognosis (object recognition) (Banus et al. 1979).

Touch, pain, and temperature are predominant sensations in the newborn, while position and movement sense develop later (Peiper 1963). The capacity to generate tactile stimulation independently is limited for the first few months because of the immaturity of the visual system, the presence of reflexive rather than voluntary grasp, and the strong Avoiding Responses. Discrete tactile sense and voluntary movements increase simultaneously at 4 and 5 months as withdrawal patterns (which were necessary for self-protection) are modified and vision begins to monitor reaching movements. Because the visual system and the tactile system mutually reinforce each other, impressions gained by one stimulate associations from the other. Stereognosis, the ability to recognize an object by touch, is first developed by both visual and tactile cues. Later, visual cues alone recall manual impressions or vice versa.

Proprioceptors in muscles, tendons, and joints are first stimulated through vestibular sensations of rocking by caregivers, then later self-generated. For example, the 6-month-old baby deliberately practices rolling, which requires orientation of the head in space and prepares for independent sitting and standing. Position sense and awareness of body parts in space must precede successful motor planning for manipulation activities (Coley 1978).

These sensory mechanisms mature at the same time as motor skills but cannot be easily separated from them for purposes of evaluation in the first 15 months. Since the infant cannot report sensations verbally, the only indication of sensory thresholds and experiences is overt motor behavior. When a motor response to pain or touch is elicited, the neonate cannot localize or identify the stimulation, because the cortex is responsible for accurate discrimination.

Even when specific localization is first well-established, the higher centers are not yet integrated enough to permit adequate appraisal of and a meaningful response to the situation (McGraw 1969). In other words, the progressively better use of sensory impressions cannot generally be attributed to improved function of the sensory organs, but rather to the better evaluation of sensory impressions in the brain (Peiper 1963). Furthermore, sensory deficits in the child with brain damage are caused not only by lesions to sensory areas in the brain, but also by inadequate or abnormal feedback due to lesions in the motor areas (Trombley and Scott 1977).

Joanne

The lack of mobility during her first year had deprived Joanne of not only the sensory exploration of textures, shapes, sizes, and weights, but also the proprioceptive awareness of how her body moved through space. The important role of the head, shoulders, and arms in righting the body when the center of gravity is shifted is seen even in prone, supine, and sidelying positions, when normal children are rolling, crawling, and tumbling on the floor. When Joanne finally learned to sit up, she lacked Protective Extensor Thrust of the arms to protect her head when falling over, an important automatic movement normally appearing at 6 months and becoming stronger and more consistent as imperfect balance elicits the response.

During a therapy session when Joanne was being tossed forward from the therapist's lap to stimulate the protective reactions, she bumped her nose because of a sluggish arm response. When this "accident" was followed by a repeated thrust instead of comforting, Joanne's arm response was much stronger and more immediate. Her delay in reaching antigravity postures meant that she had experienced few balance-threatening situations. Simulation of a realistic situation in which loss of balance resulted in a mild "injury" elicited an appropriate survival response.

Another example of the importance of proprioceptive awareness gained from experience but linked to cognitive learning was illustrated by Joanne's first attempt to drink from a cup in a floor-sitting position instead of supported sitting in a high chair. She tilted her head backward to drink, realized that her sitting balance was insufficient, regarded the cup, then the floor, and decided to lie down supine to solve the problem (reversion to earlier postural set). She reclined, tilted the cup, and received a very surprising splash of water in her face. A second cup of water handed to her resulted in new behavior modified by experience. She remained sitting but, still aware of her disequilibrium, pivoted herself against a wall for support while drinking.

Once Joanne became able to bear weight on open hands, which is necessary to prepare for the normal reaching pattern, the next logical step appeared to be learning to crawl. Our fastidious attention to accepted sequences of motor skills motivated us to facilitate what we expected to be crawling but instead became "bunny-hopping." Because the Symmetrical Tonic Neck Reflex was not yet integrated, Joanne learned to use it for locomotion purposes. As her arms extended forward bilaterally and her head raised, both flexed legs followed. This pattern, because it became extremely efficient and rapid with practice, interfered with the development of reciprocal arm and leg movements, not only in crawling but in walking as well. The repetition of evolutionary history is not always appropriate for an individual child. Even reciprocal crawling was contraindicated for Joanne because of the prolongation of knee and hip flexor activity and the danger of contractures (Bobath 1971).

The importance of axial or proximal control preceding appendicular or distal control to ensure patterns as nearly normal as possible was considered when Joanne was introduced to prewriting activities. Shoulder

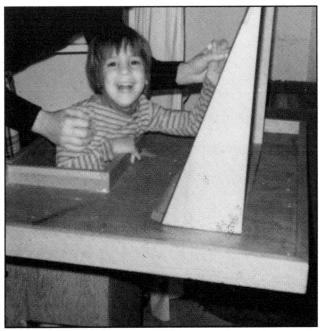

Figure 1.3. Assisted arm movement to develop shoulder control for chalkboard activities at a standing table (photo by author)

control was established first in a supported standing position at a large chalkboard (figure 1.3). The palmar-supinate grasp of the chalk afforded the most visual and motor control. Basic directional lines and shapes were achieved before attempting the more mature digital-pronate grasp. A problem arose when Joanne's increased spasticity with effort caused hyperpronation, wrist flexion, and ulnar deviation, obliterating her view of her work as well. Many children with cerebral palsy become fixed at this stage and are not able to progress to the tripod posture, or they may carry over the previous atypical patterns to that posture. Joanne's predominant flexor tone was difficult to overcome.

Another example of reversion to earlier patterns was observed when an adapted spoon was given to Joanne before hand-to-mouth patterns were well established in finger feeding. The added stress of grasping and manipulating the spoon produced increased spasticity in the form of shoulder elevation, internal rotation, adduction and flexion of the arms, and fisting of the opposite hand. The presence of these developmentally inappropriate patterns, which did not resolve within a reasonable length of time, indicated premature presentation rather than merely a state of disequilibrium.

Fisting of the right hand (associated reactions) was a continual concern as Joanne relied more and more on her more skillful left hand (figure 1.4). The discrepancy between the developmental levels of each hand threatened to widen as she grew older. In order to help Joanne improve the use of her left hand, it was necessary to provide activities typical of both the bilateral and unilateral stages of hand use (figure 1.5).

Sensory perception, which normally develops from the physiological prerequisites of dense innervation of the volar pads integrated with a wealth of sensorimotor experience, was extremely delayed for Joanne. Her manipulation of doll clothes, for example, could not take place successfully until a high level of fine motor skill was achieved and coordinated with tactile and proprioceptive information. Social development also needed to be at a stage where doll play, imitative play, and dressing activities were linked to appropriate language and cognitive motivation, not chronological age.

Joanne's intervention program was based on the concept that normal development is understandable and predictable and that if conditions causing atypical patterns can be altered or corrected, normal development can be resumed (Maier 1969). Additionally, if the child with brain injury is seen as the victim of abnormal sensorimotor experiences because of the persistence of primitive reflexes and abnormal muscle tone, special handling is needed to inhibit the reflexes and facilitate normal tone (Bobath 1967). The neuro-developmental therapist, then, needs to consider normal motor development in terms of postural control against gravity, the specific pathology (abnormal tone and atypical patterns) of each child with cerebral palsy, the range of treatment techniques, and, most important, how to adapt the techniques to the individual child at each particular stage of development (Bobath 1971).

The author's motivation for application and acceptance into the basic eight-week Neuro-Developmental Treatment (NDT) certification course in London, England, in 1977, arose from dissatisfaction with the limited knowledge of the Bobath methods available through short workshops, journal articles, and books.

References

Annett, M. 1970. The growth of manual preference and speed. *British Journal of Psychology* 61:545-58.

Ayres, A. J. 1973. *Sensory integration and learning disorders.* Los Angeles: Western Psychological Services.

_____. 1974. Ontogenetic principles in the development of arm and hand functions. In *The development of sensory integrative theory and practice: A collection of the works of A. Jean Ayres,* compiled by A. Henderson, E. Gilfoyle, L. Lorens, C. Myers, and S. Prevel, 3-13. Dubuque, IA: Kendall/Hunt.

Banus, B. S., C. A. Kent, Y. Norton, D. R. Sukiennicki, and M. L. Becker. 1979. *The developmental therapist.* Thorofare, NJ: Charles B. Slack.

Bobath, B. 1967. The very early treatment of cerebral palsy. *Developmental Medicine and Child Neurology* 9:373-90.

_____. 1971. Motor development, its effect on general development, and application to the treatment of cerebral palsy. *Physiotherapy* 57:526-32.

Bower, T. G. R. 1979. *Human development.* San Francisco: W. H. Freeman.

Campbell, B. G. 1966. *Human evolution.* Chicago: Aldine.

Coley, I. L. 1978. *Pediatric assessment of self-care activities.* St. Louis, MO: C. V. Mosby.

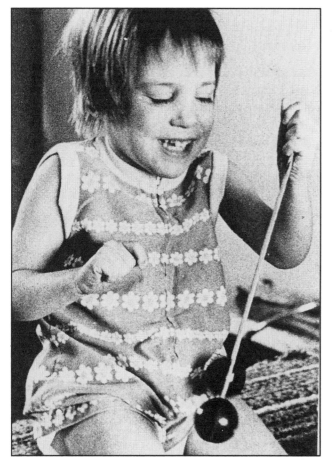

Figure 1.4. Fisting of the right hand (associated reactions) during left-hand play with "clackers" (photo by Harry Jennings, courtesy of *The Forum*)

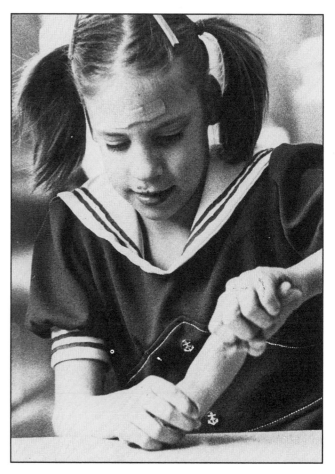

Figure 1.5. Clay activities used for bilateral as well as unilateral hand use (photo by Colburn Hvidston III, courtesy of *The Forum*)

Connolly, K., and J. Elliott. 1972. The evolution and ontogeny of hand function. In *Ethological studies of child behavior,* edited by N. Blurton-Jones, 329-83. Cambridge, MA: University Press.

Crinella, F. M., F. W. Beck, and J. W. Robinson. 1971. Unilateral dominance is not related to neuropsychological integrity. *Child Development* 42:2033-54.

Erhardt, R. P. 1974. Sequential levels in development of prehension. *American Journal of Occupational Therapy* 28:592-96.

Field, J. 1977. Coordination of vision and prehension in young infants. *Child Development* 48:97-103.

Flavell, J. 1963. *The developmental psychology of Jean Piaget.* Princeton, NJ: Van Nostrand.

Gesell, A., and C. S. Amatruda. 1969. *Developmental diagnosis.* 2d ed., revised and enlarged. New York: Harper and Row.

Gesell, A., and L. B. Ames. 1947. The development of handedness. *Journal of Genetic Psychology* 70:155-75.

Gibson, E. J. 1972. The development of perception as an adaptive process. In *Readings in child behavior and development,* edited by C. S. Lavatelli, 231-43. New York: Harcourt Brace Jovanovich.

Halverson, H. M. 1931. An experimental study of prehension in infants by means of systematic cinema records. *Genetics Psychology Monographs* 10:107-286.

Heinlein, J. H. 1930. Preferential manipulation in children. *Comparative Psychology Monographs* 7:1-121.

Illingworth, R. S. 1970. *Development of the infant and young child.* Baltimore, MD: Williams and Wilkins.

Jackson, J. H. 1932. Evolution and dissolution of the nervous system. In *Selected writings of John Hughlings Jackson,* vol. 2, edited by J. Taylor, 3-118. New York: Basic Books.

Johnson, K., and M. J. Cohen. 1975. *The hand atlas.* Springfield, IL: Charles C. Thomas.

Johnson, M. K. 1973. *The hand book.* Springfield, IL: Charles C. Thomas.

Maier, H. W. 1969. *Three theories of child development.* New York: Harper and Row.

Marquis, P. 1979. Therapies for cerebral palsy. *American Family Physician* 19:101-05.

McGraw, M. B. 1969. *The neuromuscular maturation of the human infant.* New York: Hafner.

Napier, J. R. 1956. The prehensile movements of the human hand. *Journal of Bone and Joint Surgery* 38B:902.

Paine, R. S. 1962. On the treatment of cerebral palsy. *Pediatrics* 4:605-16.

Peiper, A. 1963. *A cerebral function in infancy and childhood.* New York: Consultants Bureau.

Piaget, J. 1952. *The origins of intelligence in children.* New York: International University Press.

Rosenbloom, L., and M. E. Horton. 1971. The maturation of fine prehension. *Developmental Medicine and Child Neurology* 13:3-8.

Skerik, S. K., M. W. Weiss, and A. E. Flatt. 1971. Functional evaluation of congenital hand anomalies. *American Journal of Occupational Therapy* 25:98-104.

Swinyard, C. A. 1967. Developmental aspects of neurological structure relevant to cerebral palsy. *Developmental Medicine and Child Neurology* 9:216-21.

Trombley, C. A., and A. D. Scott. 1977. *Occupational therapy for physical dysfunction.* Baltimore: Williams and Wilkins.

Twitchell, T. E. 1970. Reflex mechanisms and the development of prehension. In *Mechanisms of motor skill development,* edited by K. J. Connolly, 25-38. London: Academic Press.

White, B., P. Castle, and R. Held. 1964. Observations on the development of visually-directed reaching. *Child Development* 35:349-64.

Chapter Two
Patrick

The Bobaths and the Neuro-Developmental Approaches

The performance of functional skills such as feeding, dressing, and writing requires very complex and selective patterns of muscular coordination. These depend on an intact and mature central nervous system and a background of basic motor patterns that children with normal development profiles acquire during the first few years of life. Understanding the basic concepts of the function of the central nervous system with respect to the organization of normal motor activity is necessary to explain the nature of cerebral palsy and the rationale for the Bobath approach (Bobath and Bobath 1972).

The Postural Reflex Mechanism

The central nervous system's function is integration. In every motor act, a large and varying part is automatic and outside consciousness. The ratio of "most automatic" to "least automatic" movement is greatest in the newborn, gradually reversing as cognitively directed volitional movements increase. As the infant begins to move, especially against gravity, muscles are immediately coordinated in constantly changing patterns.

The highly complex mechanism that regulates the delicate changes of muscle tone needed to maintain balance is called the postural reflex mechanism, consisting of important automatic reactions serving two purposes: (1) maintenance of equilibrium when the body position changes or parts of the body change in relation to other parts, and (2) fixation of body parts for support of moving parts.

Postural control develops as the child lifts the head against gravity, improves righting reactions, gains rotation within the body axis, and experiences compensatory shifts of muscle tone to maintain or restore balance. This background of automatic postural control, which develops in a definite sequence in babies who are progressing normally, is needed as a preparation for functional skills and all future voluntary movements.

Reciprocal Innervation

Studies of decerebrate animals show that during reflex activity at the spinal level, agonist muscles are excited and totally contracted, while simultaneously antagonists are totally inhibited and relaxed (reciprocal inhibition). In normal humans, however, the higher brain centers inhibit antagonists in a gradual and adapted manner, in step with the contracting agonists. Synergic muscle groups also steady and fix other joints to provide optimal mechanical conditions for the interplay of these opposing muscular forces. For example, as finger and thumb flexors contract to grasp an object, the extensors gradually relax, but synergists also raise the wrist, stabilizing it in extension. Reciprocal innervation, then, is the dynamic state of agonists and antagonists in simultaneous contraction (Bobath 1974).

Inhibition and Differentiation

While the postural reflex mechanism and reciprocal innervation are becoming refined, another maturation process takes place as the early total synergies of muscular coordination are gradually broken up to allow for increasingly selective and differentiated movements (B. Bobath 1971; K. Bobath 1971). The child learns to use only parts of total patterns and to combine them in various new ways. For example, after first learning to grasp an object, holding it close to the body, the child must learn to grasp while reaching with extended arm. Then the child must retain grasp while moving the arm above the head, sideward, or any other position. The first grasp is with the whole hand and all the fingers, but later, to pick up crumbs or other small objects, the child must restrict grasp to thumb and index finger, keeping the other fingers out of the way.

This modification process is achieved by gradual inhibition of those parts of the movement that are unnecessary and disturbing to the performance of a specific task. Thus, inhibition is an important factor in coordination of fine, selective movements. Associated movements, mirroring, or overflow into the other hand are frequently seen during most of the first year, as well as in older children and adults during stressful activities such as lifting or squeezing. As the child matures, these associated movements are largely inhibited (Bobath 1959). Table 5 describes arm and hand activities in terms of their importance in the development of the normal postural mechanism and in the elaboration of the primitive total synergies by increase of inhibitory control.

Primitive and Pathological Patterns

The normal child learns new skills by trial and error, just as adults do. When the basic, well-coordinated motor patterns have to be used in different combinations of patterns for new and more advanced tasks, temporary regression occurs to less selective and more primitive motor activity. These movements are clumsy and slow, requiring excessive effort and increased muscle tension. Adaptation and repetition make the performance more automatic and smoother, requiring less effort. Because of the mixture of primitive (normal) and pathological (abnormal) patterns in cerebral palsy, the child reinforces the abnormal elements by repetition instead of adaptation, and prolongs the period of regression. Increased muscle tone, clumsiness, and slowness may then be incorporated into the new skill as a permanent pattern (B. Bobath 1971).

Primitive patterns are those present in a normal baby in the first four months, while pathological patterns are never seen in any developmental stage (Bobath and Bobath 1972). In babies with cerebral palsy and older children who are mildly affected, primitive patterns predominate, but pathological patterns are more frequent in older and/or more severe cases. Pathological components may coexist with primitive movements if tone is abnormal (hypertonic, hypotonic, or

Table 5. Stages of Motor Development

Age	Activities of Arms and Hands
3-4 months	Abduction-flexion limb patterns, forearm support in prone; arms flexed and hands together in midline in supine; hands clutch, pull, pluck.
4-5 months	Beginning of extension-abduction limb patterns, arms either forward in prone for nearly extended support, or retracted and flexed, hands off surface, support on one forearm in prone while reaching for toys; hands engage in supine in midline while rolling to side; arms retracted and flexed in insecure sitting; bilateral hand approach, whole-hand voluntary grasp (bottle).
6 months	Strong extension-abduction limb patterns, weight bearing on both extended arms in prone, reaching with one, supporting on the other; reaching with extended arms in supine, playing with feet; sitting with arm support briefly; transfers objects, feeds self finger foods, bangs, pats objects.
8 months	Rotation around body axis, moving from prone to sitting by pushing up with arms; reciprocal crawling on belly; sitting with arm support forward and sideward; uses hands to pull up to standing; finger-thumb opposition, index finger approach, beginning of release.
10 months	Improved balance, crawls on hands and knees or hands and feet; arm support backward in sitting; neat pincer grasp, pokes with index finger, releases objects into containers.

The material in this table is based on B. Bobath (1971).

Developmental Hand Dysfunction

fluctuating), movements are stereotyped and invariable, or other skills are missing from the same stage of development. For example, grasping may be possible only with flexed, pronated arms and head and trunk flexion; the hands may open only when the entire arm is extended; forearms may always be pronated, never supinated; elbow extension may always be associated with internal rotation of the arm; or grasping may be done with one hand only (Bobath 1974).

Regressive Patterns

Milani, however, does not consider any patterns pathological, since he observed many so-called abnormal movements in the normal fetus through his ultrasound research (Milani-Comparetti 1980). His "competition of patterns" concept explains "regressive patterns" traced to a prenatal central nervous system insult and then persisting in the postnatal period, because the tyranny of those patterns allows no alternatives. Often a slight intrauterine lesion may damage the baby enough to prevent the baby's full cooperation in the birth process (fetal propulsion), prolonging labor and causing respiratory distress and a secondary insult.

Tonic Reflexes

Brain lesions that disturb the postural reflex mechanism and reciprocal innervation also release primitive tonic reflexes from the suppression normally exercised by the higher centers (Bobath 1974). These early reflexes, which are usually integrated by 4 or 5 months of age, affect shoulder and arm patterns as well as hand movements. For example:

- The persistence of the Tonic Labyrinthine Reflex (TLR) causes increased extensor tone in supine and shoulder retraction that prevents hands from coming to midline in preparation for transferring objects from one hand to the other.

- The Asymmetrical Tonic Neck Reflex (ATNR), causing increased flexor tone on the skull-side arm and increased extensor tone on the face-side arm when the head is rotated, interferes with midline orientation and eye-hand coordination.

- The Symmetrical Tonic Neck Reflex (STNR), causing increased extensor tone in arms when the head is raised and increased flexor tone when the head is lowered, interferes with differentiation of head and arm movements (Fiorentino 1981).

The tonic reflexes gain in strength instead of disappearing, often dominating the motor activity of the child with cerebral palsy (Bobath and Bobath 1956). Higher-level responses, such as the Protective Extensor Thrust (arms automatically extending when falling), may not emerge. The intelligent child, particularly, will adapt primitive reflexes for functional use, internalizing and reinforcing abnormal patterns (Bobath 1967).

Grasping Reactions

Specific reflexes affecting the development of voluntary prehension were studied by Twitchell (1965, 1970), who maintained that early reflex grasping cannot be isolated from the total flexion pattern of the upper extremity traction response. In fact, he insisted that the usual contact stimulation in the newborn's palm alone will elicit only an Avoiding Response and that proprioceptive stimulation (passive stretch of the arm adductors and flexors) is necessary to produce a strong reflex grasp at that age. By 2 or 3 weeks of age, synergistic flexion, which includes hand grasp, can be evoked more easily by contact stimulation (deep and pressing, not light), and the ability to elicit it proprioceptively begins to decline. The fully developed Grasp Reflex, consisting of "catching and holding" against traction, is freed from synergistic flexion of fingers and thumb (Twitchell 1965).

Early attempts at voluntary prehension occur simultaneously with the emergence of the Instinctive Grasp Reactions, which develop automatic palpating and adjusting responses without visual direction (Twitchell 1970). Orienting movements of the hand are seen first as slight supination following contact stimulation of the radial side. Later, pronation can be obtained from stimulation of the ulnar border. As the child matures, the range of movement increases, and groping movements of the entire hand toward the stimulus appear. The final stage of the Instinctive Grasp Reaction consists of trapping or finally grasping the stimulus, again without any visual component (Twitchell 1965).

The Avoiding Response interfaces with these other grasping reactions even in the newborn, when a light contact stimulus evokes a slight withdrawal consisting of dorsiflexion and abduction of the fingers. By 1 or 2 months, a facile response is evidenced by strong finger extension and abduction, as well as wrist extension and pronation, elbow flexion, and shoulder retraction. Thus, a baby at that age will reflexively grasp an object placed in contact with the palm but will subsequently drop the object if it touches the fingertips and activates the Avoiding Response. For the next few months, these competing reactions result in alternate opening and closing of fingers, intermittent grasp strength, and spontaneous dropping of objects (Twitchell 1970).

In the development of voluntary prehension, each successive stage in the evolution of automatic grasping reactions is associated with increasingly complex volitional grasp (Twitchell 1965). The delay in voluntary prehension in children with congenital encephalopathies can be traced to a failure of integration of the reflex substrata described above (Twitchell 1959). If the sequence of reflex maturation is derailed at any stage, the residual reactions may hypertrophy and become exaggerated. For example, the traction response component of reflexive grasp interferes with the normal reaching pattern of extended elbow, wrist, and fingers. As the arm partially extends with great difficulty and the fingers close, the wrist also flexes, thus weakening the grip by imposing a mechanical disadvantage to full flexion of the fingers.

If certain automatic responses (such as the Instinctive Grasp Reactions) do not develop, the hand does not orient or adjust to the shape of an object and visual guidance becomes essential, thus requiring more cognitive attention. In certain instances in which the Grasp Reflex has been unopposed by the Avoiding Response, flexion predominates, and the fingers release an object with great difficulty. The maturity of prehension depends on the equilibration of Avoiding Responses with Grasping Responses (Twitchell 1970).

The most common method of classifying the various types of cerebral palsy has been according to muscle tone. Table 6 compares spastic, athetoid, and flaccid conditions in terms of muscle tone, reflexive influences, reciprocal innervation, and postural patterns affecting arm and hand function.

Patrick

Patrick had always wanted to move, roll over, crawl, reach for and play with toys, sit up, and stand. Children with athetosis, however, because of the strong influence of exaggerated tonic reflexes, fluctuating muscle tone, and faulty reciprocal innervation, do not develop a normal postural reflex mechanism. The basic motor patterns acquired during the first year lack the large automatic component so important as a foundation for later functional skills such as feeding, dressing, and writing.

The Tonic Labyrinthine Reflex contributed to the extreme arching of Patrick's back when he lay in supine and to his shoulder retraction, especially on the right

Table 6. Classification of Cerebral Palsy Affecting Arm-Hand Movement Patterns

Type	Reflexive Influences	Reciprocal Innervation	Postural Patterns
Spastic	ATNR, TLR, STNR, Grasp Reflex	Excessive co-contraction, simultaneous contraction of agonists and antagonists, flexors predominating, motion limited in range and speed, excessive effort	Abnormal, stereotyped patterns, poverty of movements, lack of selectivity, total flexion or total extension, voluntary use of reflex patterns for purposive movements, asymmetrical
Athetoid	ATNR, STNR, TLR, Grasp Reflex, Avoiding Response	Lack of co-contraction, excessive extension or flexion, unmodified reciprocal innervation, contraction of agonists results in excessive relaxation of antagonists, poor synergistic control	Extreme ranges of movement, poor midrange control, asymmetrical, disorganized movements, lack of selectivity, poor fixation, dystonic spasms interfere with postural control
Flaccid	TLR, Avoiding Response	No co-contraction, very low muscle tone, intermittent extensor spasticity when handled or on voluntary effort to move	Full range but not used because of low tone, hypermobile joints, early patterns resemble premature child, never had physiological flexion of full-term newborn

The material in this table is based on Bobath (1967), Bobath (1974), and Twitchell (1965, 1970).

Developmental Hand Dysfunction

(figure 2.1). His "flying hand" also originated from effects of the Asymmetrical Tonic Neck Reflex. Since Patrick's left hand was much more efficient than his right, he reinforced the reflex by turning his head to watch his left arm reach out into extension as his entire right arm moved into obligatory flexion.

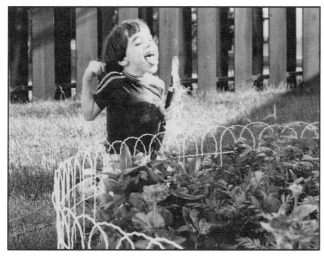

Figure 2.1. The shoulder retraction pattern persisting in upright as well as supine positions (photo courtesy of Sallie and John Mooneyham)

As Patrick tried to move from prone to hands and knees, he used a total flexor pattern to pull his knees under his abdomen, with head down, then lifted his head, using the Symmetrical Tonic Neck Reflex (STNR) to get arm extension. In order to gain stability despite his fluctuating tone, he internally

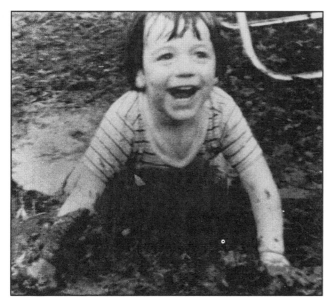

Figure 2.2. Use of the STNR for W sitting during play (photo courtesy of Sallie and John Mooneyham)

rotated his arms, locked his elbows into extension, and bore his weight on fisted hands, sitting between his flexed legs on a wide base of support (figure 2.2).

Hand reflexes interfering with prehension included the Grasp Reflex, especially the traction component, and the Avoiding Response. When well supported in a chair at a table and trying to feed himself, Patrick first used the ATNR to extend his left arm to reach the spoon, while his right arm pulled back into flexion. In order to maintain grasp on the spoon, bend his left arm to bring the spoon to his mouth, and keep his head in midline, he used a total flexion pattern, including head and trunk (figure 2.3). If he tried to stabilize the dish with his right hand, the light contact immediately activated the Avoiding Response, which, combined with the ATNR influence, resulted in retraction of the entire arm.

These reflexes could be counteracted and more normal patterns achieved if Patrick's right hand grasped a C-clamp placed at the edge of the table during spoon feeding with the left hand (figure 2.4). The C-clamp could be conveniently taken to his preschool, to restaurants, or to friends' homes. This same concept was effective during drawing activities, using

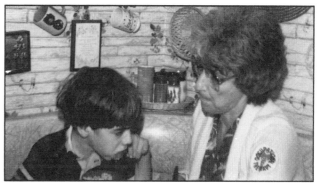

Figure 2.3. Use of the flexor synergy for spoon feeding (photo by author)

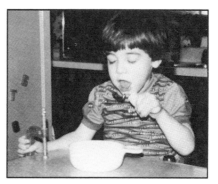

Figure 2.4. Use of the C-clamp to achieve more normal patterns during feeding (photo by author)

a permanent dowel in his desk (figure 2.5). To help Patrick integrate the ATNR, his head was maintained in midline, and his face limb was prevented from going into extension as he reached actively to pull off pieces of paper taped to his opposite shoulder (figure 2.6)

Because Patrick's athetosis was mixed with spasticity, he attempted to compensate for poorly regulated reciprocal innervation by excessive co-contraction at proximal joints (such as the shoulders) or distal joints (such as the hands and feet). When throwing a ball from a rather unstable vertical kneeling position, for example, his shoulders were elevated and his arms flexed and adducted (figure 2.7). His postural reflex mechanism could not develop normally, since righting and equilibrium reactions cannot be activated unless muscle tone is near normal. Intermittent dystonic spasms (sudden involuntary contractions) caused dramatic losses of balance, and without well-developed Protective Extensor Thrust of the arms, Patrick frequently bumped his head badly, especially backward.

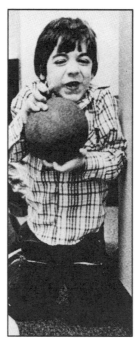

Figure 2.7. Unstable posture in vertical kneeling contributing to excessive co-contraction throughout upper body (photo by Dave Wallis, courtesy of *The Forum*)

Total flexion or extension synergies lingered during Patrick's developmental process, instead of breaking up to form combinations of movements and more selectivity. When trying to poke his extended index finger into a toy telephone hole, Patrick could not inhibit extension of the other three fingers. Drawing with his left hand always caused fisting, or associated reactions, in his right hand.

Learning new skills always produced some excess muscle tone (spasticity) throughout Patrick's entire body and increased if he happened to be in an unstable position, such as sitting unsupported or with feet dangling instead of planted firmly on the floor (figure 2.8). Unless he was provided with more stability, through positioning or with manual support, his repetition of new skills only reinforced these labored, slow, clumsy movements, his only sensorimotor experience.

During the long, tedious process of determining appropriate medication combinations and dosages for Patrick's uncontrolled seizures, his posture and movement patterns, as well as his behavior, were negatively affected by drug side effects.

The importance of stability in order to gain mobility was addressed at an NDT Refresher

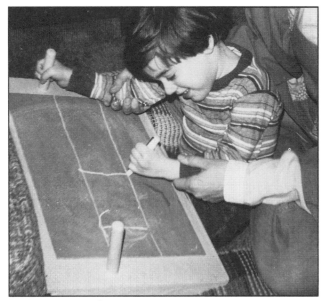

Figure 2.5. Use of the dowel to achieve more normal patterns during drawing activities (photo by Sheldon Green; desk courtesy of Courtney Rotzien)

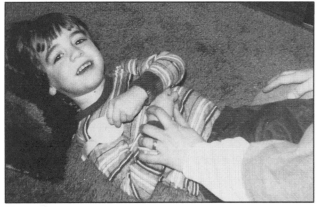

Figure 2.6. Integrating the ATNR by pulling off paper taped to the opposite shoulder, while head is maintained in midline (photo by author)

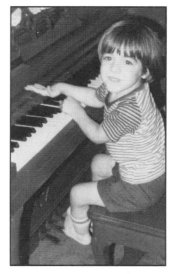

Figure 2.8. Lack of postural stability (feet dangling from piano bench) contributing to atypical hand patterns (photo courtesy of Sallie and John Mooneyham)

Developmental Hand Dysfunction

Weekend in Chicago in 1980 (Alexander, Cupps, and Haebig 1980). By analyzing the interrelationship of gross motor, fine motor, and respiratory-feeding-phonation development during the first 12 months of life, the baby's search for stability was dramatically illustrated. An NDT Baby Treatment certification course in New York in 1981 provided the author with more intensive knowledge about normal development, the importance of early intervention to prevent what were then termed abnormal "blocks" or "fixes," and special handling techniques incorporated into daily living activities such as feeding, bathing, dressing, lifting, carrying, and playing (Quinton et al. 1981) (figures 2.9, 2.10).

References

Alexander, R., B. Cupps, and R. Haebig [Boehme]. 1980 (October). Developmental kinesiology. Presented at Neuro-Developmental Treatment (NDT) Refresher Weekend. Chicago, Illinois.

Bobath, B. 1967. The very early treatment of cerebral palsy. *Developmental Medicine and Child Neurology* 9:373-90.

_____. 1971. Motor development, its effect on general development, and application to the treatment of cerebral palsy. *Physiotherapy* 57:526-32.

Bobath, B., and K. Bobath. 1956. The diagnosis of cerebral palsy in infancy. *Archives of Diseases in Childhood* 31:408-14.

_____. 1975. *Motor development in the different types of cerebral palsy.* London: William Heineman Medical Books.

Bobath, K. 1959. The neuropathology of cerebral palsy and its importance in treatment and diagnosis. *Cerebral Palsy Bulletin* 1:13-33.

_____. 1971. The normal postural reflex mechanism and its deviation in children with cerebral palsy. *Physiotherapy* 57:515-25.

_____. 1974. *The motor deficit in patients with cerebral palsy.* Suffolk: Lavenham Press.

Bobath, K., and B. Bobath. 1972. Cerebral palsy. In *Physical therapy services in the developmental disabilities,* edited by P. H. Pearson and C. E. Williams, 31-185. Springfield, IL: Charles C. Thomas.

Fiorentino, M. 1981 (May). A basis for sensorimotor development—Normal and abnormal. Presented at Continuing Education Programs of America. Minneapolis, Minnesota.

Milani-Comparetti, A. 1980 (October). The prenatal development of movement: Implications for developmental diagnosis. Presented at Professional Development Programs. St. Paul, Minnesota.

Quinton, M., L. Bly, F. Stern, and E. Danella. 1981 (June). Presented at Neuro-Developmental Treatment Association (NDTA) Baby Course. Roosevelt, New York.

Twitchell, T. E. 1959. On the motor deficit in congenital bilateral athetosis. *Journal of Nervous and Mental Diseases* 129:105-32.

_____. 1965. The automatic grasping responses of infants. *Neuropsychologia* 3:247-59.

_____. 1970. Reflex mechanisms and the development of prehension. In *Mechanisms of motor skill development,* edited by K. J. Connolly, 25-38. London: Academic Press.

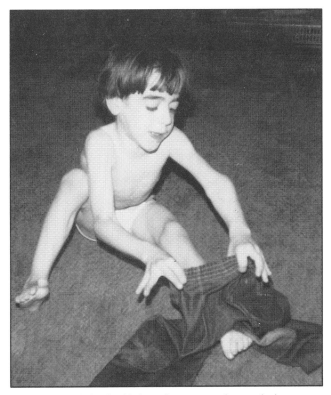

Figure 2.9. "Fixing" with jaw, fingers, and toes during dressing (photo by author)

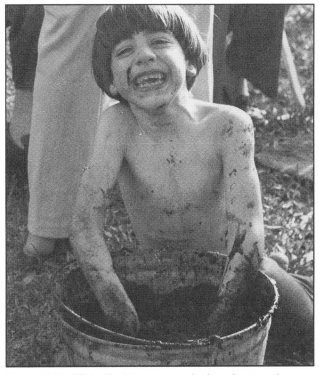

Figure 2.10. "Fixing" with asymmetrical neck extension, right shoulder elevation, and arm internal rotation during play (photo courtesy of Sallie and John Mooneyham)

Chapter Three
Kristy

The Search for Stability

Arm and hand patterns of the normal newborn are influenced by the prevailing uterine physiological flexion posture, which is passive rather than active. This strong flexor tone prevents full range of extension when the baby is at rest and allows random arm and hand movements with some components of extension only during the Moro (startle) Reflex or during total involuntary stretching patterns (Alexander, Cupps, and Haebig 1980). The Moro Reflex itself may be the baby's reaction to reaching back toward the uterine wall, not finding it there, and feeling lost in space. The physiological flexion is necessary to "keep the baby together" and to help integrate the very primitive central nervous system; it also serves an important purpose in limiting the amount of body surface receiving tactile stimulation, so that it can be comfortably interpreted as self-regulation of the baby's own responses if learned gradually. Otherwise, the baby may "shut down" the system to avoid overload.

This predominance of flexor tone at the natal stage of development provides stability in the head and shoulder area. The scapula and humerus are one unit, not differentiated, so the arms are usually flexed, adducted, and internally rotated in supine, prone, and supported sitting positions. Because the shoulders are elevated, the baby appears to have no neck, and no differentiation is present between the head and shoulder girdle. Table 7 traces the development of movement at the neck and shoulder by describing the gradual decrease of physiological flexion, the interaction of primitive reflexes with active movements, differentiation of head from shoulders and shoulders from arms, and the increase of mobility from points of stability (Alexander, Cupps, and Haebig 1980; Quinton et al. 1981).

Prenatal Considerations

Physiological flexion, present in the normal newborn, develops during the last 2½ months in utero. The 6-month fetus is completely hypotonic if born prematurely. Flexion begins in the hips at 6½ months and appears in the knees at 7 months, with the legs appearing somewhat frog-like at 7½ months. Not until 8 months do the upper extremities begin to gain more than minimal flexor tone, which increases gradually until the very hypertonic posture of 9 months is achieved (Amiel-Tison 1968).

As intensive care nurseries provide increasingly specialized medical services, many premature babies whose central nervous systems are essentially intact survive the stress of early birth and are able to function normally by 18 months (Quinton et al. 1981). Others, whose low muscle tone persists, do not try to move or respond to environmental stimulation at first. The lack of resistance to passive movement results in very little discomfort in positions that would normally be uncomfortable. Therefore, the baby has no desire to move or change position.

The usual posture of the floppy baby is on the back with widely abducted and externally rotated lower limbs flexed at hips and knees. The arms are also abducted, externally rotated, and flexed at the elbows. The neck and shoulders are retracted, pulled back against the surface by gravity, without the counterbalance of anterior flexor control. The baby rarely looks at the hands or engages in body play and never reaches for objects. Several months or even a year later, when reacting to stimulation and handling, postural tone develops, but it is not sufficient to withstand gravity. The baby begins to go into exaggerated

Table 7. Development of Movement at the Neck and Shoulders

Age	Supine	Prone	Sitting
Natal	Physiological flexion: shoulders elevated to ears; arms flexed, adducted, and internally rotated; elbows, wrists, fingers flexed, thumbs inside or outside; upper extremities may extend in total pattern of stretching or Moro Reflex.	Physiological flexion: shoulders elevated to ears; arms flexed, adducted, and internally rotated under body; hands fisted and pronated, thumbs inside; asymmetrical neck hyperextension used to lift head.	Pull to sit: head lag not total because of physiological flexion; no differentiation between neck, shoulders, arms.
1 month	Physiological flexion inhibited by more random movements; because of scapular adduction, arms more abducted against surface for stability to move head, legs; shoulder and arm not differentiated, so hands can't come to midline; ATNR helps first visual fixation on hand.	More extension, abduction, and external rotation; ATNR provides stability as neck extends asymmetrically, face-side arm extends, skull-side arm flexes; shoulder internally rotates, and arm flexes.	Pull to sit: head lag because passive flexion decreased and active flexion against gravity not yet present; shoulders elevated, neck hyperextended to gain head control.
2 months	More hypotonic with more extension and abduction of arms; shoulders less elevated; asymmetrical extension of neck replaced by asymmetrical neck flexion against gravity; more finger extension, thumbs outside.	Elbows still behind shoulders, but more weight on forearms, ulnar side of opening hands; arms more abducted and externally rotated, away from body; shoulders elevate and hands fist during head raising.	Pull to sit: uses asymmetrical flexion to lift head; momentary control, shoulders elevated.
3 months	Midline orientation and symmetry, less ATNR; differentiation of humerus and scapula allows shoulders lower than ears; arm flexion forward with internal rotation allows hand clasping in midline, hands loosely closed; hands to mouth, hand-watching.	Elbows still slightly behind shoulders, which are lower than ears, weight bearing on forearms; some weight shifts when head turns allows unsuccessful reaching; neck develops active control in flexion-extension; hands open at rest, fisted during head raising.	Pull to sit: more flexor control, less head lag, assists with upper extremities, not abdominal muscles; some co-contraction of neck flexors and extensors; still asymmetrical.
4 months	Strong symmetry and controlled flexion; abdominals help get hands to knees; hands together in space; bilateral reaching with ulnar grasp; mouthing fingers and objects.	Arms forward under shoulders with shoulder depression; good co-contraction between back extension and trunk flexion; weight on forearms and palmar surface of hands; no successful reaching.	Pull to sit: neck flexors assist, arms pull, abdominals begin; more symmetry; hands to mouth, hands together; tries to sit with shoulder retraction.
5 months	Rotation between shoulder and pelvis; hands to feet, feet to mouth; arms reaching forward.	Weight shifting on forearms, trying to reach with one arm; weight bearing on extended arms, radial-palmar surface of hands.	Pull to sit: chin tucks, arms and legs flex, active abdominals; less neck hyperextension; stable shoulders allow arms reaching forward.
6 months	Increased pelvic stability allows shoulder control and mobility; reaching with one or both hands, transferring objects; head lifting.	Weight bearing on extended arms more in midline; successful reaching with one arm while weight bearing on forearms.	Sits with arms propped, shoulders depressed, begins to reach with one arm.
7 months	Does not tolerate supine position; rolls to prone or sidelying.	Reaching while weight bearing on extended arm.	Moves from sidesitting or hands and knees to sitting, reaches freely with both arms.

The material in this table is based on Alexander, Cupps, and Haebig (1980) and Quinton et al. (1981).

Developmental Hand Dysfunction

extension, overuse reflex patterns, and fix, usually at the neck and shoulder area, searching for stability (Bobath 1974). These movement patterns resemble some of the decreasing physiological flexion postures of the 1-month-old baby, whose shoulders are elevated, whose neck is hyperextended, and who uses the ATNR to gain stability during asymmetrical head raising (Alexander, Cupps, and Haebig 1980). Since muscle tone is spotty (a mixture of basic hypotonus and fluctuating hypertonus), the process of normal adaptation is interrupted. Fixation, or repetition of purposeless lower-level movement patterns, results in regression and developmental disability (Gilfoyle, Grady, and Moore 1981).

Milani's work with the ultrasound scanner revealed a large quantity as well as a variety of prenatal movements, supporting his hypothesis that all elements of motor behavior are present in the fetus. Constant movements are seen during all 24 hours, with no more than a few minutes of inactivity at a time. By 2 months, when the embryo becomes a well-established fetus, the vermicular, trembling movements of the unstable neuromuscular system are being replaced by exploratory motions and the beginning of vital reflex patterns such as sucking and grasping. Milani prefers his term "primary motor patterns" to "primitive reflexes," since the pure stimuli-responses are modified by competitive patterns and are available for functional use in utero, during infancy, and throughout adult life. As the fetus grows and becomes too long for the uterus, attempts to enlarge the space result in extending and thrusting movements. Fetal locomotion (climbing, rolling over, and even somersaulting) enables the full-term baby to find the best position in preparation for presentation. Fetal propulsion (pushing with the legs against the uterine wall) is needed for normal labor in collaboration with contractions of the uterus.

Some floppy full-term babies, whose birth histories are reported as normal, may have had a CNS insult before 6 months gestation age. Characteristic postures and movement patterns at that level or earlier levels may be perpetuated, blocking further development. Vermicular tremors may persist, and the neuromuscular system remains unstable and immature. Muscle tone may remain low instead of gradually increasing to the normal hypertonus of the normal newborn. Unable to participate as fully as possible in the birth process, some of these babies could suffer a secondary asphyxia because of prolonged labor. Movement patterns observed

in children with developmental disabilities could therefore be termed regressive rather than abnormal (Milani-Comparetti 1980).

The correlation of etiology to different types of cerebral palsy is complicated by the high incidence of mixed characteristics in most cases. In one study of 190 children with cerebral palsy, 33 showed normal birth histories, 36 were premature, and the remainder listed a variety of perinatal problems (Bobath and Bobath 1956). Table 8 presents fetal postures, muscle tone, and reflexes from 6 months gestation age to the full term of 9 months.

Kristy

Kristy's mother was convinced that this second pregnancy was different from the first. The baby's first movements appeared normally at approximately 4 months but were less vigorous than she remembered. For several days during the fifth month, very little movement occurred. When the baby did become active again, the quality of movement had changed. Instead of total body movements, only smaller twitching motions were felt, combined with tremulous shivers, which continued until Kristy was delivered spontaneously at full term.

A seizure was observed on Kristy's second day of life. She then developed pneumonia, was given intravenous antibiotics, and was kept in an incubator until she was discharged when about 2 weeks old. Seizure medication needed to be increased at 3 weeks of age when more seizures appeared, but after 3 months, medication was gradually eliminated with no recurrence of problems.

Although the cause of Kristy's cerebral palsy has not been determined, a hypothetical inference drawn from prenatal, perinatal, and postnatal history can be useful in identifying a true motor development age for intervention purposes. Reversion to primitive, tremor-type movements and fixation at the floppy stage of muscle development could have resulted from damage to the central nervous system during the fifth month of pregnancy.

Without normal physiological flexion and mature sensory regulatory mechanisms as a protection against overwhelming tactile and proprioceptive stimulation, Kristy may have reacted by partially "shutting down"

Table 8. Fetal Posture, Muscle Tone, and Reflexes

Gestation Age	Posture	Return to Flexion of Forearms	Grasp	Moro
6 months	Completely hypotonic	Upper limbs very hypotonic, limbs lying in extension	Good finger grasp and reaction through upper limb, but not strong enough to lift from surface	Weak, elicited once, not every time
6½ months	Some hip flexion			
7 months	More hip flexion		Stronger	Complete reflex
7½ months	Frog-leg position	Beginning of weak flexion of forearms	Stronger	Complete reflex
8 months	Flexion of all four limbs	Strong return to flexion, but flexor tone inhibited if forearm maintained 30 seconds in extension	Strong enough to lift body weight	Complete reflex
8½ months	Hypertonic	Strong return to flexion, forearm returns promptly after 30 seconds in extension	Strong enough to lift body weight	Complete reflex
9 months	Very hypertonic	Same as above	Strong enough to lift body weight	Complete reflex

The material in this table is based on Amiel-Tison (1968).

the system. She was comfortable in almost any position, demonstrating very little desire to move. She had a significantly higher threshold of pain and touch than other babies. This reduced awareness and lack of mobility allowed some tactile recognition and repetition, but very little assimilation, accommodation, or adaptation. Kristy scratched at clothing and sometimes her body, repeating the activity, but she did not reach out and assimilate the movements to many other materials; she did not accommodate her hand to the form of new objects; and thus she did not adapt and learn new positions and movements.

Because her shoulders were elevated and arms retracted from the gravity pull of supine lying and from the stress of maintaining head control in supported sitting, the secondary schemata of vision and prehension were not coordinated. Her hands were seldom within her visual field, a prerequisite for voluntary reach and grasp (figures 3.1, 3.2).

Since physiological flexion provides the baby's first stability in developing posture and movement against gravity, Kristy's lack of proximal co-contraction was a major factor in her limited mobility. When attempting to lift her head in prone, she used total extension patterns, hyperextending the neck, back, and arms,

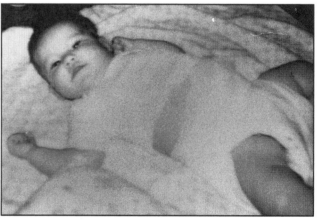

Figure 3.1. Arm retraction in supine preventing eye-hand coordination (photo courtesy of Carmon and Mike Cymbal)

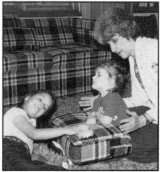

Figure 3.2. Inability to use downward gaze and reach for the toy her sister is presenting, despite therapist's support in sitting (photo by author)

with extension-abduction of the legs (figure 3.3). Without the push of the flexed arm against the surface, however, she could not roll from prone to supine. The development of head control and weight bearing on forearms, therefore, was a primary goal to prepare for rolling, as well as sitting (figure 3.4).

The use of total extension movements to gain stability and mobility could have begun in utero, assuming that Kristy's fetal propulsion contributed to normal labor and delivery. If fetal behaviors represent important components of Kristy's present motor skills, they must be included not only in the theoretical base for a practical theory of prehension but in the considerations for assessment and treatment as well.

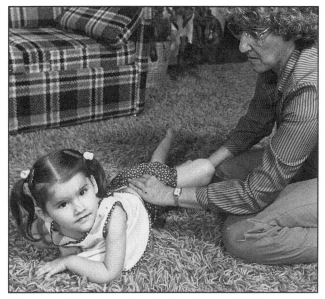

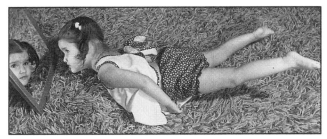

Figure 3.3. Extensor synergy used for head lifting in prone (photo by Sheldon Green)

Figure 3.4. Therapy to develop head control during weight bearing on forearms (photo by Sheldon Green)

References

Alexander, R., B. Cupps, and R. Haebig [Boehme]. 1980 (October). Developmental kinesiology. Presented at Neuro-Developmental Treatment (NDT) Refresher Weekend. Chicago, Illinois.

Amiel-Tison, C. 1968. Neurological evaluation of the maturity of newborn infants. *Archives of Disease in Childhood* 43:89-93.

Bobath, K. 1974. *The motor deficit in patients with cerebral palsy.* Suffolk: Lavenham Press.

Bobath, K., and B. Bobath. 1956. The diagnosis of cerebral palsy in infancy. *Archives of Disease in Childhood* 31:408-14.

Gilfoyle, E. M., A. P. Grady, and J. C. Moore. 1981. *Children adapt.* Thorofare, NJ: Charles B. Slack.

Milani-Comparetti, A. 1980 (October). The prenatal development of movement: Implications for developmental diagnosis. Presented at Professional Development Programs. St. Paul, Minnesota.

Quinton, M., L. Bly, F. Stern, and E. Danella. 1981 (June). Presented at Neuro-Developmental Treatment Association (NDTA) Baby Course. Roosevelt, New York.

Chapter Four
The Architect

The Maturity of Prehension

The compilation and comparison of developmental norms of prehension from nine literature sources revealed a significantly consistent sequence of behavior components from birth to 15 months (Erhardt, Beatty, and Hertsgaard 1981). A videotaped study of hand development in normal babies during the same period supported the compiled norms in developmental ages as well as sequences (Erhardt and Pullen 1981).

Because essential components of prehension are developed and functional at approximately 15 months, further refinements, increased skill, and the use of tools (such as the pencil, brush, or knife) are the result of learned experiences. Thus, the 15-month level can be considered the maturity of prehension. Primitive reflexes such as the ATNR, Grasping Reactions, and Avoiding Responses, necessary physiological substrata for complex voluntary hand movements, are well integrated by that age, and voluntary patterns of approach, grasp, manipulation, and release have been perfected. The arm demonstrates a direct, unilateral approach, with extended elbow, wrist, and fingers. Grasp can be delicately limited to the tips of two or three fingers. Manipulation has replaced mouthing and is possible without visual monitoring. Release into small containers is precise. Pencil grasp, which develops in stages from the ages of 1 to 6 years, becomes perfected through experience (Erhardt, Beatty, and Hertsgaard 1981).

Adult Reversion to Earlier Patterns

In times of stress or to achieve high levels of skill, the normal adult has access to the repertoire of previously integrated primitive reflexes and early positions of stability. Thus, the architect, needing to achieve a perfect production of a rendering which cannot be erased, automatically seeks a position of greater stability: he elevates his shoulders and internally rotates and adducts his non-dominant arm, bearing weight on the forearm and fisted hand, reminiscent of the 3-month baby in prone (figure 4.1).

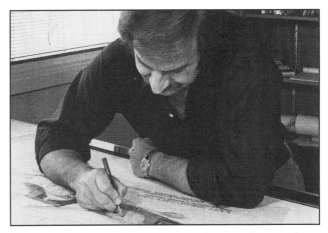

Figure 4.1. Seeking postural stability for a perfect production (photo by Sheldon Green)

When he knife-cuts poster board, he gains strength and accuracy by assuming the 2-month-level ATNR position: head rotated toward the extended arm holding the board in place, while the flexed arm uses a palmar-supinate grasp, typical of the 1- to 2-year-old pencil grasp (figure 4.2). For large lettering, he changes his total body position by walking around the table to orient himself for as many vertical lines as possible, the first drawing stroke achieved by children at 2 years of age as they pull the crayon down on paper or wall (figures 4.3, 4.4).

The effects of stress are also dramatically illustrated in one of Auguste Rodin's famous sculptures of the human adult hand, *The Left Hand,* which bears a remarkable resemblance to the typical spastic pattern of flexed wrist, hyperextended metacarpophalangeal (knuckle) joints, and flexed fingers.

Further Postural Considerations

As previously stated, many variables influence the normal adult's choice of body position as well as type of grasp. The nature of the activity, convenience, and the requirements of speed, precision, and strength do not always elicit the most appropriate sitting and standing postures, however, and certain work-related injuries may result from persistent physiologically unfavorable working conditions. Architects and draftsmen, for example, have historically suffered from kyphosis, scoliosis, backaches, and headaches, due to sitting or standing at horizontal rather than elevated inclined drawing boards (figure 4.5).

Visual problems such as increased myopia (nearsightedness) can occur as the eyes consistently accommodate to the reduced distance between eyes and board, caused by leaning on the elbow. With presbyopia

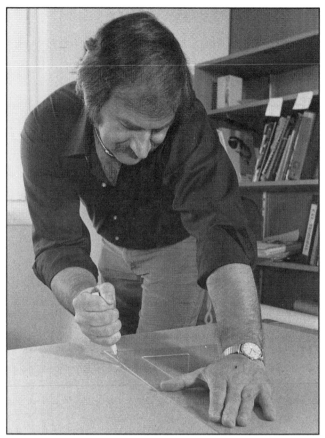

Figure 4.2. Achieving strength and accuracy with the ATNR position and palmar-supinate grasp (photo by Sheldon Green)

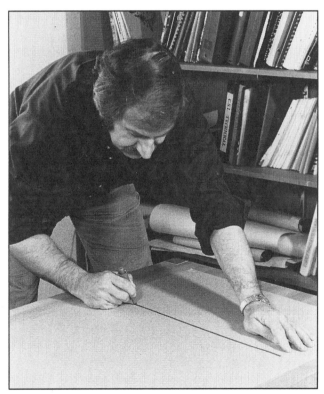

Figure 4.3. Positioning for vertical line downward (photo by Sheldon Green)

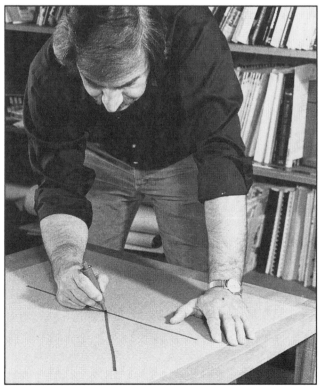

Figure 4.4. Repositioning to maintain orientation of vertical line downward (photo by Sheldon Green)

Developmental Hand Dysfunction

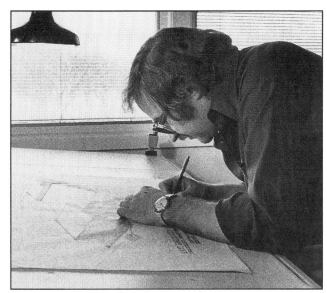

Figure 4.5. Horizontal surface contributing to kyphosis (photo by Sheldon Green)

(farsightedness) caused by increasing age, the need for focusing the eyes in a direction perpendicular to the board is even more necessary, not only to avoid distortion of the image but also because the range and speed of accommodation become more limited. The normal eye perceives details most clearly in a range of 25 to 35 centimeters, the average length of an adult's forearm (Kuhlmann and Mueller 1980). This is corroborated by research done by the Winterhaven Lions Club Project on Perceptual Training, which defines the Harmon Distance as that distance from the child's nose to the paper equaling the length of the forearm (from elbow to first knuckle). A 20° sloped board rather than a flat surface was recommended for children as well (Harmon 1958).

Adjustable work stations including chairs as well as tables are needed to adapt to the variety of human dimensions such as upper and lower leg length, arm length, and elbow height. Focal length and eye height are affected by the use of bifocal or trifocal lenses, indicating the need for a lower position than the usual 15° below the horizontal line of sight (Hollerith 1980).

New types of stools and chairs have alleviated many problems by allowing a variety of adjustments in seating height, seat and back inclinations, and rotation. The need for dynamic motion as well as static postures is also addressed in sales literature by manufacturers. Their opinions are similar to those of Bobath, who insisted that no one correct sitting posture exists because no position is constant, nor should it be. The normal adult is programmed for movement and needs

many different sitting positions to avoid discomfort, just as the child with a disability who remains in one position risks contractures and deformities (Polsky 1981; Bobath 1977; Finnie 1975) (figures 4.6, 4.7).

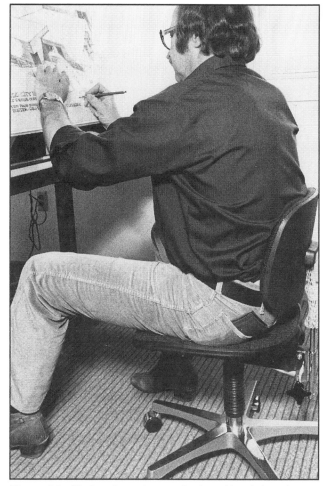

Figure 4.6. Chair adjusted to vertical position (photo by Sheldon Green; chair courtesy of Mathison's)

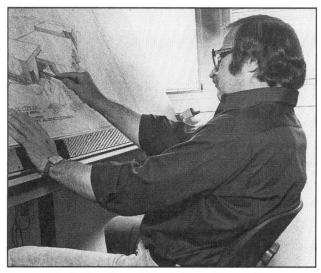

Figure 4.7. Chair adjusted for slight inclination (photo by Sheldon Green; chair courtesy of Mathison's)

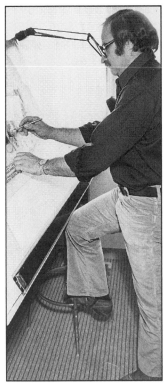

Figure 4.8. Standing position with one foot elevated (photo by Sheldon Green; chair courtesy of Mathison's)

The architect may need to work in a standing position to reach distal areas of large drawings or to use more efficient and comfortable head movements when transferring information from reference material to the board. Lower back strain can be avoided if one foot is elevated (figure 4.8).

The problems of adult posture are exaggerated in children with developmental disabilities. Because Joanne worked on shoulder control and large arm movements for drawing skills in a supported standing position, she did not develop the flexed and kyphotic posture typical of many children with spasticity (figure 4.9). Patrick's 25° tilt of his custom-made desk facilitated visual perception (figure 4.10). Seating systems should support without restricting movement, and should be modified to decrease support as the child improves. Creative thinking and problem-solving skills are required for the ongoing process of individualizing each child's seating system.

The Creative Process

Theories of development addressed thus far have included those from the fields of medicine (orthopedic, pediatric, and neurologic), education, psychology, and anthropology. The synthesis of developmental theories and their subsequent use for purposes of assessment and treatment cannot occur without the catalyst of the creative process, inherent in the field of architecture.

The fundamental characteristic of the self-actualized persons studied by Maslow was their creativity, which was the impetus to use fully their talents, capacities, and potentialities (Maslow 1971). Maslow and Toffler were convinced that in an era undergoing changes

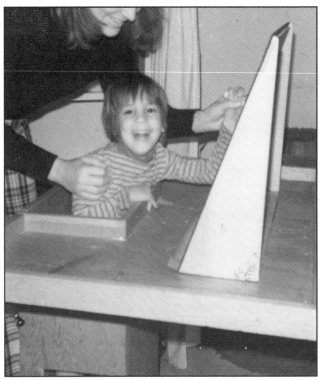

Figure 4.9. Drawing activities in supported standing (photo by author)

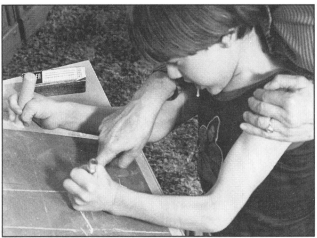

Figure 4.10. Inclined surface to bring surface parallel to face and eyes (photo by Sheldon Green; desk courtesy of Courtney Rotzien)

more rapidly than any previous one in history, a new kind of human being was needed (Toffler 1971). The creative, improvising, adapting, problem-solving person could anticipate, enjoy, and be challenged by change.

Maslow (1956) believed that people are born with innate potentialities for creativity, spontaneity, caring for others, and yearning for truth, often stifled and lost because of the influence of acculturation, especially the pressures to conform.

Developmental Hand Dysfunction

Frank Lloyd Wright, who vigorously shared the opinion of many who considered him the world's greatest living architect, believed that contemporary education sought to condition rather than enlighten human beings. For individuals to preserve their own integrity, they must pay attention to their inner vision and inner voice, maintain their own convictions, and cultivate the resources in themselves that contribute to their vision (Wright 1966).

Throughout his autobiography, Wright described his repeated stubborn refusals to relinquish many of his own ideas, for fear that he would lose that which he recognized as preciously unique (Wright 1932). And yet, he realized that the architect had an obligation to explore the nature of everything he encountered, in order to uncover the essential truth of rock, flower, building, tool, client. His ideal, the organic building, represented unity and harmony in every aspect, but it was never reached, nor did it need to be, because the process was more important than the finished product.

By being a *relentless observer*, the therapist, as well as the architect, becomes first a scientist, curious, investigating, analyzing separate units of phenomena. Then, as an artist, the therapist relates these units to the whole, a fundamental order waiting for discovery and expression. Again, understanding the process of development, rather than a preconceived notion of the final goals, is the vital key to therapeutic intervention.

Because Frank Lloyd Wright also realized that constant change was an inherent part of all things—that houses needed to perform new functions as families grew, decreased, or diversified—his designs anticipated and provided for continuous change. His term *plasticity* means that materials flow or grow into the form instead of joining or attaching. With perfect correlation of parts, form and function are unified (Twombly 1973).

His narrative, "Designing Unity Temple," is a classic example of the creative process in action. Wright began with the philosophy of the structure. What was the purpose of the building? A room was worship, simple, beautiful, natural. What shape, what form, what style? The shape depended on the material. Why not concrete, which was cheap? How to form it? The geometric form of the cube denoted integrity. The style wasn't chosen; it was created from the sense of order and the love of beauty—an exciting moment to the architect as the first rough plan emerged.

Wright let the ideas simmer. Later, he applied concentrated attention to perfecting design and details. The character or sense of the Room came through as the soul of the design. Therefore, the sketch came after the building was designed as a whole, not before.

One biographer was critical of what he perceived as Wright's singular belief that the architect knows what is best for the client, seeking very little consultation with those primarily affected (Twombly 1973). The clients themselves, writing about the process of working with Wright, gave him their list of guidelines and "absolute requirements," but they soon found themselves fired with enthusiasm as they listened to his charming and persuasive descriptions of his own innovative plans for them. A series of letters, however, illustrated that even Wright accepted his clients' desired changes, which they cogently but tactfully justified (Jacobs and Jacobs 1978).

The Problem-Solving Process

Therapists, too, need to use others fully in the decision-making and problem-solving processes. The team can, and often does, involve professionals such as the occupational therapist, physical therapist, speech therapist, nurse, teacher, psychologist, social worker, physician, and counselor. But equally important are lay persons such as parents, grandparents, siblings, friends, and, of course, the child.

The team must perceive the child's motor, cognitive, language, and social milestones evolving from the consequences of logical, orderly development. Only when the nature of a problem (disorder) is understood can the solution emerge. The creative process begins with intense curiosity. What is happening?

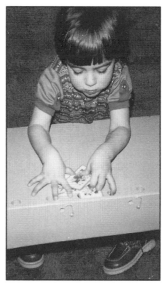

Figure 4.11. Atypical hand pattern common in individuals with cerebral palsy (photo by author)

Patrick grasps with flexed, pronated wrist, hyperextended MCP joints (knuckles), and subluxed proximal thumb joint (figure 4.11). Why? What information concerning development must be considered?

An idea appears, a single image, then a cluster of images.

- Wrist flexion and pronation and thumb adduction are normal up to the 5-month level, when the child uses a palmar grasp of a cube (fingers pressing cube into center of palm, thumb adducted, not opposed, wrist flexed and pronated).

- Grasp of the pellet is unsuccessful in the normal baby until 7 months, when the adducted thumb and extended fingers rake it into the center of the palm.

- Use of the thumb in opposition to grasp the pellet does not appear until almost 9 months, when the child begins to finger feed dry cereal, for example.

- Excessive extension of the fingers during approach, linked with overreaching, is normal from 6 to 10 months

Various hypotheses are proposed. At Patrick's chronological age of 6 years, his cognitive and social levels motivate him to attempt some tasks above certain of his current motor levels, resulting in a combination of developmental patterns that appear atypical or inappropriate (flexed, pronated wrist, hyperextended MCPs, adducted proximal thumb joint, and extended distal thumb joint).

Since each developmental pattern prepares for the next sequential pattern, missing patterns force inappropriate combinations (maladaptations). Thus, filling in certain developmental gaps can allow development to proceed in a more normal sequence, reducing the need for atypical compensatory patterns. This germ of an idea begins to develop. By the collaborative process of discussion and experimentation involving therapist, parent, teacher, child, and others, the idea is enlarged, altered, and enriched. This pleasurable process of discovery begins with the intrigue of putting certain related information together, proceeds with the gradual illumination of the concept, and culminates in the arrival at a solution (or solutions) that everyone recognizes, sharing in the excitement (Rufrin 1981).

Therapeutic intervention, then, by all team members can be the art and science of directing the individual's response to the environment, as well as adapting the environment to foster the individual's potential for self-actualization.

Maslow (1970) refuted both polarized positions in the debate on the role of heredity versus environment.

He was more concerned with the power of the environment to diminish genetic potential rather than creating or even increasing it. Therefore, he felt that the role of the environment should be to nurture and foster the psychological potentials needed for self-actualization (Maslow 1959).

Gilfoyle (1980) defined *caring* as a process to help another gain self-actualization and achieve more independence. Caring as a philosophy of occupational therapy practice integrates the methods of the science of therapy into a humanistic focus: the art of therapy. Through the caring, therapeutic relationship, the application of scientific principles to purposeful activity can be a process of mutual growth and collaboration between therapist and child. Parents, teachers, and others who form the child's human environment can all participate in a multidimensional series of shared learning experiences from which problem-solving skills arise.

Practice of the Art

The knowledge, skills, and attitudes necessary to practice the art of therapy are components of the creative process that can be compared to those of the architect practicing the art of his profession.

Knowledge

The architect gathers data for the building project. He examines the site, investigates the functional and aesthetic needs of the client, and determines the parameters. He reviews the materials and processes that may be used in construction and begins considering types of original designs.

The therapist needs to know and understand general and specific information about the child's medical condition. Therapeutic methods and techniques that may apply to that condition must be considered in terms of the child's own special abilities, limitations, and needs. The child is always realized as a unique individual, not a stereotype.

Skills

The architect presents a building program to the client, sketches some tentative designs, and receives feedback from the client, which leads to refinements relating to the design itself and/or to the budget.

The therapist evaluates the child, plans a treatment program, and continually assesses it, learning from previous experiences with this child and with other children, adapting and modifying treatment in response to continual feedback from the child and others.

Attitudes

The architect learns to develop *patience* throughout the long process of design and construction. When compromises are necessary, he must somehow reconcile them with his own standards of quality in order to be *honest* with himself. *Trust* in his co-workers, engineers, and construction crew must be tempered by his basic responsibility, which requires his involvement in all steps of the building process. A *humble* awareness of the need for continual learning to keep up with new products and processes is coupled with the *courage* to try new ideas and approaches and the *hope* that each new structure is more beautiful and unique than the last.

The therapist displays *patience* by enabling children to grow at their own rate and within their own particular style. *Honesty* involves seeing children as they really are and not as we wish they were. When children are encouraged to become independent rather than dependent, they begin to *trust* their own abilities as others trust them. An attitude of *humility* is consistent with the therapist's realization that much more needs to be learned about individual children and how to help them. The therapist's willingness to try new things supports children in developing *courage* of their own. Finally, by setting realistic expectations for children, *hope* is affirmed.

References

Erhardt, R. P., P. A. Beatty, and D. M. Hertsgaard. 1981. A developmental prehension assessment for handicapped children. *American Journal of Occupational Therapy* 35:237-42.

Erhardt, R. P., and D. Pullen. 1981. *Normal hand development: Birth to 15 months,* videotape. Moorhead, MN: Moorhead State University TV Production Center. (Available from Erhardt Developmental Products, 2379 Snowshoe Court, Maplewood, MN 55119.)

Finnie, N. 1975. *Handling the young cerebral palsied child at home.* New York: E. P. Dutton.

Gilfoyle, E. M. 1980. Caring: A philosophy for practice. *American Journal of Occupational Therapy* 34:517-21.

Harmon, D. B. 1958. *Notes on a dynamic theory of vision:* Vol. 1, 3d revision. Austin, TX: D. B. Harmon.

Hollerith, R. 1980. People are different, so why not their work stations? *The Office,* November 63-66.

Jacobs, H., and K. Jacobs. 1978. *Building with Frank Lloyd Wright.* San Francisco: Chronicle Books.

Kuhlmann, F., and H. Mueller. 1980. *Investigation into layout in the drawing office.* Houston, TX: Kuhlmann-Impex, Inc.

Maslow, A. H. 1956. Self-actualizing people: A study of psychological health. In *The self,* edited by C. E. Moustakes, 165-87. New York: Harper Brothers.

_____. 1959. Psychological data and value theory. In *New knowledge in human values,* 119-36. New York: Harper Brothers.

_____. 1970. *Motivation and personality.* New York: Harper and Row.

_____. 1971. *The farther reaches of human nature.* New York: Viking Press.

Polsky, N. 1981. Discovery in office seating systems through the 1990 paperless office. Kansas City: Fixtures FMC Ltd., December 9.

Rufrin, J. 1981. *Uncommon women.* Piscataway, NJ: New Century Publications.

Toffler, A. 1971. *Future shock.* New York: Bantam Books.

Twombly, R. C. 1973. *Frank Lloyd Wright.* New York: Harper and Row.

Wright, F. L. 1932. *An autobiography of Frank Lloyd Wright.* New York: Longmans, Green and Company.

Wright, O. L. 1966. *Frank Lloyd Wright: His life, his work, his words.* New York: Horizon Press.

Chapter Five
A Synthesized Theory of Prehension

The Taxonomy of Learning

Bloom's taxonomy of educational objectives for the cognitive domain describes the various levels of learning as Knowledge, Comprehension, Application, Analysis, Synthesis, and Evaluation (Bloom 1956). This study of prehension began by listing theories of human development and defining the terms used to describe the theories. The basic Knowledge (Level One) was presented concurrently with Comprehension (Level Two), which reviewed and discussed the theories, recognizing their relevancy to hand function. Application (Level Three) was achieved by illustrating each theory with specific examples from the case studies of the three children and an adult. Analysis (Level Four) was also interwoven with the interpretation of the theories by comparing normal and abnormal (atypical) prehension development, noting similarities and differences among the children, and relating adult reversion to primitive patterns. Synthesis (Level Five) necessarily involves the creative process, which relates not only to development of a new theory but also to its practical use for assessment and treatment.

Characteristics of a Theory

A different taxonomy of levels of performance for theory building was proposed by Rogers, who viewed professional practice based on a knowledge of order, disorder, and change (Rogers 1982).

Order, an image of the normal state of man, must be known well by the practitioner who seeks to establish, maintain, or enhance it. Disorder, which is judged in relation to order and includes phenomena disrupting

order, must also be recognized. Change stems from the knowledge of both, allowing the practitioner to prescribe a course of action converting disorder to order. The field of occupational therapy views competence in self-care, work, and play as developing through occupation, active participation in meaningful physical, mental, and social activities. Performance, which relates to a continuum of competence, may be facilitated or hindered by hereditary and environmental factors. Therefore, intervention is designed to maximize the individual's productivity. In the case of children, their work is play; their occupation is student or learner, always in the process of development.

The usefulness of a theory in any practice discipline depends on the effectiveness of its remedial measures; that is, its ability to convert disorder into order. In addition, a theory should be easily explained, distinguished from others, allow scientific elaboration and refinement, and possess a unifying concept that can be applied to specific situations (King 1978).

In order to further scientific knowledge, a theory provides (1) a method of organizing and categorizing information, (2) explanations of past events, (3) understanding of what causes events, (4) predictions of future events, and (5) potential for control of events.

Development of a Theory

The *exploratory* stage of theory construction has been described as a period when huge amounts of data are collected and analyzed. A commitment is made to acquire a thorough knowledge of existing related theories, without being bound to them as the only and final explanation (Reynolds 1971). This early fact gathering may begin as a random, casual activity, restricted to the data available, with no effort to be critical. As interest grows, the subject matter becomes engrossing, and the challenge of solving a puzzle in a new or better way becomes a motivation for research.

During the *descriptive* stage of theory construction, more selection, definition, and direction occur as tentative hypotheses arise. Procedures for classifying phenomena are conceptualized. Unrelated information drops out, and some causal processes are considered. Comparisons of various theories reveal that phenomena described and interpreted differently by different people begin to lose their divergence. Significant facts are determined and matched with existing theories and grouped into similar sets (Kuhn 1970). Terminology may be redefined and updated to reflect current standards of acceptability (for example, "atypical" replacing "abnormal").

Actual theory construction begins during the *explanatory* stage, when an explicit theory is tested, reformulated, reconstructed, retested, and so on (Reynolds 1971).

Typical research methods used for this study of prehension included historical documentation (case study data), experimental research (an interrater reliability study and informal field studies), interviews, and observational methods (videotapes) (Compton and Hall 1972).

The evolution of a theory of prehension has embraced both the scientific research process and the creative process. The long period of preparation—the years of studying, reading, experiencing, writing, and talking with others—was the important "soaking-up" process. It was intermingled with the "simmering" stage, when the work was put aside, not consciously attended, but nevertheless thought about at odd times. When inspiration began to lead to sudden solutions, new relationships appeared and ideas came rapidly. Thinking was still difficult but enjoyable, and goals began to take shape. Verification and revision of ideas required objective data, continued observation, and additional reading (Engle and Snellgrove 1979). This empirical work finally resulted in articulation of the theory, resolution of ambiguities, and development of rules enabling the theory to be applied to other situations.

The only remaining strategy was the development of a representational or visual model. Interviews with the architect, who served as the example of adult prehen-

sion patterns, led to discussions of the creative process and to a comparison of the professions of occupational therapy and architecture. As the process of designing and implementing a therapy program was compared to designing and building a structure, a visual representation of prehension development began to emerge.

Developmental Prehension Sequence Clusters

The consistent sequence of prehension pattern components compiled from developmental norms in the literature had been organized and refined through research already described. These pattern components could logically be arranged in vertical stacks of cubes, which indicated age levels. These stacks, or buildings, were termed *developmental prehension sequence clusters* and were grouped into three sections:

- Section 1. Primarily involuntary arm-hand patterns (positional-reflexive)

- Section 2. Primarily voluntary movements of approach, grasp, manipulation, and release (cognitively directed)

- Section 3. Prewriting skills (pencil grasp and drawings)

Shaded areas would indicate Norms (permanent patterns emerging at various age levels and continuing throughout life). Figure 5.1 presents these developmental prehension sequence clusters.

A Theory of Inappropriate Prehension Patterns

According to Reynolds (1971), a theory is a collection of statements, not only a set of laws (well-supported empirical generalizations) and axioms (definitions and propositions), but also a causal process (effects of independent variables on dependent variables). In reviewing theoretical statements presented in earlier chapters, the importance of their relevance to a causal process is apparent.

Gesell saw neuromotor readiness influencing maturation more than environmental factors and function developing by expansion of the reflex system, gradually becoming voluntary. Children changed at a different rate but in the same sequence (Gesell and Amatruda 1969).

Developmental Hand Dysfunction

DEVELOPMENTAL PREHENSION SEQUENCE CLUSTERS©

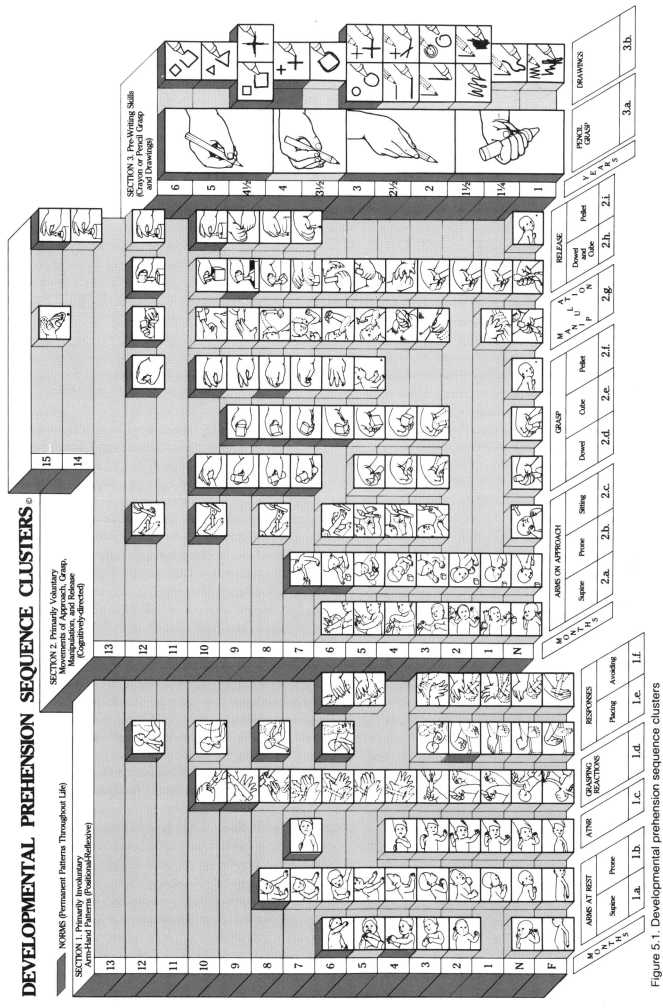

Figure 5.1. Developmental prehension sequence clusters

Piaget's view of the reflex system proceeding toward adaptive behavior considered external experiences important in the repetition and modification process. Disequilibrium or disorganized, clumsy behavior was typical during transition periods to higher levels (Piaget 1952).

Ayres stated that although innate phylogenetic patterns are inherited, individual expression depends on ontogenetic experience, as the environment demands interpretation of sensory stimuli and adaptive responses (Ayres 1974).

Bobath explained the process of inhibition and differentiation as total synergies are broken up to allow more selective movement. Increased tension during the learning of new skills and temporary regression to more primitive motor activity occurs in the child who is developing normally, but with repetition and adaptation, the performance becomes more automatic and smooth. The child who has cerebral palsy, however, with a mixture of primitive and pathological patterns, reinforces the abnormal elements because of poor adaptation, often incorporating them into the new skill as a permanent pattern (Bobath 1971).

The spatiotemporal theory of adaptation developed by Gilfoyle, Grady, and Moore (1981) described the effects of environmental demands that exceeded the child's functional capacities. Reversion to lower-level behaviors, a direct result of sensory input occurring at an inappropriate rate, intensity, and/or duration, may persist, unmodified by the normal adaptation process, causing developmental dysfunction.

Awareness of this causal process, inherent and clearly stated in these reviewed theories, led to the formulation of a theory of prehension necessarily related to assessment and intervention.

Developmental hand dysfunction poses a difficult problem for the professional because of the scarcity of evaluation instruments that are both quantitative and qualitative. Assessment methodology that is quantifiable allows tracking of development over time, demonstrating change and accountability. Qualitative attributes are particularly important for planning and implementing appropriate intervention. Reasons for dissatisfaction with available tests include lack of objectivity, insufficient items, failure to assess quality of performance, inappropriateness of design for severely involved and very young children, and limited use for structuring treatment programs. Global development scales, such as the Bayley Scale of Infant Development and the Denver Developmental Screening Test, although useful in assigning developmental levels, possess limitations related to the size of steps between the behavioral sequences leading to emerging skills, the rate of skill acquisition, and the influence on one skill by the acquisition of others (Erhardt, Beatty, and Hertsgaard 1981).

Developmental testing does provide an awareness of the quality of movements, because what is appropriate (normal) for a 1-month-old child (flexed wrist and fisted hand, for example) is not appropriate (atypical) for a 7-month-old child. In other words, the fisted hand is not really an abnormal pattern unless it is developmentally inappropriate. Some movements appear to be abnormal because they are never seen in children who are developing normally (flexed wrist and hyperextended metacarpophalangeal joints, for example). That particular pattern, however, is a combination of two normal patterns: the flexed wrist (appropriate during rest, body play, approach, grasp, and release) and excessive finger extension (appropriate at 6 to 8 months during approach). Thus, the term "abnormal" is redefined as "atypical" or "developmentally inappropriate."

Each pattern can be described as a primary developmentally inappropriate pattern in a child who is 12 months old. When the two patterns are combined, the resulting atypical pattern can be described as a secondary developmentally inappropriate pattern, evolving because of environmental demands that have exceeded ability level. Therefore, combinations of primary normal patterns may produce secondary atypical patterns when development has not proceeded in a sequential manner, and quality of movement really can be assessed with a developmental approach.

Analysis of the visual representation of normal prehension development in figure 5.1 (developmental prehension sequence clusters) reveals the intricate yet logical ways that each developmental pattern prepares for the next sequential pattern as control is first gained at the more proximal joints, through total synergies, and by stabilization on a surface. Figure 5.2 illustrates a theory of inappropriate prehension patterns relating to developmental hand dysfunction.

Developmental Hand Dysfunction

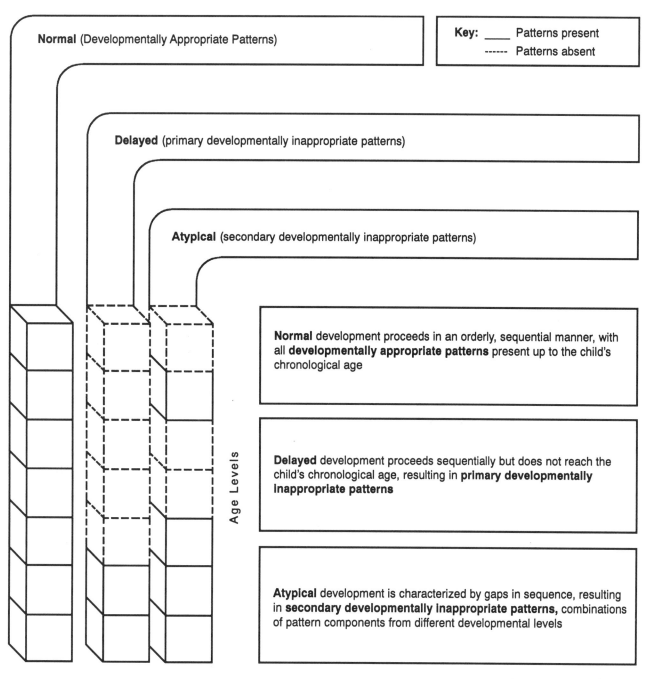

Key: _____ Patterns present
------ Patterns absent

Normal (Developmentally Appropriate Patterns)

Delayed (primary developmentally inappropriate patterns)

Atypical (secondary developmentally inappropriate patterns)

Age Levels

Normal development proceeds in an orderly, sequential manner, with all **developmentally appropriate patterns** present up to the child's chronological age

Delayed development proceeds sequentially but does not reach the child's chronological age, resulting in **primary developmentally inappropriate patterns**

Atypical development is characterized by gaps in sequence, resulting in **secondary developmentally inappropriate patterns,** combinations of pattern components from different developmental levels

Figure 5.2. A theory of inappropriate prehension patterns relating to developmental hand dysfunction

Use of the Theoretical Model for Evaluation and Treatment

Figure 5.3 analyzes a common atypical grasp of the cube, well established in many older children with cerebral palsy. The wrist is flexed, thumb adducted with excessive effort, fingers accommodating to the shape of the object in a maladaptive manner. Although many normal components are present at the 3-, 5-, and 9-month levels, a key element is missing: the 7-month radial-palmar grasp, one of the most stable of all grasps, because the palm, all fingers, and thumb are shaped securely around the object. Because of this stability, less effort is required. The wrist no longer needs to flex to reinforce finger flexion, and the web space begins to enlarge as the thumb comes out of the palm and fully participates in grasp.

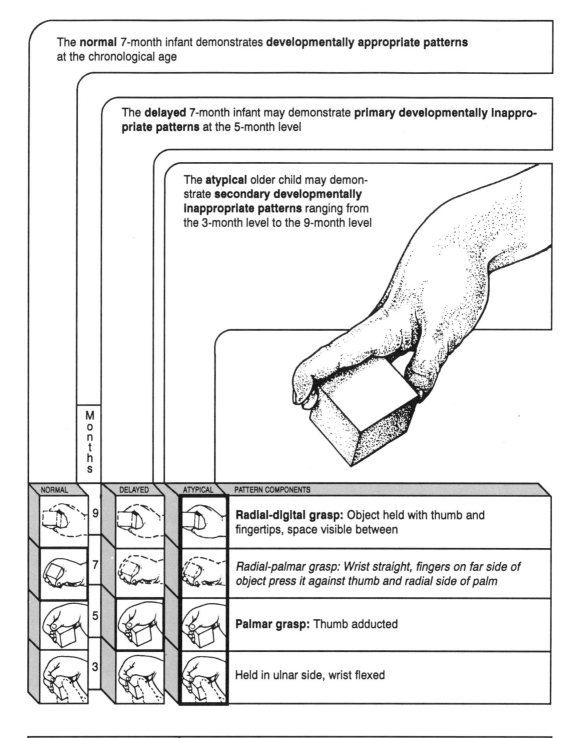

The **normal** 7-month infant demonstrates **developmentally appropriate patterns** at the chronological age

The **delayed** 7-month infant may demonstrate **primary developmentally inappropriate patterns** at the 5-month level

The **atypical** older child may demonstrate **secondary developmentally inappropriate patterns** ranging from the 3-month level to the 9-month level

Months

NORMAL		DELAYED	ATYPICAL	PATTERN COMPONENTS
	9			**Radial-digital grasp:** Object held with thumb and fingertips, space visible between
	7			*Radial-palmar grasp: Wrist straight, fingers on far side of object press it against thumb and radial side of palm*
	5			**Palmar grasp:** Thumb adducted
	3			Held in ulnar side, wrist flexed

Key: _____ Patterns present
------ Patterns absent

Current developmental level

Present normal pattern components combining to form atypical patterns

Italics indicate absent normal pattern components needed to fill sequential gaps

Figure 5.3. A comparison of normal, delayed, and atypical prehension development and a treatment model: Grasp of the cube

Figure 5.4 illustrates another familiar atypical pattern in children who begin early to attempt difficult fine motor tasks. Proximal thumb joint instability results in subluxation during voluntary hand use. The missing components of the 8-month scissors grasp provide important sensorimotor experience as the child uses the surface to stabilize, either resting the curled index finger and sliding the thumb to capture the pellet, or resting the thumb and sliding the curled index finger toward it.

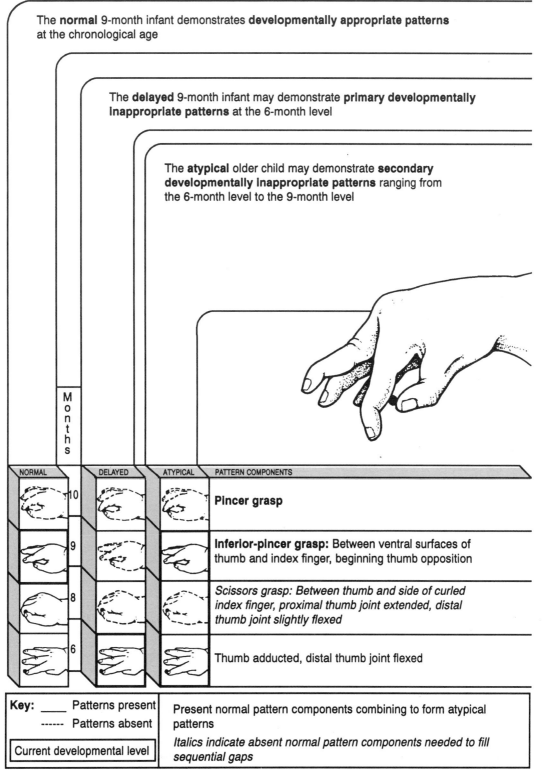

The **normal** 9-month infant demonstrates **developmentally appropriate patterns** at the chronological age

The **delayed** 9-month infant may demonstrate **primary developmentally inappropriate patterns** at the 6-month level

The **atypical** older child may demonstrate **secondary developmentally inappropriate patterns** ranging from the 6-month level to the 9-month level

NORMAL	Months	DELAYED	ATYPICAL	PATTERN COMPONENTS
	10			**Pincer grasp**
	9			**Inferior-pincer grasp:** Between ventral surfaces of thumb and index finger, beginning thumb opposition
	8			*Scissors grasp: Between thumb and side of curled index finger, proximal thumb joint extended, distal thumb joint slightly flexed*
	6			Thumb adducted, distal thumb joint flexed

Key: ____ Patterns present
------ Patterns absent

Current developmental level

Present normal pattern components combining to form atypical patterns

Italics indicate absent normal pattern components needed to fill sequential gaps

Figure 5.4. A comparison of normal, delayed, and atypical prehension development and a treatment model: Grasp of the pellet

Figure 5.5 examines a distorted digital-pronate grasp of the pencil, with some elements of the static tripod posture. The slight pronation and ulnar deviation normally present at 2 to 3 years is exaggerated because of insufficient stability, normally developed by the missing palmar-supinate grasp of 1½ years.

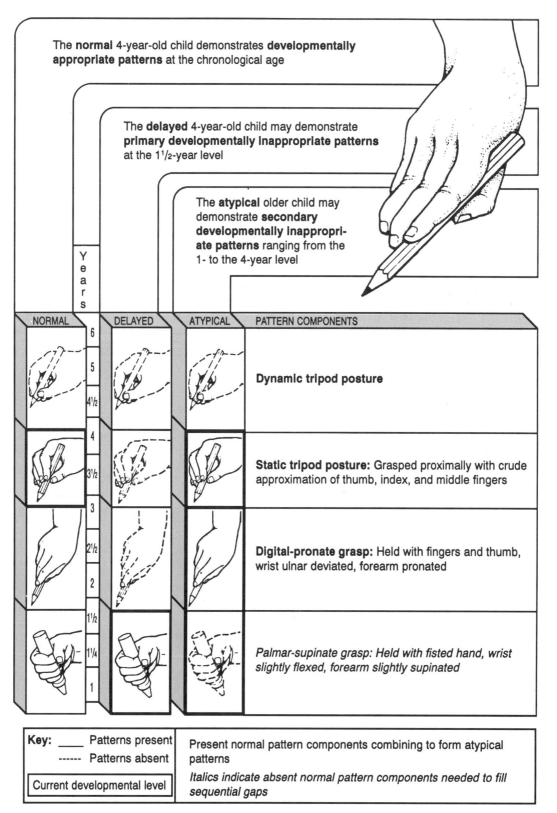

The **normal** 4-year-old child demonstrates **developmentally appropriate patterns** at the chronological age

The **delayed** 4-year-old child may demonstrate **primary developmentally inappropriate patterns** at the 1½-year level

The **atypical** older child may demonstrate **secondary developmentally inappropriate patterns** ranging from the 1- to the 4-year level

NORMAL	Years	DELAYED	ATYPICAL	PATTERN COMPONENTS
	6, 5, 4½			**Dynamic tripod posture**
	4, 3½, 3			**Static tripod posture:** Grasped proximally with crude approximation of thumb, index, and middle fingers
	2½, 2			**Digital-pronate grasp:** Held with fingers and thumb, wrist ulnar deviated, forearm pronated
	1½, 1¼, 1			*Palmar-supinate grasp: Held with fisted hand, wrist slightly flexed, forearm slightly supinated*

Key: ____ Patterns present
------ Patterns absent

☐ Current developmental level

Present normal pattern components combining to form atypical patterns

Italics indicate absent normal pattern components needed to fill sequential gaps

Figure 5.5. A comparison of normal, delayed, and atypical prehension development and a treatment model: Crayon or pencil grasp

Developmental Hand Dysfunction

References

Ayres, A. J. 1974. Ontogenetic principles in the development of arm and hand functions. In *The development of sensory integrative theory and practice: A collection of the works of A. Jean Ayres,* compiled by A. Henderson, E. Gilfoyle, L. Lorens, C. Myers, and S. Prevel, 3-13. Dubuque, IA: Kendall/Hunt.

Bloom, B. 1956. Taxonomy of educational objectives. In *Handbook 1: The cognitive domain.* New York: David McKay.

Bobath, B. 1971. Motor development, its effect on general development, and application to the treatment of cerebral palsy. *Physiotherapy* 57:526-32.

Compton, N. H., and O. A. Hall. 1972. *Foundations of home economics research.* Minneapolis, MN: Burgess.

Engle, T. L., and L. Snellgrove. 1979. *Psychology.* New York: Harcourt Brace Jovanovich.

Erhardt, R. P., P. A. Beatty, and D. M. Hertsgaard. 1981. A developmental prehension assessment for handicapped children. *American Journal of Occupational Therapy* 237-42.

Gesell, A., and C. S. Amatruda. 1969. *Developmental diagnosis.* 2d ed., revised and enlarged. New York: Harper and Row.

Gilfoyle, E. M., A. P. Grady, and J. C. Moore. 1981. *Children adapt.* Thorofare, NJ: Charles B. Slack.

King, L. J. 1978. Toward a science of adaptive responses. *American Journal of Occupational Therapy* 32:429-37.

Kuhn, T. S. 1970. *The structure of scientific revolutions.* Chicago: University of Chicago Press.

Piaget, J. 1952. *The origins of intelligence in children.* New York: International University Press.

Reynolds, P. D. 1971. *A primer in theory construction.* Indianapolis, IN: Bobbs-Merrill.

Rogers, J. C. 1982. Order and disorder in medicine and occupational therapy. *American Journal of Occupational Therapy* 36:29-35.

Chapter Six
New Theoretical Concepts

The previous chapters represent traditional concepts which contributed to the development of a synthesized theory of prehension. This chapter will include new clinical insights gained during consultation and evaluation of children with cerebral palsy, sharing ideas with colleagues, attending national and regional conferences, and reviewing recent literature. The new approaches do not replace older theories but supplement them as new research always adds to and builds on previous knowledge.

Originally perceived as an orthopedic disorder with a neurological basis, cerebral palsy has been recognized as a multihandicapping condition, a major disorder in development, and a disability emerging as a child grows (Scherzer and Tscharnuter 1990).

The terms *impairment, disability,* and *handicap* are defined in the World Health Organization manual (1980).

- *Impairment* represents disturbance at the organ level.

- *Disability* describes the consequence of impairment for function and activity.

- *Handicap* expresses the disadvantage experienced by the individual as a result of impairment and disability, thus reflecting the individual's interaction with and adaptation to the environment.

Professionals working with children who have cerebral palsy need to be aware of these terms when planning assessment procedures and intervention programs. Thus *impairments* are determined by assessing performance components, *disabilities* will affect occupational performances, and *handicaps* can be overcome by attention to role performances.

The occupational therapy profession has historically developed around the concept of helping persons with *disabilities* interact successfully within their environment by trying to remediate their *impairments.* New federal legislation, by ensuring the rights of all people to be part of the mainstream of life, will play a major part in reducing their *handicaps.* Chapter 8, Application of Assessment Data to Treatment in Functional Environments, will discuss these legislative changes and the impact on transitions from childhood to adulthood.

Sensation and Manipulation

Tactile information is a major source of information about the environment and the effect of motor responses on the environment. As a person moves, sensory information is continuously assimilated to guide the movement. This tactile perception integrates with information from proprioceptors to achieve well-controlled, coordinated movements in which muscle agonists and antagonists work in smooth synergy. This is particularly important for higher-level skills involving in-hand manipulation, necessary for many daily living activities in the domestic, vocational, leisure, and community domains.

When a person manipulates an object within the hand, finger movements are responsive to and refined by the sensory properties of the object. Praxis, dependent upon tactile discrimination, is required when a task is unfamiliar, and conceptualization of a motor plan is needed before it is executed. Dyspraxia is a neurologically based disorder of motor planning abilities. Children with tactile discrimination deficits may compensate by using other sensory systems (such as vision) to accomplish efficient manipulation. Therapy to remediate these problems needs to focus on tactile awareness and the functional use of tactile information (Case-Smith 1991).

Exner (1993) defines in-hand manipulation as the process of using one hand to adjust an object in that hand for more effective placement prior to use or release. The current version of her In-Hand Manipulation Test (IMT), containing approximately 50 test items, can be used with children 18 months or older to measure the quality and efficiency of these skills. Some examples of in-hand manipulation skills include picking up and fanning a handful of playing cards, grasping several coins and moving one of them to the fingertips to insert into a vending machine, and picking up and adjusting a pencil so that fingers and thumb are closer to the writing end. A key factor for in-hand manipulation is the stability/mobility mechanism, since one object may be moved within hand while another object is stabilized, usually by the ulnar fingers. Most individuals with developmental disabilities use inappropriate points of stability; thus movement patterns are inefficient (Exner 1992).

The mastery of buttons, zippers, shoelaces, scissors, and other tools requires the most complex distal movement patterns of manipulation. These fine motor blends are a combination of simple patterns performed sequentially and concurrently to complete a functional task (Boehme 1988).

Joanne

At the age of 24 years, Joanne enjoys playing card games with her niece and nephew. She demonstrates clever compensations for her lack of in-hand manipulative skills. To cope with her difficulty picking up playing cards and shifting them within either hand, she uses the table as an intermediary by placing the card on it and sliding it off the edge of the table, where it is easier to grasp. She also uses intense visual fixation to monitor her hands to compensate for her decreased tactile discrimination.

Patrick

At the age of 16 years, Patrick uses a computer for most of his academic work at school and for assignments at home. Grasping a floppy disk and positioning it correctly in his hand for insertion into the disk drive is a challenge because of inadequate in-hand manipulation skills. He usually uses his other hand to reposition the disk.

Sensorimotor Measurement of Cognitive Disability

Sensory cues, sensorimotor associations, and motor actions are measured within a cognitive frame of reference described by Allen (1992). She describes those three dimensions of thought, stages within an information-processing model, which are assessed at each of six hierarchical cognitive levels: (1) reflexive, (2) movement, (3) repetitive actions, (4) end product, (5) variations, and (6) tangible thought. The relative difficulty of specific activities can be determined in terms of information-processing demands. Thus therapists can modify the structure of activities at the appropriate level to enable completion of the task.

Kristy

At the age of 14 years, Kristy is nonverbal and has no apparent receptive language. She responds appropriately, however, to some gestures and to social interactions. At level 1, reflexive, she is highly motivated by sensory cues such as hunger, thirst, taste, and smell, which are alerting stimuli, sensorimotor associations. Her motor actions of spoon feeding are spontaneous.

At level 2, movement, self-feeding is initiated quickly when the spoon is placed in her hand (proprioceptive sensory cues), and she is able to reduce the discomfort of hunger (sensorimotor associations). She can also imitate approximate gross movements (motor actions).

Kristy demonstrates level 3, repetitive actions, when she responds to tactile sensory cues by manipulating the spoon in a repetitive hand-to-mouth action, again recognizing the effect of her movements (sensorimotor association). Her motor actions are spontaneous and repetitive.

Level 4, end product, relies on visual cues to initiate goal-directed actions. Kristy does indeed reach for a spoon when it is presented in her visual field (sensory cues) but is not able to adapt her spontaneous motor actions to orient her wrist and hand to grasp the spoon independently and achieve her goal (sensorimotor associations).

Kristy does not demonstrate behaviors at level 5, variations, and level 6, tangible thought, which require sensory cues of concrete and abstract relationships between objects, two- or three-step imitative behaviors, and exploratory or preplanned motor actions. Her therapists need to analyze Kristy's activities in terms of how her sensorimotor system processes cognitive information.

Sensory Integration Theory

Sensory integration therapy is a treatment approach developed by occupational therapist Dr. A. Jean Ayres and defined as the organization and processing of sensory information from the different sensory channels and the ability to relate input from one channel to that of another in order to emit an adaptive response. Information from three basic senses (touch, movement, and position) is used to plan and sequence movements, to coordinate both sides of the body, to develop balance, to coordinate eye and hand movements, and to develop body awareness.

Many children with cerebral palsy as well as those with learning disabilities have problems receiving and processing sensory input, resulting in hypersensitivity or hyposensitivity to touch (the tactile system), gravitational insecurity (the vestibular system), and motor planning problems (dyspraxia). They may also have difficulty regulating and processing sensory information from visual, auditory, gustatory, and olfactory channels. Certain medications may stimulate cortical areas of the brain to help CNS organization. However, children with seizures who need CNS depressants may experience side effects that influence posture, movement, and behavior, fluctuating from day to day when the seizures are not well regulated by the medication.

Treatment techniques for *tactile* and *vestibular* problems focus on providing a combination of exploration and structured play experiences which will assist in sensory modulation for the child who is overreacting or underreacting to tactile stimulation. Activities may include firm, deep pressure through weight bearing on different parts of the body and movement through all planes of space at different speeds.

Children with *dyspraxia* have trouble planning movements and putting them into complex sequences, which affects their ability to move from one position into another, construct a drawing, or manipulate buttons (Foltz, DeGangi, and Lewis 1991). Therapy aims to increase registration and integration of sensory input, develop mature postural control and movement patterns, and improve body scheme. This is achieved by providing constantly changing activities which require the child to be adaptive and goal-directed. Ideation and organization can be improved in a dressing activity, for example, by encouraging the child to verbalize (talk through the movement sequences).

Treatment principles for sensory integrative deficits include normalizing sensory input, considering development in terms of the stability/mobility spiral process, determining effectiveness by the child's response, and requiring the child to be an active participant, responding appropriately while achieving mastery over movement and the environment (Dunn 1987).

Joanne

A favorite recreational activity for Joanne is swimming in a warm therapeutic pool, where she has recently learned to float and move independently while wearing a life jacket. This activity, which provides significant tactile and vestibular input, helps her improve adaptive motor skills in supine, prone, sidelying, sitting, and standing positions.

Patrick

By the time Patrick reached his teenage years, he was found to have a learning disability in addition to his diagnosis of cerebral palsy. Processing of visual information was so difficult for him that he was an extremely slow reader and poor speller. Comprehensive testing, however, revealed that he was a strong auditory learner. In the ninth grade his reading skills clustered between first and second grade levels, while his listening comprehension was *above* the twelfth grade level, according to the Woodcock-Johnson Psycho-Educational Battery (Woodcock and Johnson 1990).

With the help of a special tutor who used an auditory phonics approach, Patrick began to read well within three months and made rapid strides in all his academic classes. He began to use a tape recorder regularly in school. By the tenth grade, his reading had reached the fourth-grade level. Another contributing factor to his academic success was the reduction and, finally, elimination of all seizure medication since Patrick had been seizure-free for several years. The effects of medications which depress the CNS can be illustrated by Patrick's comment after they were discontinued: "I feel like my brain is racing. I can't keep up with everything I'm thinking."

Patrick now completes all his class assignments independently with the help of a powerbook computer and software programs such as Co-Writer (word prediction) and Write Outloud (voice output) (both available from Don Johnston Developmental Equipment, Inc., P.O. Box 639, Wauconda, IL 60084-0639). Patrick, his teachers, and his family are realizing that the computer will be a key factor as he considers future occupational choices.

Kristy

To compensate for tactile hyposensitivity during her early development, Kristy learned to rely on visual and oral exploration of her environment and objects in it. In therapy sessions, with vision occluded, her hands become significantly more active in manipulating objects.

Spatiotemporal Adaptation

The theory of spatiotemporal adaption is expanded in the second edition of *Children Adapt* (Gilfoyle, Grady, and Moore 1990). Updated principles are listed here.

- Development is a function of nervous system maturation, occurring through person-environment adaptation.

- Adaptation depends upon active participation within spatiotemporal dimensions of the environment to provide sensory feedback about self and environment.

- Occupations are purposeful, meaningful experiences motivating higher-level adaptive responses.

- Adaptation spirals through primitive, transitional, and mature developmental phases, linking strategies to skilled performance.

- Stressful situations elicit previously acquired strategies which are also adapted to the present situation.

- Spatiotemporal distress provokes dysfunctional behaviors which are maladaptive and not linked to higher-level behaviors, resulting in regression.

- Flexibility or plasticity of the nervous system enhances the capability for sensorimotor adaptation which then facilitates nervous system modification, such as formation of new synapses.

- Intervention providing appropriate sensory input, motor output, and sensory feedback, and employing the spiraling process of linking strategies and sequences, will influence neural organization and facilitate maturation.

Motor Learning and Motor Control Theory

Motor control, learning, and development represent three approaches to understanding motor behavior. For motor control, the question is, "How is the control organized?" For motor learning, the question is, "How are skills acquired through experience and practice?" For motor development, the question is, "How does motor behavior change during age-related growth?" (VanSant 1991).

Principles of motor learning support a treatment approach that emphasizes practice of movement patterns and components of patterns in relation to functional tasks. Skill acquisition depends on both the type of task and the subject's stage of learning. Feedback, facilitation, and practice are important instructional variables. Tasks can be categorized as closed or open. In closed tasks, objects and people in the environment are stationary and timing is unspecified (grasping a spoon), but some objects are variable as to size and shape (different spoons at home, school, or community). In open tasks, objects and/or people are in motion, either consistent (lifting furniture) or unpredictable (maneuvering a power chair in a mall). Open tasks require quick adaptation to the changing environment, so automatic movement is not possible because of that uncertainty.

The stages of motor learning are cognitive (inconsistent performance, must be thought out), associative (more refinement, errors are used to correct performance during practice), and automatic (little cognitive processing, less susceptible to distractions).

Developmental Hand Dysfunction

Feedback can be intrinsic (sensory input from receptors) or extrinsic (external source such as a therapist, used to augment impaired intrinsic feedback).

Many types of practice methods have been studied to determine which are the most effective.

- massed practice (rest time less than practice)
- distributed practice (rest time greater than practice)
- blocked practice (same order)
- random practice (different order)
- variable practice (different conditions)
- constant practice (same conditions)
- part practice (subset of components)
- whole practice (entire task)

Research has shown that random and variable practice produce better learning and generalization for tasks such as feeding, which may take place under different conditions. Part practice is more efficient for complex tasks such as dressing. Whole practice is important for integrated timing.

Facilitation includes verbal instruction, demonstration, and manual guidance, always within the context of the whole task (Poole 1991).

Joanne

Joanne's job at a pizza restaurant requires her to clean and stack booster seats, an open task which is predictable. She is presently functioning at the associative stage of motor learning and needs extrinsic feedback from her job coach, as well as verbal reminders and some manual guidance during the whole task.

Patrick

When Patrick goes shopping in a mall, he drives his three-wheel scooter, an unpredictable open task which is not automatic and requires concentration while ignoring visual and auditory distractions. His feedback is now intrinsic, and he needs few verbal reminders after many years of practice driving battery-operated vehicles (toy car, power wheelchair, scooter).

Kristy

Grasping a spoon is a closed task for Kristy and always predictable for her, because the same spoon is used at home, school, and community. Kristy completes certain components automatically (spoon to mouth) but needs manual guidance for accurate scooping because she does not adapt cognitively nor motorically to locating food on the plate.

Model of Human Occupation and Play

Kielhofner's model of occupation (1985) describes how people function in an open system that organizes and changes over time because of constant interaction with the environment. The four phases of this system are:

- intake (the delivery of new information)
- feedback (responses from previous output)
- throughput (performance, habituation, and volition)
- output (occupational behavior)

Throughput performance includes communication, perceptual-motor, and process. Habituation results in productive habits. Volition is the energy invested in exploring and mastering the environment to develop interests, values, and the sense of accomplishment. This model of occupation contends that maladaptive behaviors are caused or made worse by environmental factors. Therefore, therapeutic structure and reinforcement can provide positive intervention for learning of life tasks (Kielhofner 1985).

A primary occupation of childhood, play is characterized by fun and spontaneity. It involves exploration, experimentation, imitation, and repetition (Florey 1981). Most therapists intuitively incorporate play into treatment sessions, but play and leisure are finally being recognized as viable occupations for adults as well. Valid and reliable measures of play are being developed so that interventions can include appropriate elements of playfulness, a term used by Bundy (1993). Playfulness can be applied to all persons participating in recreational and leisure activities throughout their lifespans. Unlike self-care and work, play is an activity in which the player is in control and can express an individual style for interacting with the environment. The three elements of play—intrinsic motivation, internal control, and the freedom to suspend reality—can be measured as traits viewed on a continuum of playfulness or nonplayfulness.

Play deprivation is common in children with physical disabilities because of many different forms of barriers. These include limitations imposed by caregivers, who are overprotective and fear injury; physical limitations of the child, whose lack of mobility has prevented exploratory play with household objects; environmental barriers in homes, schools, and community; and social barriers, due to limited interaction with nonhandicapped peers (Missiuna and Pollock 1991).

By integrating play into therapy sessions, therapists can promote interaction with the environment and mastery of new skills, and develop risk-taking, problem-solving, and decision-making abilities (Reilly 1974). Skills learned from playing with a switch-adapted, battery-operated toy can serve as preliminary training for operation of a powered chair, as well as computers, augmentative communication devices, and environmental control systems (Williams and Matesi 1988).

Integrating play into Neuro-Developmental Treatment (NDT) can be particularly effective, because patterns of movement can be promoted and atypical postural reactions can be prevented while the child is engaged in functional, purposeful activities. NDT aims to produce automatic movement patterns without placing conscious attention on the process and eliciting excessive effort. A child absorbed in play is not focused on the specific motor demands of the activity and can be stimulated to use therapeutically appropriate movements to improve control of head, trunk, and arms during manipulation of toys. The occupational therapist's task analysis skills are used to continually adapt size, shape, or consistency of materials; rules and procedures; position of child or materials; and nature and degree of personal interaction (Anderson, Hinojosa, and Strauch 1987).

Joanne

Video games are intrinsically motivating for Joanne because she is in control and is able to achieve a sense of accomplishment as she plays alone or with friends. The activity has helped improve fine motor skills such as thumb isolation in both hands.

Patrick

Playing basketball with his brother is a sport that provides Patrick with opportunities for social interaction and skill achievement. He demonstrated his creativity and decision-making skills by adapting the ability

to ensure success while building strength and improving accuracy. He began by throwing the ball into a large trash can, then gradually moved it further away, and finally aimed for the basket overhead.

Kristy

Because of delayed hand development, Kristy had very limited control of her environment. An adapted switch has enabled her to operate television, a favorite leisure activity. It can be generalized for other uses, such as a call-for-help switch.

Current NDT Concepts

Berta Bobath and her husband Dr. Karel Bobath originated Neuro-Developmental Treatment in the early 1940s. At a symposium in the United States in 1985, she reviewed the changes in NDT during the past 40 years. She stressed that while the emphasis on various aspects has shifted, and much was learned from other professionals such as Kabat, Rood, and Peto, the basic concept remained the same. The most significant changes were related to the need for more direct transition of treatment into functional activities. This was best accomplished by observing the child during everyday activities to assess abilities and disabilities, and treating the child in functional situations in home and school to ensure carryover (Bobath 1985).

NDT theory is still undergoing dramatic changes. The original model based on the concepts of the Bobaths is incorporating newer theories of nervous system organization and function. New motor control theories encompass a contemporary systems approach that is more holistic and task-oriented than traditional ones. The heterarchy of motor behavior is considered just as important as the hierarchy of developmental central nervous system organization. Hierarchy means a traditional developmental sequence, with each step following a predetermined previous one. Heterarchy means that task-oriented, controlled behavior is a result of interactions and adaptations of many body systems and between the person and the environment.

Developmental milestones are important to serve as a guide for treatment, but always in the context of age-appropriate skills. For example, activities of daily living could include transitional movements within a developmental sequence, such as achieving prone weight bearing on the arms in an older child while standing at a table, or getting the hands-to-feet pattern in an adult while pulling on socks in sitting instead of supine.

The child/adult determines which task is most important. True motor learning can then be achieved because posture and motor synergies are organized around specific functional tasks. Thus the therapist's first responsibility is to create an environment which allows the individual to initiate and organize purposeful movement. Correct alignment can then be provided through handling techniques that allow muscles to work in normal synergies. Traditional theory stressed the proximal-distal developmental progression. New thinking realizes that movements may also have a distal-proximal progression, at times more functionally oriented (for example, the type of weight bearing on the hands affects forearm and shoulder postures).

Feedforward is now considered just as important as feedback because a growing reference base can be used to give more anticipatory control. That reference base can be expanded by providing toys and other materials with a great variety of textures, shapes, weight, and so on. Although atypical movement occurs because of the damaged CNS, sensory input which is correctly interpreted can improve motor learning through adaptation and regulation. Therefore, normal development varies with personal characteristics and environmental factors, and new movement patterns are best learned in functional contexts. Motivation produces goal-directed actions, within occupational roles (Bly 1992).

In a study of progress in patients receiving NDT, changes were observed across many developmental areas, despite emphasis on motor function. Gains in gross and fine motor domains as well as cognition, communication, and social-emotional skills appeared to be related to the meaningful activities and interactions facilitated by skillful therapists (DeGangi 1993).

The importance of selecting functional treatment goals is also stressed in the second edition of *Early Diagnosis and Therapy in Cerebral Palsy* (Scherzer and Tscharnuter 1990). Emphasis on achieving specific components of movement and automatic responses has changed because of the realization that children were not always able to spontaneously integrate those components into functional activities. Achieving postural organization is a *means* to achieve functional skills.

These newer approaches also place less emphasis on motor patterns and more priority on the perception of sensory input which precedes motor activity. Atypical patterns, especially hypertonicity, are viewed as an expression of compensatory postural stability. Creating an efficient base of support during weight bearing provides the tactile and proprioceptive input needed for postural alignment and postural control. The arms can be used freely for reaching and manipulation only when the lower extremities form that support, dynamic and in all positions, and the child is always aware of the relationship between the center of gravity and the base of support.

Important upper extremity skills develop initially during activities in weight bearing in prone, where the child gradually develops the ability to shift weight through the trunk and pelvis, in lateral as well as posterior directions. This developmental progression affects positions of the head, shoulders, arms, and hands in prone during rest, head raising, and approach. If primitive patterns are retained, arms may be posterior to the shoulders and internally rotated, and hands may be fisted, with thumbs inside palms. Consequently, dissociation of movement between head and shoulders, and between shoulders and arms, does not develop. Also missing is stability at all upper extremity joints, which develops from weight-bearing proprioceptive input. Accurate reaching and fine graded manipulative skills are impeded. During facilitation, control should be sought first in both end ranges of movement (flexion and extension), which developmentally precedes midrange control (Scherzer and Tscharnuter 1990).

The role of occupational therapy in NDT emphasizes upper body control and acquisition of hand skills for self-care, academics, leisure, and community activities, leading to as much independence as possible. Handling techniques are designed to obtain postural alignment throughout the entire body and prepare upper and lower extremities for weight bearing, weight shifting, and function (Foltz, DeGangi, and Lewis 1991).

NDT has also been combined with sensory integration (S.I.) treatment, since both approaches address adaptive responses of the individual and utilize sensory input to produce the motor response. Main differences are that NDT focuses on the motor output, the production of motor control, while S.I. focuses on the sensory processing aspect (Blanche and Burke 1991).

Joanne

Joanne's current occupational therapy assessment recommends the resumption of NDT-oriented intervention, because of her need for better midrange control during gross motor transitions and fine motor reaching and manipulation. Some of her functional problems include knocking over objects inadvertently, difficulty rising from the floor after falling, and using her hands together (for example, knife and fork). NDT principles which are applicable to Joanne's needs include:

- providing her with an efficient base of support (distal as well as proximal, when appropriate)

- emphasis on sensory input preceding movement, to ensure correct postural alignment over her center of gravity

- self-initiated, goal-directed activities within functional contexts

Patrick

Weightlifting at a local health club is a recreational activity that provides Patrick with opportunities for social interaction and risk taking, as well as skill acquisition. He is highly motivated, since weekly written documentation of pounds lifted gives him tangible proof of his increasing strength. To ensure correct alignment for muscles to work in normal synergies and to avoid atypical patterns due to excessive effort, his therapist consults with Patrick's personal trainer. For example, she observes hyperextension of his lower back as he does arm curls sitting at one of the machines, corrects it with her hands, and places a belt in the same place to maintain the position as he continues independently.

Kristy

Although Kristy had developed excellent head control through intensive therapy in her preschool years, prone weight bearing was a significant area of deficit. At age 14 her arms were still internally rotated in prone, with elbows posterior to the shoulders instead of straight forward with elbows directly under the shoulders. Insufficient stability at wrist, elbow, and shoulder joints (both scapular and glenohumeral) interferes with accurate reaching into space in all positions, as well as weight bearing when side-sitting independently. Her therapy program places emphasis on activities in various prone positions, with correct alignment facilitated by her therapist.

Motor Operations for Eye-Hand Coordination

The coordination of hand and eye depends first on the control of the head, enabling the eyes to monitor the task of the hands. A stable shoulder girdle then dictates the effectiveness of the arm in transporting the hand to its task and maintaining it during manipulation (Penso 1990). The relationships between external/internal and proximal/distal stability have important clinical implications. High-level manipulation skills and writing require adequate external support in children of *normal* abilities. Children with cerebral palsy who lack some developmental components, regulate muscle tone poorly, and don't use automatic points of stability such as the other arm on the surface or the feet on the floor, will revert to more primitive patterns due to stress (Hirschel, Pehoski, and Coryell 1990).

Functional motor operations for goal-directed arm and hand movements are listed here:

- Eye-head orientation which leads to identification of the object is organized at the midbrain level around the superior colliculus.

- Arm mobilization which localizes the object following a triggered ballistic movement prescribing in advance the direction and distance of travel depends upon brainstem structures.

- Grasping movement which adjusts the terminal guided approach is primarily under cortical control.

Each of these motor patterns receives and uses sensory information, especially visual feedback loops that have processed size and shape cues, calibrated gaze orientation, and guided arm trajectory and orientation of hand grip. After contact, tactile cues shape the grasp and assist in manipulation (Paillard 1990).

During early use of writing implements, only the pencil tip touches the page as arm and hand move unanchored through space. Trunk and shoulder are providing internal stability for arm mobility. Later, the elbow and ulnar side of the hand rest on the writing surface (external stabilization) as forearm mobility depends on elbow stability. Next, the wrist stabilizes on the surface and the hand moves. Finally, with maturity, the hand itself stabilizes, allowing finger movement dissociated from the metacarpophalangeal (MCP) joints. This developmental progression of the stabilizing point of control from proximal to distal joints has been correlated with that of immature to mature pencil grips (Erhardt 1982).

The role of vision is to reinforce accidental efforts, slow down movements during attempts to guide them visually, and keep the child's attention on the task by sustained visual tracking of the hand. Visual feedback is used more efficiently in older children. For example, in a study by Schneck and Henderson (1990), older children slowed down when coloring near the edge of a circle, while younger children achieved accuracy by changing to a less mature but more stable grip.

In school, functional eye-hand skills are important for recreational activities such as team sports and prevocational activities such as keyboard use, as well as writing. Scribbling, coloring, and drawing have provided the visual-motor experiences which are necessary for complex writing tasks. These tasks are learned by tracing (eyes direct hand to follow the visual representation), imitating (eyes watch and remember another's action in order to repeat the same action and production), and copying (eyes alternate glances between visual representation and own production in process).

The normal hand is usually held in a position of approximately 45° supination with the wrist in slight extension for handwriting and drawing, a task requiring static grasp of the pencil at the same time as dynamic movement of the arm. For operating a keyboard, the hands are usually held in a pronated position with wrists in slight extension. The hand postures of individuals with cerebral palsy typically have limitations of wrist supination and extension which interfere with these skills for written communication (Penso 1990). Additionally, visual monitoring of the hands is often inconsistent because of inadequate head control and/ or the persistence of primitive reflexes.

Strategies to accommodate these problems include positioning of the individual in appropriate seating systems, adjustment of the work surface with inclines or easels, and the use of adaptations for crayons, pencils, pens, or markers such as grips of plastic, foam rubber, or thermoplastic material in triangular, cylindrical, ball, or customized shapes, useful for other utensils and tools, also.

Games and sports require even higher levels of eye-hand coordination for efficient throwing, catching, and hitting a variety of balls. Keyboards and computers which make specific demands on the visual-motor system at school and home also offer some occupational choices for the child growing into adulthood. Functional skill requirements involving tools contain components of abilities that are innate but also must be practiced to reach a safe level of competency (Starkes 1990).

Joanne

Although lacking in finger strength to grasp a conventional bowling ball, Joanne is able to participate in this life-long recreational sport by using an adapted ball with a retractable handle. A current therapy goal is to increase range of motion at the shoulder joint in her bowling arm. Her eye-hand coordination continues to improve as she practices bowling regularly on outings with the two other young women who live with her in their adult foster care home.

Patrick

Adaptations of materials, work surfaces, and positioning make oil painting a successful activity for Patrick. He uses an inclined easel parallel with his face for better eye-hand coordination. He keeps his large-handled brushes in a vertical holder to facilitate grasp. Adapted handles are also used for other tools, such as his toothbrush and certain eating utensils.

Kristy

Stimulating computer graphics programs are motivating to Kristy because they access her strongest sensory channels: visual and auditory. She is learning the cause-and-effect power of her adapted switch to control these programs, leading to communication and learning programs at her cognitive level.

The Rehabilitation Frame of Reference and Adaptive Equipment

A truly functional approach must consider the rehabilitation frame of reference which teaches patients to compensate for underlying deficits that cannot be remediated. Specific adaptive devices and modified procedures provide the link to functional outcomes. These devices may be simple low-tech aids, such as adapted handles, or high-tech electronic equipment.

A major challenge for professionals and family members assisting the person with handicaps is identifying strategies to enable oral and written communication skills to develop. Persons with slow or unintelligible speech require alternative methods to communicate and thus act upon and control events in their own lives. Technology has dramatically increased these opportunities in recent years, with a variety of commercial communication boards, voice output communication aides (VOCA), and accessibility switches. Transdisciplinary evaluations determine exactly which devices and which components of each device are appropriate for each individual, by identifying visual needs, the most effective body part movement, and the cognitive and language levels, as well as projected potential. Activation of a single switch must consider placement for hand access and pressure required. Computer-assisted instruction (CAI) has also expanded within the educational system, with new equipment that may be accessed through keyboards, single or multiple switches, touch panels, touch windows, voice input, and voice output. The large variety of adapted software programs with graphics and voice feedback are highly motivating. They can be used with very young children for simple cause-and-effect activities, and with older children and adults who are reinforced by the interactive processes allowing self-controlled learning. An individualized computer system for a person with severe handicaps can include a communication program, environmental control, and social-leisure activities (Fraser, Hensinger, and Phelps 1990). Virtual reality software can also be used for motor training (such as operating a powered wheelchair).

References

Allen, C. A. 1992. Cognitive disabilities. In *Cognitive rehabilitation: Models for intervention in occupational therapy,* edited by N. Katz, 1-21. Boston: Andover Medical Publishers.

Anderson, J., J. Hinojosa, and C. Strauch. 1987. Integrating play in Neuro-Developmental Treatment. *American Journal of Occupational Therapy* 41(7):421-26.

Blanche, E. J., and J. P. Burke. 1991. Combining neuro-developmental and sensory integration approaches in the treatment of the neurologically impaired child, Part I. *Sensory Integration Quarterly* 19:1-5.

Bly, L. 1992 (May). What's happening with NDT theory. Paper presented at the Fifth Annual NDTA Conference. Denver, Colorado.

Bobath, B. 1985 (May). Changing trends in NDT. In *Symposium in Neuro-Developmental Treatment.* Conducted at the meeting of the Neuro-Developmental Treatment Association (NDTA). Baltimore, Maryland.

Boehme, R. 1988. *Improving upper body control.* Tucson, AZ: Therapy Skill Builders.

Bundy, A. C. 1993. Assessment of play and leisure: Delineation of the problem. *American Journal of Occupational Therapy* 47(3):212-22.

Case-Smith, J. 1991. The effects of tactile defensiveness and tactile discrimination on in-hand manipulation. *American Journal of Occupational Therapy* 45(9):811-18.

DeGangi, G. A. 1993 (September). Therapists' perception of gains made when using Neuro-Developmental Treatment. *NDTA Network* 1, 5, 7, 9, 11.

Dunn, W. 1987 (May). Sensory integration. Lecture presented at the NDT OT Instructor Course. Akron, Ohio.

Erhardt, R. P. 1982. *Developmental hand dysfunction: Theory, assessment, and treatment.* 1st ed. Tucson, AZ: Therapy Skill Builders.

Exner, C. E. 1992. In-hand manipulation skills. In *Development of hand skills in the child,* edited by J. Case-Smith and C. Pehoski, 35-45. Rockville, MD: The American Occupational Therapy Association.

_____. 1993. Content validity of the In-hand manipulation test. *American Journal of Occupational Therapy* 45(6):505-13.

Florey, L. L. 1981. Studies of play: Implications for growth, development, and for clinical practice. *American Journal of Occupational Therapy* 35(8):519-28.

Foltz, L. C., G. DeGangi, and D. Lewis. 1991. Physical therapy, occupational therapy, and speech and language therapy. In *Children with cerebral palsy: A parents' guide,* edited by E. Geralis, 209-260. Rockville, MD: Woodbine House.

Fraser, B. A., R. N. Hensinger, and J. A. Phelps. 1990. *Physical management of multiple handicaps.* Baltimore, MD: Paul H. Brookes.

Gilfoyle, E. M., A. P. Grady, and J. C. Moore. 1990. *Children adapt.* 2d ed. Thorofare, NJ: Slack.

Hirschel, A., C. Pehoski, and J. Coryell. 1990. Environmental support and the development of grasp in infants. *American Journal of Occupational Therapy* 44(8):721-27.

Kielhofner, G. 1985. *A model of human occupation.* Baltimore, MD: Williams and Wilkins.

Missiuna, C., and N. Pollock. 1991. Play deprivation in children with physical disabilities: The role of the occupational therapist in preventing secondary disability. *American Journal of Occupational Therapy* 45(10):882-88.

Paillard, J. 1990. Basic neurophysiological structures of eye-hand coordination. In *Development of eye-hand coordination across the life span,* edited by C. Bard, M. Fleury, and L. Hay, 26-74. Columbia, SC: University of South Carolina Press.

Penso, D. E. 1990. *Keyboard, graphic, and handwriting skills: Helping people with motor disabilities.* London: Chapman and Hall.

Poole, J. L. 1991. Application of motor learning principles in occupational therapy. *American Journal of Occupational Therapy* 45(6):531-37.

Reilly, M. 1974. *Play as exploratory learning.* Beverly Hills, CA: Sage.

Scherzer, A. L., and I. Tscharnuter. 1990. *Early diagnosis and therapy in cerebral palsy.* 2d ed. New York: Marcel Dekker.

Schneck, C. M., and A. Henderson. 1990. Descriptive analysis of the developmental progression of grip position for pencil and crayon control in nondysfunctional children. *American Journal of Occupational Therapy* 44(10):893-900.

Starkes, J. L. 1990. Eye-hand coordination in experts: From athletes to microsurgeons. In *Development of eye-hand coordination across the life span,* edited by C. Bard, M. Fleury, and L. Hay, 309-26. Columbia, SC: University of South Carolina Press.

VanSant, A. 1991. Motor control, motor learning, and motor development. In *Motor control and physical therapy: Theoretical framework and practical applications,* edited by P. C. Montgomery and B. H. Connolly, 13-28. Hixson, TN: Chattanooga Group.

Williams, S. E., and D. V. Matesi. 1988. Therapeutic intervention with an adapted toy. *American Journal of Occupational Therapy* 42(10):673-76.

Woodcock, R. W., and M. B. Johnson. 1990. Woodcock/Johnson Psycho-educational battery—Revised. Allen, TX: DLM Teaching Resources.

World Health Organization. 1980. *International classification of impairments, disabilities, and handicap.* Geneva: WHO.

PART TWO

From Assessment to Treatment to Function

Chapter Seven
Evolution and Evaluation of the Assessment

The Need

Occupational therapists traditionally have been involved with the evaluation and treatment of hand dysfunction. As previously stated, the majority of evaluation instruments available during the early 1950s measured joint range of motion, muscle strength, coordination (usually timed tests), and activities of daily living such as feeding, dressing, grooming, and written communication.

Pediatric therapists working with developmental and/or neurological conditions such as cerebral palsy became dissatisfied with the lack of progress in those children and began to search for testing materials that would help with programming. The Gesell Developmental Schedules were more useful than the more orthopedically oriented tests because of their sequential organization, which served as a guide for treatment planning as well as assigning developmental levels. Many therapists used the Gesell material in designing their own forms, usually checklists, which met the needs of their particular caseloads and treatment programs.

The First Revisions

The first formal checklist used by the occupational therapy staff of the Easter Seal Mobile Therapy Unit in Fargo, North Dakota, for evaluation and treatment of prehension problems evolved from a chart published in 1974 in an integrated study of the theories of Gesell, Piaget, and Halverson (Erhardt 1974). This was followed by the mimeographed Developmental Prehension Assessment, which contained age levels from 4 weeks to 24 months, skill names, illustrations, a descriptive checklist, and suggested programming ideas for each age level. It was in clinical use from 1974 until 1978, when the three-page printed Erhardt Developmental Prehension Assessment was compiled by the author from the works of Gesell (Gesell and Amatruda 1969), Halverson (1931), Perlmutter (1973), and Frantzen (1957).

Limitations of the scale, especially for use with very young or severely handicapped children, led to a revised EDPA, which was copyright in 1979, printed, and distributed nationally and internationally. This eight-page booklet resulted from an extensive literature search for norms of reflexive as well as voluntary prehensile movements, pencil grasp, and drawings. Nine sources were eventually selected and compared. Items and time sequences were chosen that had a 50% or greater agreement. Test behaviors normally developing at each age level were described at four-week intervals, from neonate to 15 months, under headings of Approach, Grasp, and Release. Selected items were illustrated for clarity.

Structure and scoring of the assessment were modeled after the Gesell Developmental Schedules. The scoring system differentiated among a well-established pattern (+), an incipient pattern not fully integrated (±), a pattern not yet achieved (−), and a temporary pattern to be replaced by a more mature pattern (++). Mature permanent patterns were listed when first appearing, marked with an asterisk (*), and not repeated at higher levels, although assumed present. To facilitate determination of developmental levels, immature patterns repeated at successive levels were provided with scoring brackets when first emerging only.

Operational definitions were included, as well as a list of testing materials and scoring instructions. A separate section described the development of pencil grasp and drawing skills from the 1-year to the 6-year level. Although the EDPA was applicable for charting prehensile development of the normally developing infant from the neonate period to 15 months, it was specifically designed to describe the behaviors of the child who is delayed, atypical, or both. Since essential components of prehension are normally developed and functional at approximately 15 months, further refinements and increased hand skills after that age are primarily the result of learned experience. Therefore, the 15-month level can be considered the maturity of prehension and can be used as an approximate norm for testing older children (Erhardt, Beatty, and Hertsgaard 1981).

The EDPA was used extensively by the author in private clinical practice as consultant to school systems, special education cooperatives, child evaluation centers, and developmental activity centers for infants and preschool children with handicaps. The need to determine whether the EDPA was a reliable test of prehension for children with developmental delays, cerebral palsy, and other motor impairments led to an interrater reliability study incorporated into a two-day workshop entitled Developmental Hand Dysfunction.

Neuro-Developmental Treatment (NDT) principles learned at the basic training course in London in 1977 were interwoven into the discussions of theory and treatment at the workshop, which provided training in administration and scoring of the EDPA. During the process of preparation for the workshop, a videotape entitled *Administration of the EDPA* was produced (Erhardt 1983). The script for that videotape defined the skill components at each age level instead of listing them separately at the beginning, as in the assessment. A second revision of the EDPA followed logically as the audio script and the videotape were being edited and integrated.

The Interrater Reliability Study

Subjects

The 16 raters were registered occupational therapists whose years of pediatric experience ranged from three months to ten years. None had extensive experience with the EDPA.

Procedure

The EDPA and other informational materials were mailed to all participants one week before the workshop. Training at the workshop included:

- presentation of the theoretical basis for the EDPA: definitions and comparisons of prehension theories, stages in prehensile development, and reflexes affecting hand function

- explanation of general standardization procedures, statistical analysis, and specific procedures to be followed in the study

- observation of the videotape *Administration of the EDPA*, showing the instructor demonstrating materials, administering each test item, and recording scores

- observation of videotape segments showing the actual administration and scoring of the EDPA to a child who would not be included in the study

- practice in administering the EDPA to a workshop participant using designated materials, followed by questions and discussion

Method

Two male and two female children (identified as KM, CW, PM, and JD), ranging in age from 2 to 10 years, with diagnoses of various types of cerebral palsy (spastic, athetoid, and mixed) had been videotaped while being tested by the instructor prior to the workshop. The children were selected because they represented various levels of development as well as severity of handicap. All four had originally been given the entire EDPA, which averaged one hour for administration and included scoring both left and right hands for all 100 test items.

Because of developmental ceilings reached (KM, CW), repetition of replaced temporary patterns (CW, PM, JD), and irrelevancy of pencil grasp in the nondominant hand (CW, JD), certain segments of each child's EDPA were eliminated from the study. The children's wide range of abilities, however, allowed all 100 EDPA items to be viewed, scored, and analyzed for interrater reliability. To avoid viewer fatigue and because of workshop time restraints, the 16 raters were divided into two groups of eight for viewing videotapes of two of the four children tested by the instructor. Videotapes of KM and CW were viewed and scored by one group of eight raters; the remaining group of eight viewed and scored PM and JD.

Results

Each rater judged whether each of a series of given prehensile skills was present (+) or absent (-) for two of the four children. A comparison was made of the agreement of these judgments with the scoring of the instructor (test author).

Intraclass correlations for each child were found using all pairs of judgments for that child, including those of the test author; that is, all combinations of two of the nine raters on each skill scored for that child. These ranged from .418 to .853, and all correlations were significant at the .001 level.

Table 9 presents the major findings in terms of interrater agreements as well as interrater reliability. A very high degree of agreement was present among the various raters for two of the subjects, KM and JD. Judgments among raters for the other two subjects, PM and CW, did not have as high a degree of agreement, although intraclass correlations were still highly significant.

A test item analysis was carried out. The percentage of the eight raters agreeing with the test author for each item for each hand of each child was calculated to estimate item score objectivity in consideration of final revision of the EDPA. A given item may have been scored for a total of one, two, or three children depending on their range of abilities.

The mean percentage agreements with the test author ranged from a low of 64.78% for the left hand of PM, to a high of 96.2% for the right hand of KW. Of the total 306 judgments, which included all 100 test items, all eight of the raters agreed with the test author 142 times. On an additional 44 observations, seven of the eight raters (87.5%) agreed with the test author. Six of the eight raters agreed with the test author on an additional

38 observations. That is, on 224 of the 306 test items (73%), six or more of the eight raters agreed with the test author. Generally, the item-by-item analysis indicated a highly reliable test. Scoring of most individual items and scoring of the overall test yielded repeatable results.

Discussion

Statistical results of the single test item correlations were analyzed to differentiate high-reliability items from those with low reliability. Review of the videotapes revealed the following deficiencies in some segments: obscured or partially obscured view of hand movements; observation of movement too brief; and repetition of movement needed. Items with low correlation were also critically examined for imprecise definitions, an excessive number of components, and problems of subjective judgment.

The information was to be used to clarify or completely alter items with low reliability for the final revision of the EDPA. Although the interrater reliability procedure was intended to be helpful in developing the instrument as an aid to individual treatment planning, it should not be confused with test-retest reliability. Since the EDPA was a compilation of test items from published evaluation scales and child development literature, it could not be considered a standardized assessment tool with established validity and reliability (Erhardt, Beatty, and Hertsgaard 1981).

The 1982 Version

In July 1980 an opportunity arose to videotape the prehension development of an infant who was developing normally. Discussion of the proposed study with the director of the special education department at a

Table 9. Interrater Reliability of the EDPA

| Subject | Sex | Age (years-months) | Diagnosis | N | Percentage of Agreement | | Intraclass Correlation |
					Raters with test author	Mean for Impartial rater parts	
KM	F	2-7	Spastic quadriplegia with athetosis and cortical visual impairment	40	94.5	92.8	.85
CW	M	6-0	Athetoid quadriplegia	90	72.9	75.7	.47
PM	M	3-10	Athetoid quadriplegia with spasticity	106	71.6	70.8	.42
JD	F	10-9	Spastic quadriplegia	70	89.3	86.8	.74

N = number of items observed and scored

Source: Erhardt, Beatty, and Hertsgaard 1981.

local university led to a 16-month collaborative project of monthly videotaping involving almost 40 hours and more than 200 hours of editing, eventually including ten babies of normal ability (Erhardt and Pullen 1981).

Once again, the process of editing videotape and writing a script needed to be correlated with previous research. A new format for the EDPA arose from the integration of new information gained during 1981 from an NDT Refresher Weekend in Chicago, a workshop by Dr. Milani-Comparetti in Minneapolis, and the NDT Baby Treatment training course in New York.

A continuing review of the literature yielded current information concerning prehension as well as other areas to be considered for the EDPA, such as sensory development and dominance. Sensory functions cannot be separated from motor responses; indeed, sensory functions are expressed by motor responses rather than by verbal-cognitive reporting in the baby younger than 15 months. Therefore, sensory components were interwoven with the motor components rather than evaluated separately.

Since the development of bilateralization (using both hands together or alternating from one hand to the other) is more appropriate and relevant to function in the first 15 months than unilateralization, the testing of dominance per se was not included. Instead, unilateral and bilateral uses of the hands at every developmental level are carefully documented. Even the development of pencil grasp is marked by periods of normal ambidexterity, with definitive dominance appearing concurrently with the dynamic tripod posture at 4 to 6 years. During the testing of prewriting skills, the child's progression toward dominance is determined by hand preference and skill level in each.

The EDPA was expanded and reorganized to match the visual representation of the theoretical model entitled Developmental Prehension Sequence Clusters (figure 5.1, page 45):

- Section 1. Primarily involuntary arm-hand patterns (positional-reflexive)

- Section 2. Primarily voluntary movements of approach, grasp, manipulation, and release (cognitively directed)

- Section 3. Pre-writing skills (pencil grasp and drawings)

These three sections composed Part I, protocol sheets (developmental sequence clusters), and were to be used to record the therapist's observations of the child during the formal administration of the test. Part II, score sheets, allowed the therapist to transfer scores from the protocol sheets to determine developmental levels from each cluster. Part III, score sheet summary, provided an overview of the child's function in terms of involuntary patterns, voluntary movements, and prewriting skills.

During the early months of 1982, occupational and physical therapists from North Dakota, Minnesota, Iowa, Illinois, and Wisconsin volunteered to informally fieldtest this version of the EDPA. Their feedback and constructive criticism were carefully documented. The author was able to evaluate nearly 30 children within her private clinical practice, which included emphasis on the birth to 2-year-old population during that same period, through a consultancy contract with the state of North Dakota's Department of Human Services, Developmental Disabilities Division. Agencies such as hospitals, special education cooperatives, colleges, and human services centers in six different communities throughout this rural state were assisted in establishing and enhancing infant stimulation programs.

Finally, as detailed drawings for each pattern component were designed through many lengthy conferences with the illustrator, the EDPA was ultimately refined to ensure correlation within each cluster as well as between clusters.

The Highest Level of the Taxonomy

The taxonomy of learning begins with Knowledge and progresses through Comprehension, Application, Analysis, and Synthesis to Evaluation, the highest level in the cognitive domain. The EDPA, which "measures" and "scores" prehension development, is an instrument which in itself should be reviewed and evaluated for quality and appropriateness.

Marked deficiencies have been found in most tests measuring both fine and gross motor function, particularly in the accurate identification of different levels of function (discriminant validity) and both types of reliability (interobserver and decision-making). Discriminant validity measures the extent to which the scale discriminates between groups of children and degrees of their motor dysfunction. Interobserver or interrater reliability refers to the degree to which different persons observe the same behavior. Ideally, the observations of one should coincide with those of the others, and the observed performance should be perceived virtually identically. The interobserver reliability coefficient should exceed .80, indicating a high degree of objectivity. Decision-making reliability focuses on the consistency or dependability of the instrument.

Specific criteria useful in assessing motor scales were assembled into a checklist of questions by Berk and DeGangi (1979). The answers to these questions may serve to give a general indication of the EDPA's quality and appropriateness for use with handicapped children.

Validity

- *Is the domain of motor behaviors to be measured by the scale defined clearly? Do the items provide a representational sample?*

  Since the EDPA attempts to include nearly *all* prehension behaviors within its defined parameters, the problem of determining a representative sample is nonexistent.

- *Are the domain specifications comprehensive, are major constructs or dimensions of motor behavior identified, and is statistical evidence reported to support the structure and organization of the scale?*

  The organization and hierarchy of the EDPA are based on a sound theoretical foundation; detailed descriptions and illustrations define each pattern component; but studies are needed to provide statistical evidence of construct validity.

- *Do the items on the scale measure the motor behaviors?*

  All behaviors are included in the EDPA and thus are measured directly, by observation of the child's responses.

- *Is the scale appropriate for the intended use and population, and are cut off scores recommended for identification of degrees of motor dysfunction supported by rationale and statistical evidence?*

  Informal feedback reports indicate that the EDPA is extremely appropriate for children with developmental delays or dysfunction. Discriminant validity studies are needed, however, to identify persons for appropriate treatment programs.

Reliability

- *Is an index of interobserver or interrater reliability agreement reported?*

A complete report of an interrater reliability study is presented. Percent of agreement ranged from 70.8 to 94.5 among the raters for the various subjects.

- *Does the index indicate that the scale can be administered, scored, and interpreted objectively?*

  Intraclass correlations ranged from .418 to .853, and all correlations were significant at the .001 level.

- *Does the index indicate that decisions made with the scale would be dependable?*

  Test-retest reliability studies are needed to determine the consistency of the EDPA.

Considerations for Administration

Assessment of skills in children with significant handicaps, especially those with a slow rate of development, presents special difficulties. Their responses may be inconsistent, delayed, or performed only after considerable assistance. Very small changes must be measurable.

A developmental sequence scale which identifies a series of graded steps leading to a specific functional task allows important observations of variations in response. This scoring system is more sensitive to small changes in behavior and can be useful for evaluation of individuals functioning at very low levels (Erhardt 1982; Cole et al. 1985).

Standardized tests providing actual developmental levels are necessary for qualification for special services and quantification of subsequent gains. These data, however, have often been used to generate goals and objectives or for designing intervention programs, despite documentation of inappropriateness for those purposes. Standardized tests are not meant to provide information as to why failure occurs nor clues for facilitating success. Potential for future learning can better be assessed by measuring the zone of proximal development, described by the psychologist Vygotsky (1978) as the distance between the *actual* developmental level and the level of *potential* development when facilitated by certain interactions with people.

Intervention based on qualitative nonstandardized tests allows administrative procedures to be flexible enough to define those zones of proximal development. Those procedures include selected verbal and nonverbal cues and/or demonstrations to increase the child's problem-solving skills and thus the performance level. This method of evaluation determines the most effective approach to stimulate capacities that are actually emerging rather than absent. Assistance and facilitation can include adapted positioning to provide stability and mobility, as well as modification of materials. Any functional task that a person can accomplish with assistance but not independently can be considered within that person's zone of proximal development (Lyons 1984; Wilcox 1986).

The Current 1994 Revision

Ever since the publication of *Developmental Hand Dysfunction* in 1982, extensive feedback had been gathered from colleagues and workshop participants, as well as the author's own experience with the assessment. In 1984, during one of the reprintings of the EDPA, minor changes were made to correct a few errors and to designate as norms more test items within the developmental sequences as their functional importance throughout life was recognized. During the 10 years since the assessment was first published, the age levels had proven to be valid, but the language describing each test item needed to be clarified for more accurate recording of clinical observations. These changes were accomplished concurrently with the writing of the second edition of the book, so that the newly revised EDPA was ready to be used for the three case studies.

The EDPA-S: A Short Screening Form

The EDPA-S may be used as a quick screening test for persons from the age of 15 months through adulthood. Each cluster of the short form contains the test items designated as norms in the EDPA long form (shaded scoring boxes, under pattern components). These permanent patterns continue throughout life, as opposed to transitional patterns to be replaced by more mature patterns.

The total number of norm components is 128, compared with 341 items on the entire EDPA. If all norms in an EDPA-S cluster are scored + (well integrated, normal), then that cluster of skills can be considered intact. If any norm in a cluster is scored – (not present) or ± (emerging or inconsistent), then the entire cluster needs to be scored with the long form of the EDPA for more in-depth assessment.

This research edition of the EDPA-S is presented as a preliminary version, yet to be fieldtested. Future reliability and validity studies are planned to lead to standardization. If gaps in developmental sequences are observed in older children or adults, the test results may be used (1) to explain certain functional problems, (2) to serve as a guide for treatment, and/or (3) to provide rationale for adapted equipment and materials.

The current version of the Erhardt Developmental Prehension Assessment (EDPA) is presented in the following pages, followed by the EDPA-S (short screening form).

References

Berk, R. A., and G. A. DeGangi. 1979. Technical considerations in the evaluation of pediatric motor scales. *American Journal of Occupational Therapy* 33:240-44.

Cole, K., M. V. Swisher, M. D. Thompson, and R. R. Fewell. 1985. Enhancing sensitivity of assessment instruments for children: Graded multidimensional scoring. *Journal of the Association for Persons with Severe Handicaps* 10(4):209-13.

Erhardt, R. P. 1974. Sequential levels in development of prehension. *American Journal of Occupational Therapy* 28:592-96.

———. 1982. *Developmental hand dysfunction: Theory, assessment, and treatment.* 1st ed. Tucson: Therapy Skill Builders.

———. 1983. *Administration of the Erhardt Developmental Prehension Assessment (revised),* videotape. Fargo, ND: Snyder Film and Video. (Available from Erhardt Developmental Products, 2379 Snowshoe Court, Maplewood, MN 55119.)

Erhardt, R. P., P. A. Beatty, and D. M. Hertsgaard. 1981. A developmental prehension assessment for handicapped children. *American Journal of Occupational Therapy* 35:237-42.

Erhardt, R. P., and D. Pullen. 1981. *Normal hand development: Birth to 15 months,* videotape. Moorhead, MN: Moorhead State University TV Production Center. (Available from Erhardt Developmental Products, 2379 Snowshoe Court, Maplewood, MN 55119.)

Frantzen, J. 1957. *Toys . . . The tools of children.* Chicago, IL: National Society for Crippled Children and Adults.

Gesell, A., and C. S. Amatruda. 1969. *Developmental diagnosis.* 2d ed., revised and enlarged. New York: Harper and Row.

Halverson, H. M. 1931. An experimental study of prehension in infants by means of systematic cinema records. *Genetic Psychologic Monographs* 10:107-286.

Lyons, B. G. 1984. Defining a child's zone of proximal development: Evaluation process for treatment planning. *American Journal of Occupational Therapy* 38(7):446-51.

Perlmutter, S. 1973. *Neuroanatomy and neurophysiology underlying current treatment techniques for sensorimotor dysfunction.* Chicago, IL: University of Illinois.

Vygotsky, L. S. 1978. *Mind in society: The development of higher psychological process.* Cambridge, MA: Harvard University Press.

Wilcox, B. 1986. Still struggling with assessment. *TASH Newsletter* 12(6):2.

Erhardt Developmental Prehension Assessment (EDPA)
(Revised)

by Rhoda P. Erhardt, M.S., OTR, FAOTA   Illustrations by Gary Baune

CONTENTS

Instructions: Organization of Assessment, Materials, Procedures, and Interpretation

Part I: Protocol Sheets (Developmental Sequence Clusters)

Part II: Score Sheets (Developmental Levels)

Part III: Score Sheet Summary (Developmental Levels)

Subject _____   Examiner _____

Birth Date _____   Chronological Age _____   Test Date _____

Diagnoses _____

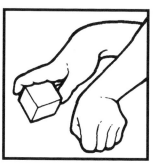

Copyright © 1994, 1989, 1982 by Rhoda P. Erhardt

Printed, published, and sold by
**Therapy
Skill Builders®** 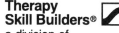 ®
a division of
The Psychological Corporation

555 Academic Court
San Antonio, Texas 78204-2498
1-800-228-0752

INSTRUCTIONS

Organization of Assessment

Part I contains Protocol Sheets, which group components of prehension into Developmental Sequence Clusters, demonstrating how transitional skills at each age level lead to those at the next. Sections 1 and 2 measure prehension from the fetal and natal period to 15 months, when the essential pattern components are developed and functional. Because further refinement, increased skill, and the use of tools are the result of learned experiences, the 15-month level can be considered the maturity of prehension, and thus an approximate norm for assessing older children and adults. Section 3 measures pencil grasp and drawings from 1 to 6 years. Age levels should be considered approximate within a varied range of normal limits.

Part II contains the Score Sheet, which presents a profile of Developmental Levels compiled from the Protocol Sheets.

Part III contains the Score Sheet Summary; approximate Developmental Levels for Section 1 (Involuntary Patterns), Section 2 (Voluntary Movements), and Section 3 (Pre-writing Skills).

Materials

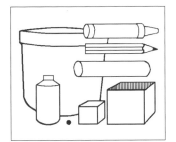

Appropriate toys and functional objects should be selected according to each subject's age, gender, cognitive, cultural, and personal interests, with enough novelty to avoid satiation or habituation.

1. Graded series of 3 dowel shapes, approximately 1 cm-2½ cm diameter
2. Graded series of 3 cube shapes, approximately 3 cm-6 cm wide
3. Graded series of 3 edible pellets, approximately 5 mm-1½ cm diameter

4. Graded series of 3 large containers (nesting boxes), approximately 5 cm-8 cm wide
5. Graded series of 3 small containers (pill bottles), approximately 1 cm-3 cm diameter
6. Pencil, 7 mm diameter, and crayon, 1½ cm diameter
7. Segments of black and white yarn and thread
8. Test kit container (plastic bucket or tote bag)

Procedures

Part I

A. Present stimuli and/or observe subject.

B. Record Pattern Component scores in small boxes according to Key B, and qualitative comments in blank page areas.

Pattern Components: Key B

+	Well-integrated normal pattern
++	Transitional pattern replaced by more mature patterns
	Norm: Permanent pattern continuing throughout life

−	Pattern not present
±	Emerging or abnormal pattern not well-integrated
⊕ ⊖ ⊕	Intervention needed
	Pattern component illustrated

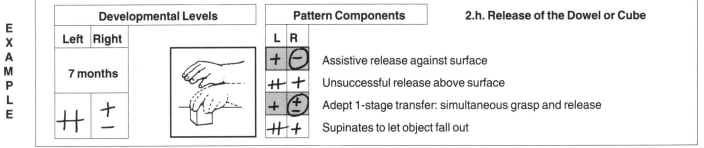

C. Determine and record Developmental Level Scores in large boxes according to Key C.

Developmental Levels: Key C

+	All pattern components present
±	Some but not all pattern components present

−	No pattern components present
++	All pattern components replaced

	NORM
+	Should be transferred as ++

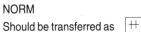

Part II

D. Transfer Developmental Level scores from the Protocol Sheets to the Score Sheet.

Part III

E. Estimate range of Developmental Levels for Score Sheet Summary.

Interpretation

Pattern Components indicate gaps in skill sequences, developmentally inappropriate patterns, and specific intervention needs.

Developmental Levels measure baseline levels, identify significant delays, and provide accountability with retesting.

Part I. Protocol Sheets (Developmental Sequence Clusters)

Section 1. Primarily Involuntary Arm-Hand Patterns (Positional-Reflexive)

Developmental Levels		Pattern Components	1.a. The Arms at Rest and During Body Play (Supine)

Left | Right

6 months

| L | R |

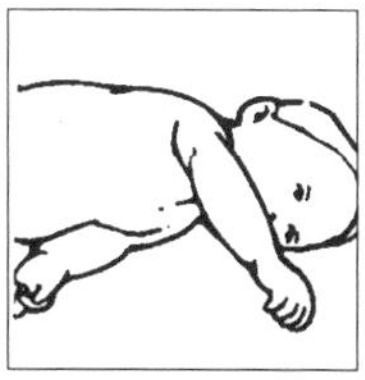

☒ Lifts **head** in midline, separately from shoulders

| L | R |

☒☐ **Rolls** to prone, upper arm adducts to help
☒☐ **Rolls** to sidelying and back to supine

5 months

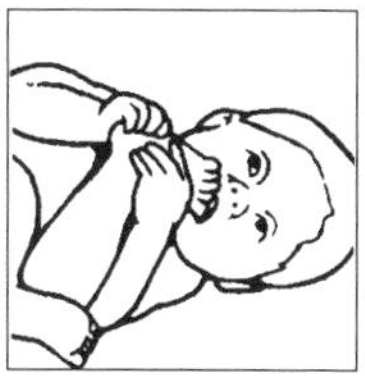

☐☐ **Hands** to foot/feet, elbows extended
☐☐ **Hands** bring feet to mouth

☐☐ **Rolls** to sidelying

4 months

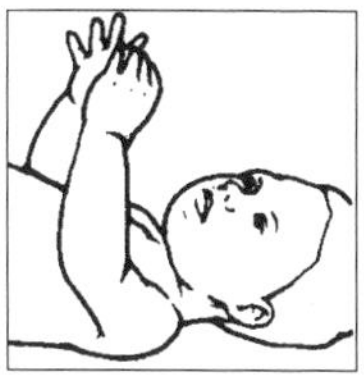

Shoulders well depressed
Neck elongated
Hands brought together in space
Wrists straight

Hands to mouth
Hands to knees
Hands open

3 months

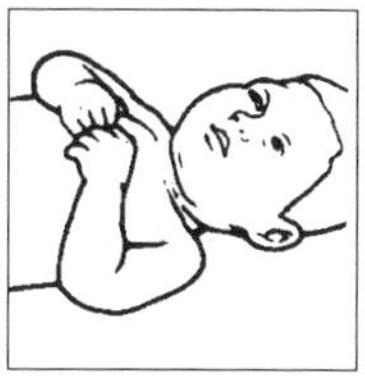

Head in midline, chin tucked
Shoulders slightly elevated
Arms internally rotated, hands clutching on chest

☐☐ **Hands** loosely closed

2 months

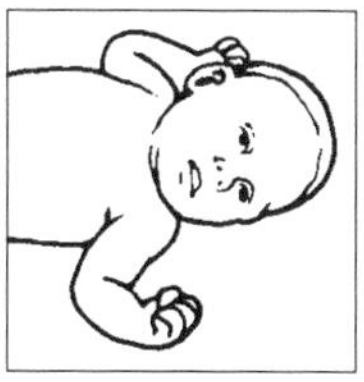

Head asymmetrically flexed
Shoulders elevated, lower than ears
Arms flexed, abducted, and externally rotated at rest

Moves in and out of ATNR position
Hands lightly fisted
Thumbs out

Natal

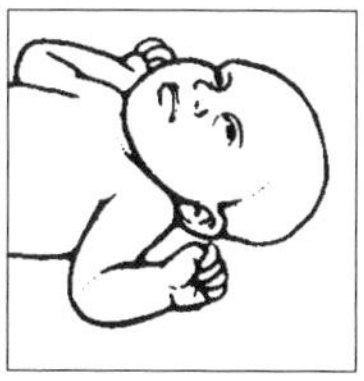

Shoulders elevated to ears
Arms physiologically flexed and adducted at rest or
Arms continually moving

Wrists flexed
Hands fisted, thumbs in and out, or Random, variable **finger** postures

Fetal

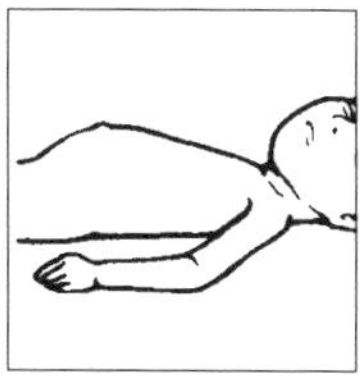

Head asymmetrically extended
Arms hypotonic

No **rolling**
No **hands** to body
Hands hypotonic

Section 1. Primarily Involuntary Arm-Hand Patterns (Positional-Reflexive)

Developmental Levels		Pattern Components	1.b. The Arms at Rest and During Head Raising (Prone)

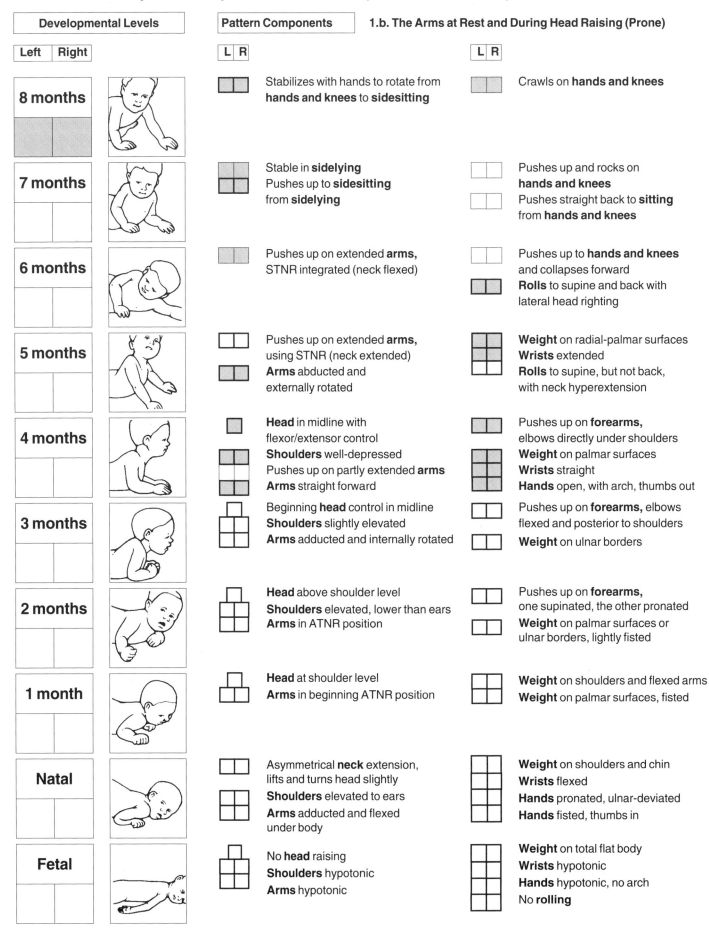

Developmental Levels (Left / Right)

8 months

L R: Stabilizes with hands to rotate from **hands and knees** to **sidesitting**

L R: Crawls on **hands and knees**

7 months

Stable in **sidelying**
Pushes up to **sidesitting** from **sidelying**

Pushes up and rocks on **hands and knees**
Pushes straight back to **sitting** from **hands and knees**

6 months

Pushes up on extended **arms,** STNR integrated (neck flexed)

Pushes up to **hands and knees** and collapses forward
Rolls to supine and back with lateral head righting

5 months

Pushes up on extended **arms,** using STNR (neck extended)
Arms abducted and externally rotated

Weight on radial-palmar surfaces
Wrists extended
Rolls to supine, but not back, with neck hyperextension

4 months

Head in midline with flexor/extensor control
Shoulders well-depressed
Pushes up on partly extended **arms**
Arms straight forward

Pushes up on **forearms,** elbows directly under shoulders
Weight on palmar surfaces
Wrists straight
Hands open, with arch, thumbs out

3 months

Beginning **head** control in midline
Shoulders slightly elevated
Arms adducted and internally rotated

Pushes up on **forearms,** elbows flexed and posterior to shoulders
Weight on ulnar borders

2 months

Head above shoulder level
Shoulders elevated, lower than ears
Arms in ATNR position

Pushes up on **forearms,** one supinated, the other pronated
Weight on palmar surfaces or ulnar borders, lightly fisted

1 month

Head at shoulder level
Arms in beginning ATNR position

Weight on shoulders and flexed arms
Weight on palmar surfaces, fisted

Natal

Asymmetrical **neck** extension, lifts and turns head slightly
Shoulders elevated to ears
Arms adducted and flexed under body

Weight on shoulders and chin
Wrists flexed
Hands pronated, ulnar-deviated
Hands fisted, thumbs in

Fetal

No **head** raising
Shoulders hypotonic
Arms hypotonic

Weight on total flat body
Wrists hypotonic
Hands hypotonic, no arch
No **rolling**

Section 1. Primarily Involuntary Arm-Hand Patterns (Positional-Reflexive)

| Developmental Levels | Pattern Components | 1.c. The Asymmetrical Tonic Neck Reflex (ATNR) |

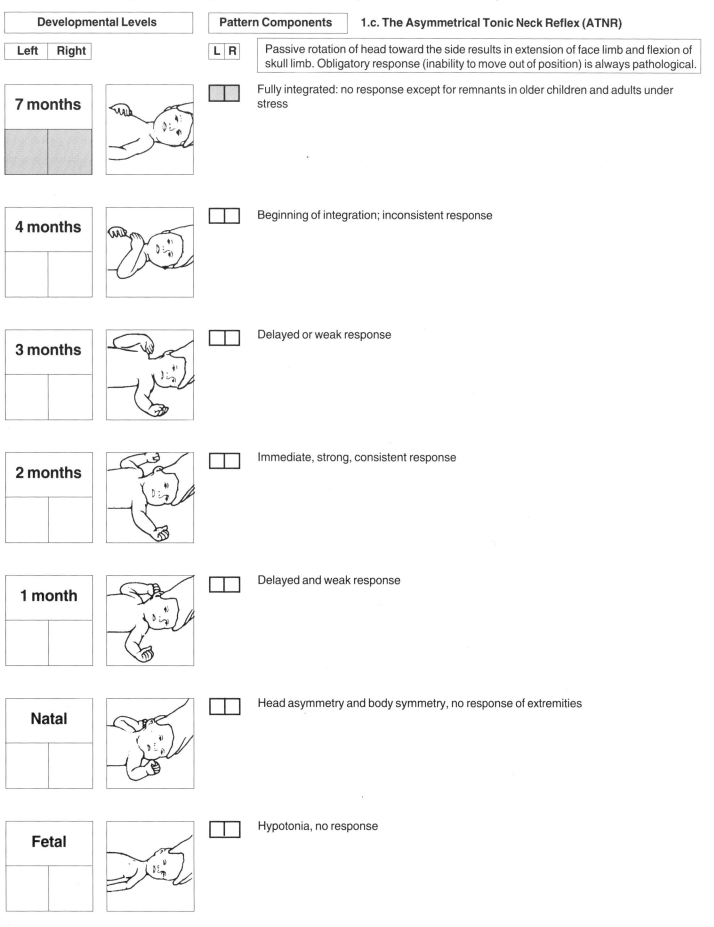

Developmental Levels

| Left | Right |

Pattern Components

| L | R | Passive rotation of head toward the side results in extension of face limb and flexion of skull limb. Obligatory response (inability to move out of position) is always pathological. |

7 months — Fully integrated: no response except for remnants in older children and adults under stress

4 months — Beginning of integration; inconsistent response

3 months — Delayed or weak response

2 months — Immediate, strong, consistent response

1 month — Delayed and weak response

Natal — Head asymmetry and body symmetry, no response of extremities

Fetal — Hypotonia, no response

Section 1. Primarily Involuntary Arm-Hand Patterns (Positional-Reflexive)

1.d. Grasping Reactions

Developmental Levels			Pattern Components		Note: Test in supine or with vision occluded to prevent contamination by voluntary movements.

Left	Right		L	R	

Instinctive Grasp Reaction: Light distally moving stimulus
Grasp Reflex: Firmly inserted stimulus

10 months					**Instinctive Grasp Reaction:** Integrated, stimulus withdrawn from **radial** side of palm results in voluntary, not involuntary movement
9 months					**Grasp Reflex:** Integrated, stimulus in **radial** side of palm results in voluntary, not involuntary grasp
8 months					**Instinctive Grasp Reaction, trapping stage:** Stimulus withdrawn from **radial** side of palm results in involuntary orienting, groping, and finally grasping
7 months					**Instinctive Grasp Reaction, groping stage:** Stimulus on **ulnar** border of hand results in involuntary pronation and movement toward stimulus
6 months					**Instinctive Grasp Reaction, groping stage:** Stimulus on **radial** border of hand results in involuntary supination and movement toward stimulus / **Grasp Reflex:** Beginning integration, weakening involuntary response to stimulus in **radial** side of palm
5 months					**Instinctive Grasp Reaction, orienting stage:** stimulus on **ulnar** border of hand results in involuntary pronation
4 months					**Instinctive Grasp Reaction, orienting stage:** Stimulus on **radial** border of hand results in involuntary supination
3 months					**Grasp Reflex:** Fully developed, stimulus in **radial** side of palm results in the **Catching phase:** Sudden finger flexion followed by the **Holding phase:** Sustained flexion when resisted
2 months					**Grasp Reflex:** Stimulus in **radial** side of palm results in thumb and all fingers flexion and adduction, followed by synergistic flexion of entire extremity
1 month					**Grasp Reflex:** Stimulus in **radial** side of palm results in thumb and index finger flexion and adduction, followed by synergistic flexion of entire extremity
Natal					**Grasp Reflex:** Stimulus in **ulnar** side of palm combined with traction results in involuntary grasp of middle, ring, little, and index fingers, and thumb in sequence, and synergistic flexion of entire extremity (lifting body weight)
Fetal					**Grasp Reflex:** Stimulus in **ulnar** side of palm results in slight or no involuntary grasp / **Instinctive Grasp Reaction:** No response to stimulus

Section 1. Primarily Involuntary Arm-Hand Patterns (Positional-Reflexive)

Developmental Levels			Pattern Components		1.e. Placing Responses
Left	Right		L	R	

Protective Extensor Thrust

12 months — Sudden movement of head and trunk **backward** results in immediate extension of elbows and hands placing on surface

10 months — Sudden movement of head and trunk **backward** results in immediate extension of arms and flexion of elbows placing on surface

8 months — Sudden movement of head and trunk **sideward** results in immediate extension/abduction of arms and fingers

6 months — Sudden movement of head and trunk **forward** and down results in immediate extension of arms and extension/abduction of fingers

3 months — Sudden movement of head and trunk **forward** and down results in arms remaining flexed or hypotonic

Proprioceptive Placing

Note: Test with vision occluded.

2 months — Fully integrated: No response to brushing back of hand lightly against table edge

1 month — Brushing back of hand lightly against table edge results in arm flexion, followed by extension and placing of **open** hand on surface

Natal — Brushing back of hand lightly against table edge results in arm flexion, followed by extension and placing of **fisted** hand on surface

Fetal — No response to stimulus

Section 1. Primarily Involuntary Arm-Hand Patterns (Positional-Reflexive)

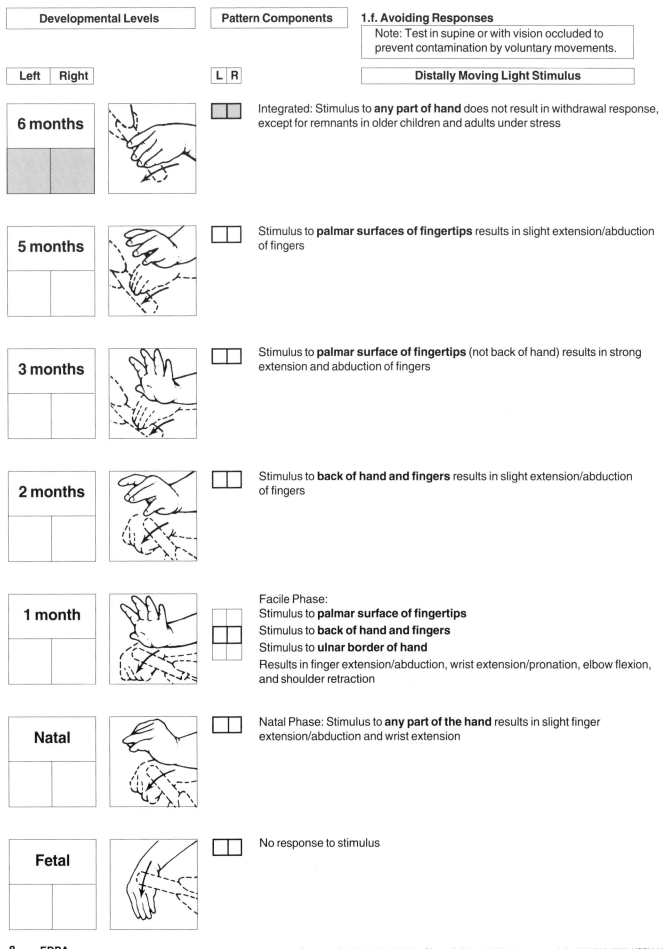

Developmental Levels		Pattern Components		1.f. Avoiding Responses

Note: Test in supine or with vision occluded to prevent contamination by voluntary movements.

Distally Moving Light Stimulus

Left	Right		L	R	

6 months — Integrated: Stimulus to **any part of hand** does not result in withdrawal response, except for remnants in older children and adults under stress

5 months — Stimulus to **palmar surfaces of fingertips** results in slight extension/abduction of fingers

3 months — Stimulus to **palmar surface of fingertips** (not back of hand) results in strong extension and abduction of fingers

2 months — Stimulus to **back of hand and fingers** results in slight extension/abduction of fingers

1 month — Facile Phase:
Stimulus to **palmar surface of fingertips**
Stimulus to **back of hand and fingers**
Stimulus to **ulnar border of hand**
Results in finger extension/abduction, wrist extension/pronation, elbow flexion, and shoulder retraction

Natal — Natal Phase: Stimulus to **any part of the hand** results in slight finger extension/abduction and wrist extension

Fetal — No response to stimulus

Section 2. Primarily Voluntary Movements (Cognitively Directed)

| Developmental Levels | | Pattern Components | 2.a. The Arms on Approach (Supine) |

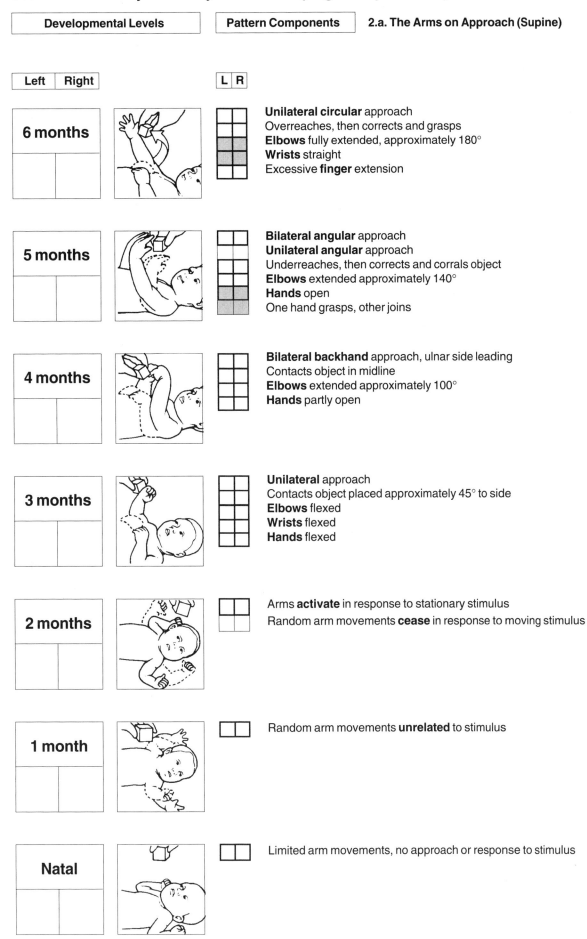

Left | Right

L | R

6 months

Unilateral circular approach
Overreaches, then corrects and grasps
Elbows fully extended, approximately 180°
Wrists straight
Excessive **finger** extension

5 months

Bilateral angular approach
Unilateral angular approach
Underreaches, then corrects and corrals object
Elbows extended approximately 140°
Hands open
One hand grasps, other joins

4 months

Bilateral backhand approach, ulnar side leading
Contacts object in midline
Elbows extended approximately 100°
Hands partly open

3 months

Unilateral approach
Contacts object placed approximately 45° to side
Elbows flexed
Wrists flexed
Hands flexed

2 months

Arms **activate** in response to stationary stimulus
Random arm movements **cease** in response to moving stimulus

1 month

Random arm movements **unrelated** to stimulus

Natal

Limited arm movements, no approach or response to stimulus

Section 2. Primarily Voluntary Movements (Cognitively Directed)

| Developmental Levels | | Pattern Components | 2.b. The Arms on Approach (Prone) |

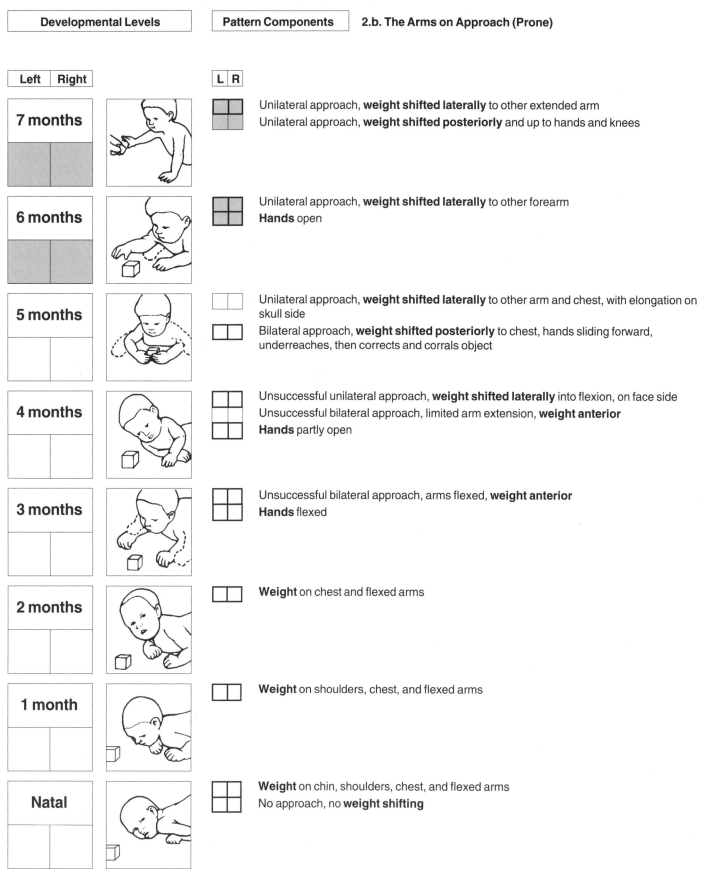

Developmental Levels — Left | Right

Pattern Components — L | R

7 months
- Unilateral approach, **weight shifted laterally** to other extended arm
- Unilateral approach, **weight shifted posteriorly** and up to hands and knees

6 months
- Unilateral approach, **weight shifted laterally** to other forearm
- **Hands** open

5 months
- Unilateral approach, **weight shifted laterally** to other arm and chest, with elongation on skull side
- Bilateral approach, **weight shifted posteriorly** to chest, hands sliding forward, underreaches, then corrects and corrals object

4 months
- Unsuccessful unilateral approach, **weight shifted laterally** into flexion, on face side
- Unsuccessful bilateral approach, limited arm extension, **weight anterior**
- **Hands** partly open

3 months
- Unsuccessful bilateral approach, arms flexed, **weight anterior**
- **Hands** flexed

2 months
- **Weight** on chest and flexed arms

1 month
- **Weight** on shoulders, chest, and flexed arms

Natal
- **Weight** on chin, shoulders, chest, and flexed arms
- No approach, no **weight shifting**

Section 2. Primarily Voluntary Movements (Cognitively Directed)

| Developmental Levels | | Pattern Components | 2.c. The Arms on Approach (Sitting) |

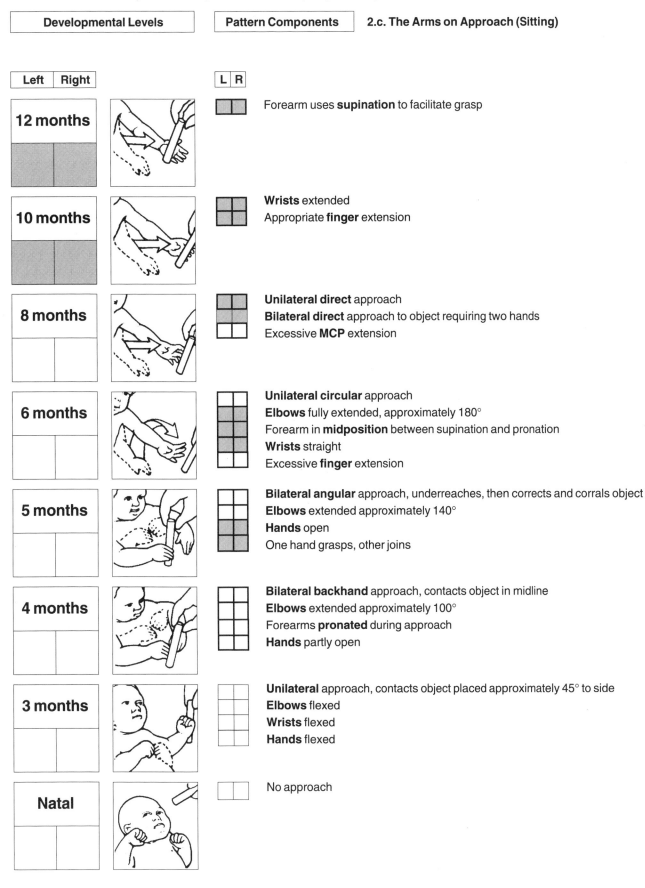

Left	Right

L	R

12 months — ▨▨ — Forearm uses **supination** to facilitate grasp

10 months — Wrists extended / Appropriate **finger** extension

8 months — **Unilateral direct** approach / **Bilateral direct** approach to object requiring two hands / Excessive **MCP** extension

6 months — **Unilateral circular** approach / **Elbows** fully extended, approximately 180° / Forearm in **midposition** between supination and pronation / **Wrists** straight / Excessive **finger** extension

5 months — **Bilateral angular** approach, underreaches, then corrects and corrals object / **Elbows** extended approximately 140° / **Hands** open / One hand grasps, other joins

4 months — **Bilateral backhand** approach, contacts object in midline / **Elbows** extended approximately 100° / Forearms **pronated** during approach / **Hands** partly open

3 months — **Unilateral** approach, contacts object placed approximately 45° to side / **Elbows** flexed / **Wrists** flexed / **Hands** flexed

Natal — No approach

Section 2. Primarily Voluntary Movements (Cognitively Directed))

| Developmental Levels | | Pattern Components | 2.d. Grasp of the Dowel (Supine, Prone, or Sitting) |

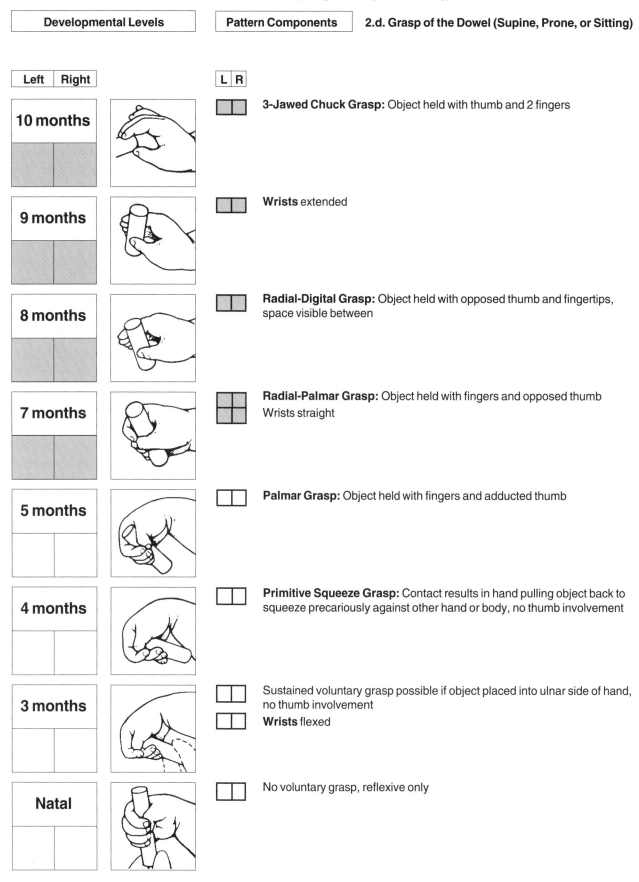

| Left | Right | | L | R | |

10 months — **3-Jawed Chuck Grasp:** Object held with thumb and 2 fingers

9 months — **Wrists** extended

8 months — **Radial-Digital Grasp:** Object held with opposed thumb and fingertips, space visible between

7 months — **Radial-Palmar Grasp:** Object held with fingers and opposed thumb
Wrists straight

5 months — **Palmar Grasp:** Object held with fingers and adducted thumb

4 months — **Primitive Squeeze Grasp:** Contact results in hand pulling object back to squeeze precariously against other hand or body, no thumb involvement

3 months — Sustained voluntary grasp possible if object placed into ulnar side of hand, no thumb involvement
Wrists flexed

Natal — No voluntary grasp, reflexive only

| Developmental Levels | | Pattern Components | 2.e. Grasp of the Cube (Supine, Prone, or Sitting) |

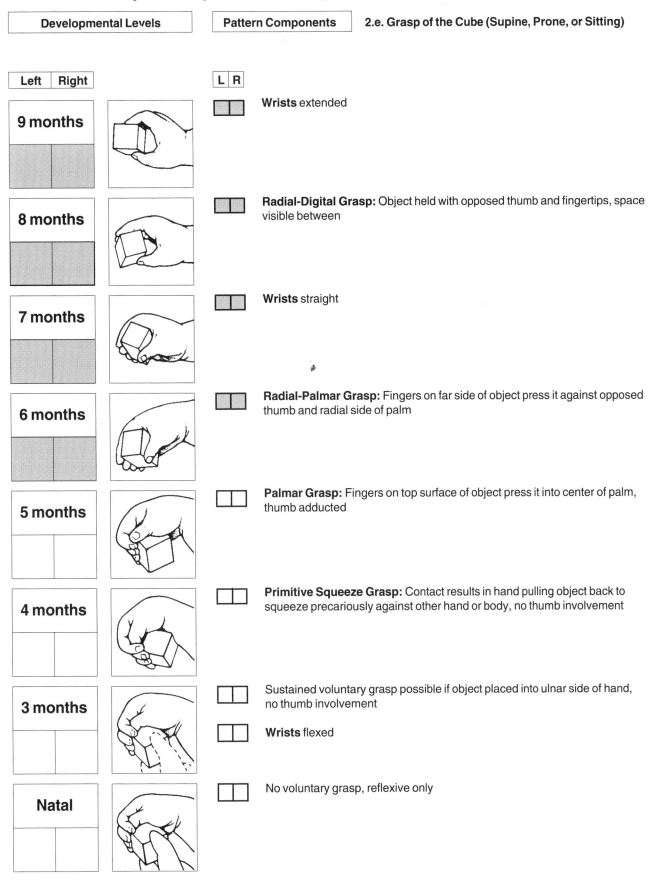

Left	Right		L	R	
9 months					**Wrists** extended
8 months					**Radial-Digital Grasp:** Object held with opposed thumb and fingertips, space visible between
7 months					**Wrists** straight
6 months					**Radial-Palmar Grasp:** Fingers on far side of object press it against opposed thumb and radial side of palm
5 months					**Palmar Grasp:** Fingers on top surface of object press it into center of palm, thumb adducted
4 months					**Primitive Squeeze Grasp:** Contact results in hand pulling object back to squeeze precariously against other hand or body, no thumb involvement
3 months					Sustained voluntary grasp possible if object placed into ulnar side of hand, no thumb involvement
					Wrists flexed
Natal					No voluntary grasp, reflexive only

Section 2. Primarily Voluntary Movements (Cognitively Directed)

| Developmental Levels | | Pattern Components | 2.f. Grasp of the Pellet (Prone or Sitting) |

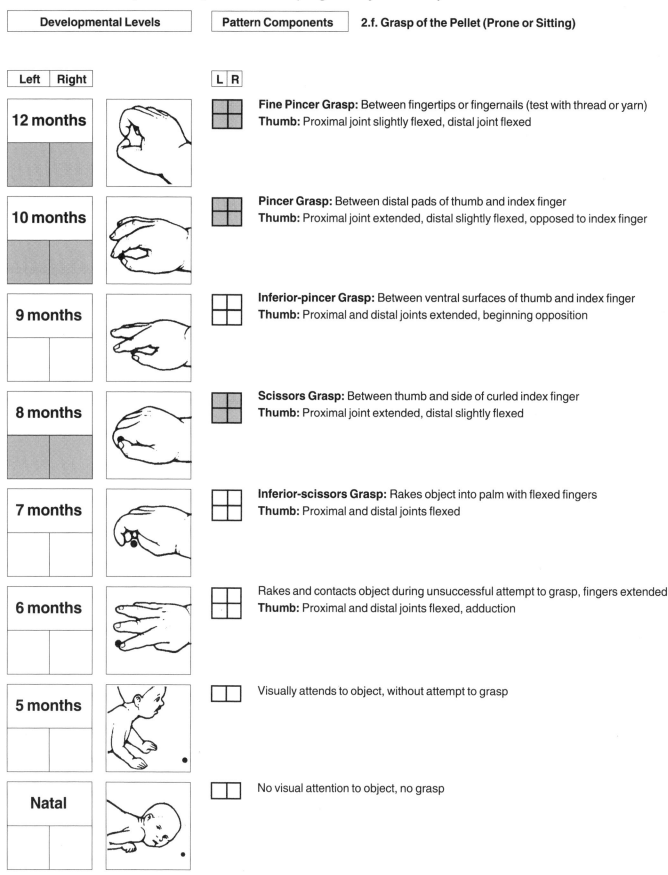

| Left | Right | | L | R |

12 months

Fine Pincer Grasp: Between fingertips or fingernails (test with thread or yarn)
Thumb: Proximal joint slightly flexed, distal joint flexed

10 months

Pincer Grasp: Between distal pads of thumb and index finger
Thumb: Proximal joint extended, distal slightly flexed, opposed to index finger

9 months

Inferior-pincer Grasp: Between ventral surfaces of thumb and index finger
Thumb: Proximal and distal joints extended, beginning opposition

8 months

Scissors Grasp: Between thumb and side of curled index finger
Thumb: Proximal joint extended, distal slightly flexed

7 months

Inferior-scissors Grasp: Rakes object into palm with flexed fingers
Thumb: Proximal and distal joints flexed

6 months

Rakes and contacts object during unsuccessful attempt to grasp, fingers extended
Thumb: Proximal and distal joints flexed, adduction

5 months

Visually attends to object, without attempt to grasp

Natal

No visual attention to object, no grasp

Section 2. Primarily Voluntary Movements (Cognitively Directed)

Developmental Levels	Pattern Components	2.g. Manipulation Skills (Prehension Schema)
Left Right	L R	L R

15 months

Inverts container to reach contents
Intentional manipulation possible without hand and object within visual field

One hand manipulates object while other holds or assists

12 months

Both hands combine objects

Tactile manipulation (rotating, squeezing, transferring) replaces **oral exploration** (mouthing)

10 months

Isolates index finger to poke, others flexed
Tries unsuccessfully to reach into small container to remove object

One hand manipulates, other hand mirrors
Shakes object with arm, elbow, and wrist motion

9 months

Tries to poke, all fingers extended
Pokes with thumb

Increased **tactile manipulation, orally explores** new objects primarily

8 months

Reciprocal Assimilation:
Watches hand and keeps it moving to make interesting sights last
Intentional manipulation possible when hand and object are within visual field
Object Permanence:
Searches for lost or removed object, ignoring new stimulus
Drops object when grasping another

Drops object
Throws object
Pushes object
Pulls object

Retains object when grasping another
Shakes one or both objects, alternating visual monitoring back and forth

7 months

6 months

Beginning of **Object Permanence:**
Searches for lost or removed object, but can be distracted by another

Alternately mouths, looks, shakes object, retaining grasp
Shakes object with arm and elbow motion

5 months

Tactile Discrimination between hand and object (bites object, not fingers)

Alternately mouths and shakes object
Shakes object with arm motion only

4 months

Mouths object or eats finger foods with insufficient **tactile discrimination** (may bite fingers by mistake)

Hand brings object to mouth, orally exploring both
Visually attends and swipes at object if within 1"

3 months

Tactile Assimilation: Hand movements extend to own face, body, clothing
Tactile Accommodation: Hands adapt to new objects, without visual attention

Tactile Recognition (eyes alert) leads to: Voluntary repetition of reflexive movements
Hand to mouth

1 month

Reflexive Movements:
Scratching and clutching

Eyes watch moving hand

Natal

Reflexive Grasp: Involuntary, without tactile awareness (eyes do not alert)
No voluntary hand movements

Visually attends to object without reaching
No voluntary hand to mouth, head/mouth move to suck on hand

Section 2. Primarily Voluntary Movements (Cognitively Directed)

Developmental Levels		Pattern Components	2.h. Release of the Dowel or Cube (Supine, Prone, or Sitting)
Left	**Right**	**L** **R**	

12 months

Precise release into **small container**
Wrists extended

10 months

Clumsy release into **small container,** rests hand on edge

9 months

Controlled release into **large container**
Wrists straight

8 months

Clumsy release into **large container** or **above surface**
Attempts unsuccessful release into **small container**

7 months

Voluntary assistive release **against surface** (stabilization)
Attempts unsuccessful release into **large container** or **above surface**
Adept 1-stage **transfer,** simultaneous grasp and release
Object falls from hand as arm extends, forearm supinates, and fingers extend

6 months

Smooth 2-stage **transfer:** One hand grasps, other joins, first hand releases
May use mouth as intermediary for **transfer**

5 months

Clumsy 2-stage **transfer:** One hand grasps, other joins, first hand releases with difficulty
Voluntary release as object is removed by another

4 months

Mutual fingering in midline, preparation for **transfer**

3 months

Involuntary release after sustained grasp, with awareness (eyes alert)

2 months

Involuntary release after retaining briefly, with some awareness (eyes alert)

1 month

Immediate involuntary release, without awareness

Natal

No voluntary release, object must be forcibly removed, or:
No grasp
Wrists flexed

Section 2. Primarily Voluntary Movements (Cognitively Directed)

| Developmental Levels | | Pattern Components | 2.i. Release of the Pellet (Sitting) |

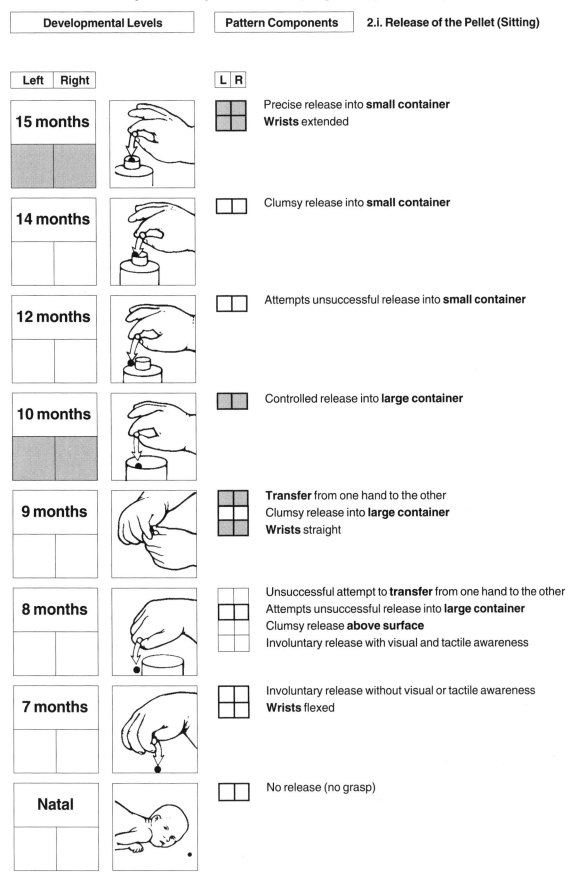

Left | **Right**   **L** | **R**

15 months
Precise release into **small container**
Wrists extended

14 months
Clumsy release into **small container**

12 months
Attempts unsuccessful release into **small container**

10 months
Controlled release into **large container**

9 months
Transfer from one hand to the other
Clumsy release into **large container**
Wrists straight

8 months
Unsuccessful attempt to **transfer** from one hand to the other
Attempts unsuccessful release into **large container**
Clumsy release **above surface**
Involuntary release with visual and tactile awareness

7 months
Involuntary release without visual or tactile awareness
Wrists flexed

Natal
No release (no grasp)

Section 3. Pre-writing Skills

| Developmental Levels | | Pattern Components | 3.a. Crayon or Pencil Grasp |

| Left | Right |

| L | R |

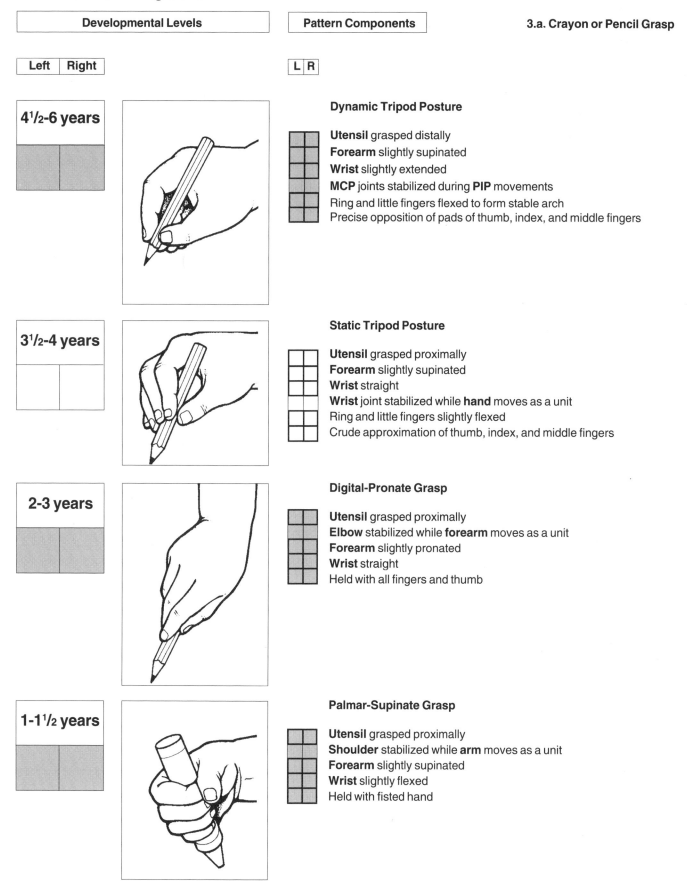

4½-6 years

Dynamic Tripod Posture

Utensil grasped distally
Forearm slightly supinated
Wrist slightly extended
MCP joints stabilized during **PIP** movements
Ring and little fingers flexed to form stable arch
Precise opposition of pads of thumb, index, and middle fingers

3½-4 years

Static Tripod Posture

Utensil grasped proximally
Forearm slightly supinated
Wrist straight
Wrist joint stabilized while **hand** moves as a unit
Ring and little fingers slightly flexed
Crude approximation of thumb, index, and middle fingers

2-3 years

Digital-Pronate Grasp

Utensil grasped proximally
Elbow stabilized while **forearm** moves as a unit
Forearm slightly pronated
Wrist straight
Held with all fingers and thumb

1-1½ years

Palmar-Supinate Grasp

Utensil grasped proximally
Shoulder stabilized while **arm** moves as a unit
Forearm slightly supinated
Wrist slightly flexed
Held with fisted hand

Section 3. Pre-writing Skills

Developmental Levels		Pattern Components		3.b. Drawings

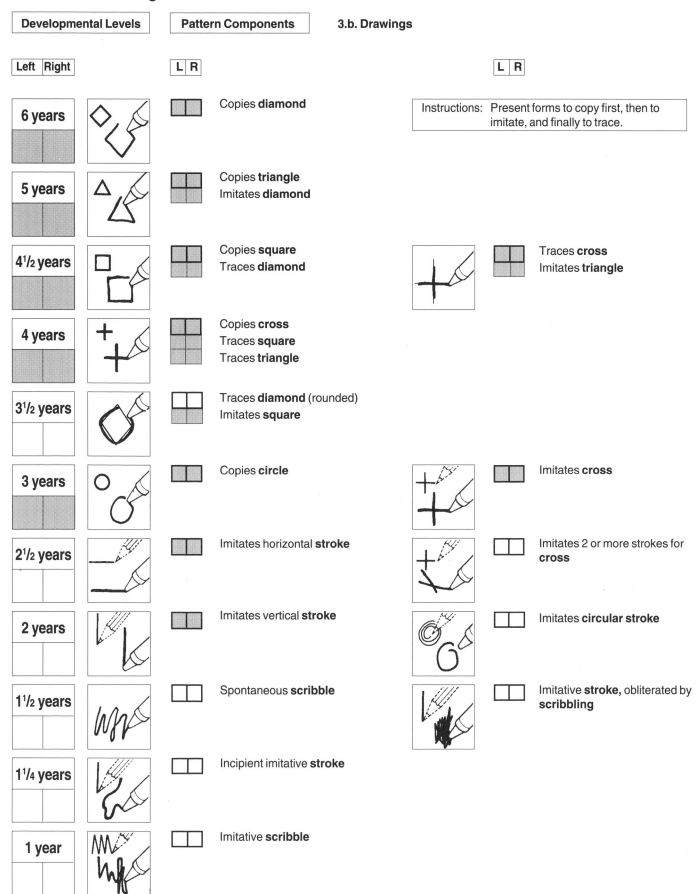

Developmental Levels

Left	Right

Pattern Components — L | R

6 years — Copies **diamond**

5 years — Copies **triangle** / Imitates **diamond**

4½ years — Copies **square** / Traces **diamond**

4 years — Copies **cross** / Traces **square** / Traces **triangle**

3½ years — Traces **diamond** (rounded) / Imitates **square**

3 years — Copies **circle**

2½ years — Imitates horizontal **stroke**

2 years — Imitates vertical **stroke**

1½ years — Spontaneous **scribble**

1¼ years — Incipient imitative **stroke**

1 year — Imitative **scribble**

Instructions: Present forms to copy first, then to imitate, and finally to trace.

L | R

Traces **cross** / Imitates **triangle**

Imitates **cross**

Imitates 2 or more strokes for **cross**

Imitates **circular stroke**

Imitative **stroke,** obliterated by **scribbling**

Part II. Score Sheet (Developmental Levels)

Section 1. Primarily Involuntary Arm-Hand Patterns (Positional-Reflexive)

Section 3: Pre-Writing Skills (Pencil Grasp and Drawings)

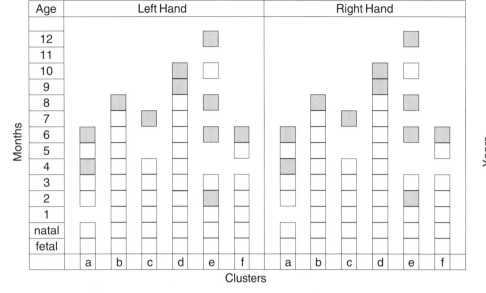

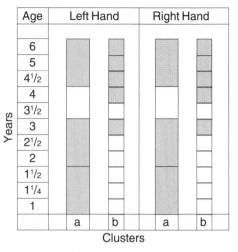

Section 2. Primarily Voluntary Movements of Approach, Grasp, Manipulation, and Release (Cognitively Directed)

Part III. Score Sheet Summary (Developmental Levels)

Subject _____   Examiner _____

Birth Date _____ Chronological Age _____   Test Date _____

Diagnoses _____

		Left Hand	Right Hand
Section 1.	Primarily Involuntary Arm-Hand Patterns	_____ months	_____ months
Section 2.	Primarily Voluntary Movements	_____ months	_____ months
Section 3.	Pre-Writing Skills	_____ years	_____ years

ISBN 0761643613

Printed in the U.S.A.

Erhardt Developmental Prehension Assessment
Short Screening Form (EDPA-S)

by Rhoda P. Erhardt, M.S., OTR, FAOTA

CONTENTS

Instructions: Materials, Administration, Scoring Procedures

Protocol Sheets

Section 1. Primarily Involuntary Arm-Hand Patterns (Positional-Reflexive)
- a. The Arms at Rest and During Body Play (Supine)
- b. The Arms at Rest and During Head Raising (Prone)
- c. The Asymmetrical Tonic Neck Reflex
- d. Grasping Reactions
- e. Placing Responses
- f. Avoiding Responses

Section 2. Primarily Voluntary Movements (Cognitively Directed)
- a. The Arms on Approach (Supine)
- b. The Arms on Approach (Prone)
- c. The Arms on Approach (Sitting)
- d. Grasp of the Dowel
- e. Grasp of the Cube
- f. Grasp of the Pellet
- g. Manipulation Skills (Prehension Schema)
- h. Release of the Dowel or Cube
- i. Release of the Pellet

Summary

Subject _____ Examiner _____

Birth Date _____ Chronological Age _____ Test Date _____

Diagnoses _____

Reproducing This Form

This form can be reproduced for administrative use (not for resale). To protect your book, make a photocopy of each reproducible page. Then use that copy as a master for photocopying or other types of reproduction.

Printed, published, and sold by

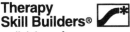

Therapy Skill Builders®
a division of
The Psychological Corporation

555 Academic Court
San Antonio, Texas 78204-2498
1-800-228-0752

The Learning Curve Design and Therapy Skill Builders are registered trademarks of The Psychological Corporation.

Printed in the United States of America

ISBN 0761643133

3 4 5 6 7 8 9 10 11 12 A B C D E

INSTRUCTIONS

Materials

Appropriate toys and functional objects should be selected according to each subject's age, gender, cognitive, cultural, and personal interests, with enough novelty to avoid satiation or habituation.

1. Graded series of 3 dowel shapes, approximately 1 cm-2$\frac{1}{2}$ cm diameter
2. Graded series of 3 cube shapes, approximately 3 cm-6 cm wide
3. Graded series of 3 edible pellets, approximately 5 mm-1$\frac{1}{2}$ cm diameter
4. Graded series of 3 large containers (nesting boxes), approximately 5 cm-8 cm wide
5. Graded series of 3 small containers (pill bottles), approximately 1 cm-3 cm diameter
6. Segments of black and white yarn and thread
7. Test kit container (plastic bucket or tote bag)

Administration

This test has been designed for subjects of all cognitive levels and chronological ages 15 months and older. Verbal directions may be given but are not required, as the subject is observed during spontaneous movement, in response to being handled, or as a stimulus is presented.

Scoring Procedures

$\boxed{+}$ Well-integrated normal pattern $\boxed{-}$ Pattern not present $\boxed{\pm}$ Emerging or inconsistent pattern

Section 1. Primarily Involuntary Arm-Hand Patterns (Positional-Reflexive)

1.a. The Arms at Rest and During Body Play (Supine)

L	R

☐ Neck elongated

☐ Lifts head in midline, separately from shoulders

☐ Head in midline, chin tucked

☐☐ Shoulders well depressed

☐☐ Rolls to prone, upper arm adducts to help

☐☐ Rolls to sidelying and back supine

L	R

☐☐ Hands brought together in space

☐☐ Arms internally rotated, hands clutching on chest

☐☐ Wrists straight

☐☐ Hands to mouth
Hands to knees
Hands open

☐☐ Thumbs out

1.b. The Arms at Rest and During Head Raising (Prone)

☐☐ Rolls to supine and back with lateral head righting

☐ Head in midline with flexor/extensor control

☐☐ Shoulders well-depressed

☐☐ Arms abducted and externally rotated

☐☐ Arms straight forward

☐☐ Purshes up on forearms, elbows directly under shoulders

☐☐ Weight on palmar surfaces

☐☐ Wrists straight

☐☐ Hands open, with arch, thumbs out

☐☐ Crawls on hands and knees

☐☐ Stabilizes with hands to rotate from hand and knees to sidesitting

☐☐ Stable in sidelying

☐☐ Pushes up to sidesitting from sidelying

☐☐ Pushes up on extended arms, STNR integrated (neck flexed)

☐☐ Weight on radial-palmar surfaces

☐☐ Wrists extended

Section 1. Primarily Involuntary Arm-Harm Patterns (Positional-Reflexive) continued

1.c. The Asymmetrical Tonic Neck Reflex (ATNR)

 Passive rotation of head toward the side results in extension of face limb and flexion of skull limb. Obligatory response (inability to move out of position) is always pathological.

☐☐ Fully integrated; no response except for remnants in older children and adults under stress

1.d. Grasping Reactions

(Test in supine or with vision occluded to prevent contamination by voluntary movements)

 Instinctive Grasp Reaction: (Light distally moving stimulus) Integrated, stimulus withdrawn from radial side of palm results in voluntary, not involuntary movement

☐☐ **Grasp Reflex:** (Firmly inserted stimulus) Integrated, stimulus in radial side of palm results in voluntary, not involuntary grasp

1.e. Placing Responses

Protective Extensor Thrust

☐☐ Sudden movement of head and trunk backward results in immediate extension of elbows and hands placing on surface

☐☐ Sudden movement of head and trunk sideward results in immediate extension/abduction of arms and fingers

☐☐ Sudden movement of head and trunk forward and down results in immediate extension of arms and extension/abduction of fingers

Proprioceptive Placing (Test with vision occluded)

☐☐ Fully integrated: No response to brushing back of hand lightly against table edge

1.f. Avoiding Responses

(Test in supine or with vision occluded to prevent contamination by voluntary movements)

 Integrated: distally moving light stimulus to any part of hand does not result in withdrawal response, except for remnants in older children and adults under stress

Section 2. Primarily Voluntary Movements (Cognitively Directed)

2.a. The Arms on Approach (Supine)   * Mature components not included in the EDPA long form

L R

☐	☐	* Unilateral direct approach
☐	☐	* Bilateral direct approach to object requiring two hands
☐	☐	* Wrists extended
☐	☐	* Appropriate finger extension
☐	☐	* Accurate approach
☐	☐	Elbows fully extended, approximately 180°
☐	☐	Wrists straight
☐	☐	Hands open
☐	☐	One hand grasps, other joins

2.b. The Arms on Approach (Prone)

☐	☐	Unilateral approach, weight shifted posteriorly and up to hands and knees
☐	☐	Unilateral approach, weight shifted laterally to other extended arm,
☐	☐	Unilateral approach, weight shifted laterally to other forearm
☐	☐	Hands open

2.c. The Arms on Approach (Sitting)

☐	☐	Forearm uses supination to facilitate grasp
☐	☐	Unilateral direct approach
☐	☐	Bilateral direct approach to object requiring two hands
☐	☐	Elbows fully extended, approximately 180°
☐	☐	Wrists extended
☐	☐	Appropriate finger extension
☐	☐	Forearm in midposition between supination and pronation
☐	☐	Wrists straight
☐	☐	Hands open
☐	☐	One hand grasps, other joins

2.d. Grasp of the Dowel (Supine, Prone, or Sitting)

☐	☐	**3-Jawed Chuck Grasp:** Object held with thumb and 2 fingers
☐	☐	**Radial-Digital Grasp:** Object held with opposed thumb and fingertips, space visible between
☐	☐	Wrists extended
☐	☐	**Radial-Palmar Grasp:** Object held with fingers and opposed thumb
☐	☐	Wrists straight

Section 2. Primarily Voluntary Movements (Cognitively Directed) continued

2.e. Grasp of the Cube (Supine, Prone, or Sitting)

L	R

☐☐ **Radial-Digital Grasp:** Object held with opposed thumb and fingertips, space visible between

☐☐ Wrists extended

☐☐ **Radial-Palmar Grasp:** Fingers on far side of object press it against opposed thumb and radial side of palm

☐☐ Wrists straight

2.f. Grasp of the Pellet (Prone or Sitting)

☐☐ **Fine Pincer Grasp:** Between fingertips or fingernails (test with thread or yarn)

☐☐ **Thumb:** Proximal joint slightly flexed, distal joint flexed

☐☐ **Pincer Grasp:** Between distal pads of thumb and index finger

☐☐ **Thumb:** Proximal joint extended, distal slightly flexed, opposed to index finger

☐☐ **Scissors Grasp:** Between thumb and side of curled index finger

☐☐ **Thumb:** Proximal joint extended, distal slightly flexed

2.g. Manipulation Skills (Prehension Schema)

☐☐ Inverts container to reach contents

☐☐ One hand manipulates object while other holds or assists

☐☐ Both hands combine objects

☐☐ Retains object when grasping another

☐☐ Isolates index finger to poke, others flexed

☐☐ **Object Permanence:** Searches for lost or removed object, ignoring new stimulus

☐☐ **Tactile Discrimination** between hand and object (bites object, not fingers)

☐☐ **Tactile Accommodation:** Hands adapt to new objects, without visual attention

☐☐ Pokes with thumb

☐☐ Intentional manipulation possible without hand and object within visual field

☐☐ **Tactile manipulation** (rotating, squeezing, transferring) replaces oral exploration (mouthing)

☐☐ Shakes object with arm, elbow, and wrist motion

☐☐ Drops objects

☐☐ Throws object

☐☐ Pushes object

☐☐ Pulls object

☐☐ Hand to mouth

☐☐ Eyes watch moving hand

Copyright © 1994 by Rhoda P. Erhardt
Published by Therapy Skill Builders, a division of The Psychological Corporation / All rights reserved.
1-800-228-0752 / ISBN 0761643133

Section 2. Primarily Voluntary Movements (Cognitively Directed) continued

2.h. Release of the Dowel or Cube (Supine, Prone, or Sitting)

L	R

☐☐ Precise release into small container

☐☐ Wrists extended

☐☐ Controlled release into large container

☐☐ Wrists straight

☐☐ Voluntary assistive release against surface (stabilization)

☐☐ Adept 1-stage transfer, simultaneous grasp and release

2.i. Release of the Pellet (Sitting)

☐☐ Precise release into small container

☐☐ Wrists extended

☐☐ Controlled release into large container

☐☐ Transfer from one hand to the other

☐☐ Wrists straight

Summary

This EDPA-S (short screening form) contains all test items in the EDPA (long form) that represent norms acquired by 15 months of age. Clusters with imperfect scores should be retested with the EDPA long form.

Key:

☐+ All scores (+)   ☐− All scores (−)   ☐± Mixture of (+), (−), and/or (±)

Score	Cluster	Score	Cluster
☐☐	1.a. The Arms at Rest and During Body Play (Supine)	☐☐	2.a. The Arms on Approach (Supine)
☐☐	1.b. The Arms at Rest and During Head Raising (Prone)	☐☐	2.b. The Arms on Approach (Prone)
☐☐	1.c. The Asymmetrical Tonic Neck Reflex (ATNR)	☐☐	2.c. The Arms on Approach (Sitting)
☐☐	1.d. Grasping Reactions	☐☐	2.d. Grasp of the Dowel
☐☐	1.e. Placing Responses	☐☐	2.e. Grasp of the Cube
☐☐	1.f. Avoiding Responses	☐☐	2.f. Grasp of the Pellet
		☐☐	2.g. Manipulation Skills (Prehension Schema)
		☐☐	2.h. Release of the Dowel or Cube
		☐☐	2.i. Release of the Pellet

Chapter Eight
Application of Assessment Data to Treatment in Functional Environments

Because of the shift in goals toward functional skills needed for adult life, more emphasis is now being placed on a top-down curriculum, in which the end goal is stated first, and objectives are designed to reach the goal, rather than on a pure developmental approach. Community-based instruction, begun during the school years, includes four domain areas: vocational, domestic, leisure, and community skills. Activities designed to build on previously learned skills, develop new ones, and increase skill levels emphasize hands-on community work experiences, functional academics, and job-seeking and retaining skills. Behavior characteristics such as self-determination, problem-solving, and persistence are especially needed for independence (Baumgart 1990; Goodwyn 1987).

Assessments need to focus on functional activities and be environmentally based, with the student observed performing in the natural environment. In this way, skills already achieved are distinguished from those needed. Intervention then concentrates on skills needed for integration into the community and should be chronologically appropriate, rather than solely developmentally appropriate.

To determine if an activity is functional, the question to be asked is: "If the student doesn't learn this skill, will someone else have to do it for the person?" If the answer is yes, the activity is functional. Choices for intervention activities should be based on the following (Flick, Shephard, and Brollier 1992):

- judgments of all team members
- the quantity of environments in which the skill will be used

- how often the skill is used during the day
- its social significance
- probability that it is achievable
- importance for health and safety

Preparation for Community Integration and Independence

Changing attitudes of society toward minority groups have benefitted persons with disabilities. New federal, state, and local legislation, promoted by advocacy groups, has meant increased integration and more appropriate health care, accessibility, housing, and transportation. Lifestyles for children and adults with moderate and severe cerebral palsy have changed from total dependence in institutional settings, to group homes, foster homes, and assisted independent living. Work opportunities have also changed from sheltered to supportive employment with job coaches, enabling the worker to function within more normal, competitive situations (Rang and Wright 1989).

However, provision of lifelong special services, which fosters dependency, can significantly interfere with the acquisition of adult life skills. The developmental tasks of adolescence include achieving emotional independence from parents, preparing for close relationships with peers, learning socially responsible behavior, and beginning vocational exploration.

These tasks are difficult when individuals are operating from a social position of passivity and helplessness, which is common in young adults with cerebral palsy because of limited mobility, few opportunities to make decisions, and dependence on others for many activities of daily living. The occupational therapist who perceives young children with cerebral palsy in the context of their entire life span will recognize the importance of encouraging them at an early age to take responsibility, be more self-reliant, and eventually become more assertive in directing their own lives (Neistadt 1987).

After the passage and implementation of the Education of the Handicapped Act, P.L. 94-142, professionals were required to work together to develop Individual Education Plans (IEPs). The process of evaluating skills, analyzing their functional importance, and selecting intervention procedures depended on the ability of those professionals to skillfully integrate all the gathered and shared information about the children, and to include the parents and the children in the decision-making process.

These children are changing as they grow, and so is the world they live in. They and their families find their priorities changing. New federal legislation for persons with disabilities now promises opportunities for increased independence through technology, funding for caregivers, and supportive employment programs. New decisions must be made that will affect their children, their siblings, and they themselves during these transitions to adulthood. The Individual Education Plans (IEPs), Individual Transition Plans (ITPs), and Individual Service Plans (ISPs) being written for these teenagers and adults place heavy emphasis on the environmental domains (domestic, vocational, leisure, and community).

Transitions

Transition is defined as the process of moving from one level of an activity to another level. In legislation pertaining to the rights of people with disabilities, *transition* has a special meaning. It refers to the establishment and implementation of a plan for helping children and young adults move to a higher level of education, employment, or other activities of adult life.

The Individuals with Disabilities Education Act (IDEA), P.L. 101-476, requires plans for transition in an IEP no later than the student's 16th birthday. IDEA also defines transition services and assistive technology services. The activities are based on the student's needs, preferences, and interests, and are chosen to increase participation in domestic, community, recreational, and vocational environments. Following completion of high school, options include further education, employment, and community living.

Transition planning also addresses recreation and leisure, community activities, and aspects of home life. These rights are now protected by the Americans with Disabilities Act (ADA), P.L. 100-336, which prohibits discrimination against the 43,000,000 Americans who have one or more physical or mental disabilities (Ellek 1991). This law covers four different areas: employment (Title I), transportation (Title II), public accommodations (Title III), and communications (Title IV).

The ADA creates a new opportunity to guide these individuals into a successful transition to a work environment, with focus on productivity in the community. In a holistic philosophy, evaluation for community employment must consider appearance (grooming and cleanliness), hand use (dexterity, bilaterality), concentration (distractibility, work habits), time responsibility (punctuality, attention to task), and social interaction (with supervisor and peers). Task analysis as well as ongoing observation and assessment of performance in the work environment is needed, especially in supported employment programs, which have a goal of community placement for every developmentally disabled adult and mandate a job coach for each individual (Herrick and Lowe 1992).

Supported employment is described as a specific strategy used to facilitate successful paid community employment for persons previously considered too disabled to work. It provides specialized training at job sites and ongoing support for the worker and employer, and stresses the importance of making the job fit the person rather than the person fit the job (Spencer 1987; Williams 1992).

The Rehabilitation Amendments of 1986 (P.L. 99-506) define supported employment as competitive work in integrated settings for (a) individuals with severe handicaps for whom competitive employment has not traditionally occurred, or (b) individuals for whom competitive employment has been interrupted or intermittent as a result of severe disability and who, because of their handicap, need ongoing support services to perform work. Supported employment is further defined in the final regulations by the refinement of its components, that is, competitive work, integrated settings, severe handicaps, and ongoing support services.

These person-centered programs should address real-life situations and give opportunities for learning. Individuals should be allowed some exposure to risks present in the community unless the person is designated as vulnerable (one who would not report abuse or neglect because of impaired physical, mental, or emotional function).

The concept of independent living supports the beliefs that control over one's life is important and that personal independence can be increased by managing one's own affairs, participating in day-to-day life, and filling a variety of roles, especially the opportunity to participate in real work. The term *least restricted alternative/environment* means access to services which enable persons to live, work, and be educated in the most natural setting with the least amount of support needed.

The spirit of these new laws and regulations is highly compatible with occupational therapy's philosophical perspective, which values functional independence, bringing all persons with disabilities into the mainstream of life, and an interactive relationship between the individual and the environment. Children learn competence and autonomy through interactions with natural environments.

In the environment-centered model for service provision (as opposed to the deficit-reduction model), the therapist has a new role as educator and consultant to individuals and businesses for alteration of materials and environments for children's and adolescents' accessibility. The therapist can promote the view of children and adolescents with disabilities as individuals striving to achieve roles and fulfill responsibilities.

Learning and taking personal responsibility is a lifelong challenge that begins in childhood. Assessment strategies are focused on environmental analysis through developmental knowledge, analysis of activities in the context of natural environments, and evaluation of the desires and abilities of the child or adolescent. Intervention requires problem solving and creativity. Activities are selected not simply because they are deficits, but because they are essential to fulfillment of a desired meaningful goal. Outcomes must directly relate to recognizable function and participation in client-determined occupations (Kalscheur 1992).

The Evaluation Report

The importance of the written report cannot be overemphasized. It serves as the vehicle of communication to all those who are involved in therapeutic intervention (Sattler 1974).

The language used in evaluation reports should be free from technical jargon and understandable to all team members—professionals from the medical and educational fields, as well as lay persons who are family, friends, and other caregivers. Medical and educational terms may be appropriately used but should be clearly defined and explained (Gilfoyle 1979). Formats of reports can vary, according to the type of evaluation, needs of the facility, and individual writing styles.

Reports which use a developmental/functional frame of reference generally include the following information:

Identifying information: name of facility, type of evaluation, name of individual, date of birth, chronological age, diagnoses, name of examiner, and date of report

Referral source: parent, physician, school, or other agency; reason for referral, concerns of parents and teachers, functional problems; and pertinent medical and educational history

General observations: where evaluation was conducted, who was there, subject's state and attitude

Findings: results of each section (narrative plus evaluation form, if desired), present level of function, clarifying information, clinical observations, summary of total performance, and conclusions

Recommendations: answers to referral questions, general recommendations, suggested community resources, and re-evaluation timelines

Signature: examiner's name and credentials, team members who will receive copies

Some reports may also include specific intervention procedures, either as part of the report or as an addendum (Coley 1978). Ongoing progress notes specifying treatment modifications can include the name of the activity, the current response, and specific recommendations.

Model for Evaluation Report

A suggested form for the Erhardt Developmental Prehension Assessment report is presented as a typical computer word-processing fill-in program. The next three chapters will show how this report form was used with the case study examples.

EDPA Report Form Example

Date:
To:
Re: (type of evaluation) for (Name)

This (age) (male/female) with a diagnosis of (diagnosis) was evaluated today (location) with the Erhardt Developmental Prehension Assessment to determine hand function relating to (specific domains, educational performance, and/or future function):

(Name) resides with (family/others), and attends (school placement/other program). (He/She) was evaluated for head, arm, and hand function in various positions: supine (on the back), prone (on the stomach), and sitting. (Persons present) contributed historical and observational information.

Section 1. Primarily Involuntary Arm-Hand Patterns (Positional-Reflexive)

1.a. The Arms at Rest and during Body Play (Supine)
Evaluation Report
   Normal patterns (developmentally appropriate):
   Delayed patterns (primary developmentally inappropriate):
   Atypical patterns (secondary developmentally inappropriate):
   Implications for function:
Treatment Program

1.b. The Arms at Rest and during Head Raising (Prone)
Evaluation Report
   Normal patterns (developmentally appropriate):
   Delayed patterns (primary developmentally inappropriate):
   Atypical patterns (secondary developmentally inappropriate):
   Implications for function:
Treatment Program

1.c. Asymmetrical Tonic Neck Reflex (ATNR)
Evaluation Report
   Normal patterns (developmentally appropriate):
   Delayed patterns (primary developmentally inappropriate):

Atypical patterns (secondary developmentally inappropriate):
   Implications for function:
Treatment Program

1.d. Grasping Reaction
Evaluation Report
   Normal patterns (developmentally appropriate):
   Delayed patterns (primary developmentally inappropriate):
   Atypical patterns (secondary developmentally inappropriate):
   Implications for function:
Treatment Program

1.e. Placing Responses
Evaluation Report
   Normal patterns (developmentally appropriate):
   Delayed patterns (primary developmentally inappropriate):
   Atypical patterns (secondary developmentally inappropriate):
   Implications for function:
Treatment Program

1.f. Avoiding Responses
Evaluation Report
   Normal patterns (developmentally appropriate):
   Delayed patterns (primary developmentally inappropriate):
   Atypical patterns (secondary developmentally inappropriate):
   Implications for function:
Treatment Program

Section 2. Primarily Voluntary Movements (Cognitively Directed)

2.a. The Arms on Approach (Supine)
Evaluation Report
   Normal patterns (developmentally appropriate):
   Delayed patterns (primary developmentally inappropriate):
   Atypical patterns (secondary developmentally inappropriate):
   Implications for function:
Treatment Program

2.b. The Arms on Approach (Prone)
Evaluation Report
Normal patterns (developmentally appropriate):
Delayed patterns (primary developmentally
inappropriate):
Atypical patterns (secondary developmentally
inappropriate):
Implications for function:
Treatment Program

2.c. The Arms on Approach (Sitting)
Evaluation Report
Normal patterns (developmentally appropriate):
Delayed patterns (primary developmentally
inappropriate):
Atypical patterns (secondary developmentally
inappropriate):
Implications for function:
Treatment Program

2.d. Grasp of the Dowel and 2.e. Grasp of the Cube
Evaluation Report
Normal patterns (developmentally appropriate):
Delayed patterns (primary developmentally
inappropriate):
Atypical patterns (secondary developmentally
inappropriate):
Implications for function:
Treatment Program

2.f. Grasp of the Pellet (Prone or Sitting)
Evaluation Report
Normal patterns (developmentally appropriate):
Delayed patterns (primary developmentally
inappropriate):
Atypical patterns (secondary developmentally
inappropriate):
Implications for function:
Treatment Program

2.g. Manipulation Skills (Prehension Schema)
Evaluation Report
Normal patterns (developmentally appropriate):
Delayed patterns (primary developmentally
inappropriate):
Atypical patterns (secondary developmentally
inappropriate):
Implications for function:
Treatment Program

2.h. Release of the Dowel or Cube
Evaluation Report
Normal patterns (developmentally appropriate):
Delayed patterns (primary developmentally
inappropriate):
Atypical patterns (secondary developmentally
inappropriate):
Implications for function:
Treatment Program

2.i. Release of the Pellet
Evaluation Report
Normal patterns (developmentally appropriate):
Delayed patterns (primary developmentally
inappropriate):
Atypical patterns (secondary developmentally
inappropriate):
Implications for function:
Treatment Program

Section 3. Prewriting Skills

3.a. Crayon or Pencil Grasp
Evaluation Report
Normal patterns (developmentally appropriate):
Delayed patterns (primary developmentally
inappropriate):
Atypical patterns (secondary developmentally
inappropriate):
Implications for function:
Treatment Program

3.b. Drawings
Evaluation Report
Normal patterns (developmentally appropriate):
Delayed patterns (primary developmentally
inappropriate):
Atypical patterns (secondary developmentally
inappropriate):
Implications for function:
Treatment Program

Summary and Conclusions

Recommendations

Signature:

The case study evaluations and reports are presented in the following chapters in a format that links the EDPA protocol sheets, evaluation reports, treatment programs, and ISP, ITP, or IEP (figure 8.1). Photographs are added for clarification. The final chapter will illustrate how progress notes are used to modify treatment through creative problem solving with family members.

References

Baumgart, D. 1990. *Career education, a curriculum manual for students with handicaps.* Frederick, MD: Aspen Publications.

Coley, I. L. 1978. *Pediatric assessment of self-care activities.* St. Louis, MO: C. V. Mosby.

Ellek, D. 1991. Health policy: The Americans with Disabilities Act of 1990. *American Journal of Occupational Therapy* 45(2):177-79.

Flick, K., J. Shephard, and C. Brollier. 1992. Key to successful transition planning: Special education. *Advance for Occupational Therapists* 5, August 10.

Gilfoyle, E. M. (ed.) 1979. *Training occupational therapy educational management in schools.* Rockville, MD: American Occupational Therapy Association.

Goodwyn, R. L. 1987. Transition and supported employment initiatives in the 1980s and beyond. *Developmental Disabilities SIS Newsletter* 10(4):3.

Herrick, J. T., and H. E. Lowe. 1992. The target—Community job placement. *Occupational Therapy Forum* 10, October 28.

Kalscheur, J. A. 1992. Benefits of the Americans with Disabilities Act of 1990 for children and adolescents with disabilities. *American Journal of Occupational Therapy* 46(5):419-26.

Neistadt, M. E. 1987. An occupational therapy program for adults with developmental disabilities. *American Journal of Occupational Therapy* 41(7):433-38.

Rang, M., and J. Wright. 1989. What have 30 years of medical progress done for cerebral palsy? *Clinical Orthopedics and Related Research* 247:55-60.

Sattler, J. M. 1974. *Assessment of children's intelligence.* Philadelphia: W. B. Saunders.

Spencer, K. C. 1987. Transition and supported employment initiatives in the 1980s and beyond. *Developmental Disabilities SIS Newsletter* 10(4):1, 6.

Williams, K. 1992. Lending a helping hand to ADA. *Advance for Occupational Therapists* 11, April 13.

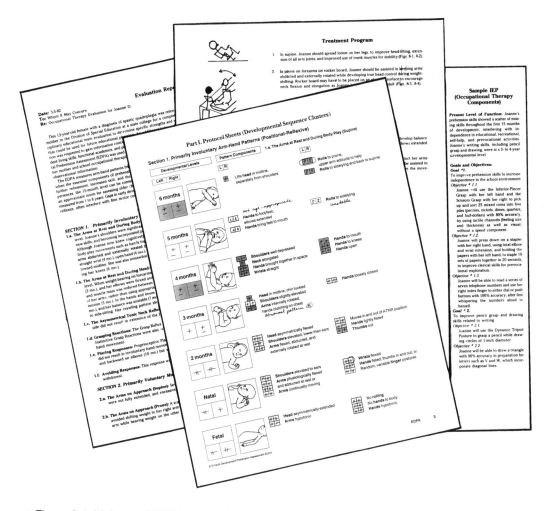

Figure 8.1. Linkage of EDPA protocol sheets, evaluation reports, treatment programs, and ISP, ITP, or IEP

Chapter Nine
Joanne
Evaluation and Treatment
Transition from Childhood to Adulthood

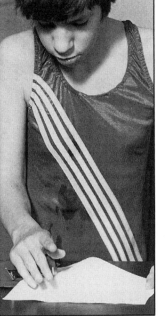

Date: 3-5-82

To: Whom it may concern

Re: Occupational therapy evaluation for Joanne D.

This 13-year-old female with a diagnosis of spastic quadriplegia was referred by her mother to the division of special education at a state college for a complete interdisciplinary educational team evaluation to determine specific strengths and weaknesses that could be used for future educational planning. An additional independent evaluation was requested to gain information concerning hand function as it relates to independent living skills, functional academics, and prevocational skills. The Erhardt Developmental Prehension Assessment (EDPA) was used to evaluate Joanne today in her home, with her mother and school occupational therapist present, contributing historical as well as observational information.

The EDPA measures arm-hand patterns from the fetal and natal periods to 15 months, when the essential components of prehension are developed and functional. Because further refinement, increased skill, and the use of tools are the result of learned experiences, the 15-month level can be considered the maturity of prehension and thus an approximate norm for assessing older children. Pencil grasp and drawings are also measured from 1 to 6 years. Gaps in early developmental sequences, especially in primitive reflexes, often interfere with fine motor coordination later in life.

After receiving the report by the college diagnostic team, Joanne's mother requested an IEP staffing to review placement and discuss related services. Recommendations from the college were that Joanne be served by an instructor for the multiply impaired/physically handicapped. According to the guidelines published by the public schools, Trainable Mentally Handicapped (TMH) placement was no longer appropriate for Joanne.

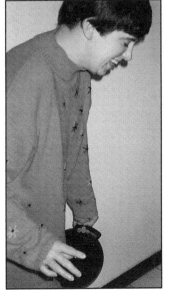

Date: 12-10-92

To: Whom it may concern

Re: Occupational therapy evaluation for Joanne D.

This 24-year-old female with a diagnosis of spastic quadriplegia was re-evaluated today in her home with the Erhardt Developmental Prehension Assessment (EDPA) to determine hand function relating to:

- home/domestic chores and personal care: meal preparation (opening packages, setting and clearing the table), cleaning (dusting, vacuuming), bed making, laundry, dressing, bathing, grooming, and eating
- recreation/leisure activities: video games, playing cards, rock 'n roll music, necklace making, telephone conversations, and community participation
- community participation: shopping, bowling, movies, restaurants, swimming, horseback riding, camping
- vocational opportunities: janitorial tasks (washing tables and windows), rolling silverware, gardening, laundry, clerical skills, stocking shelves, packaging products, and sorting large items

Joanne resides with two other women with developmental disabilities in an adult foster care home. She attends a day program which includes supportive employment in a pizza restaurant at this time.

Joanne was evaluated for head, arm, and hand function in various positions: supine (on her back), prone (on her stomach), and sitting. Her adult foster care supervisor and her job coach contributed historical and observational information.

Section 1. Primarily Involuntary Arm-Hand Patterns (Positional-Reflexive)

Evaluation Report

1.a. The Arms at Rest and during Body Play (Supine)

Joanne at 13

Joanne's shoulders were significantly elevated, a frequent early adaptation of children to the stress of attempting new skills, and becoming incorporated permanently into the new patterns. Head lifting was still accompanied by elevated shoulders. Although Joanne now knew cognitively how to bring hands to knees, according to her mother she had missed important early body play movements such as hands together on chest, hands to knees, and hands to feet and was always more comfortable with arms abducted and externally rotated (see figure 1, page 1). Her right arm lacked the mature patterns of elbow extension, straight wrist, open hand, and thumb outside the palm as she tried to internally rotate her arm when reaching toward midline. She was also somewhat unstable as she rolled from supine to sidelying and back to supine, especially when grasping her knees.

Joanne at 24

Normal patterns (developmentally appropriate): In supine Joanne was able to lift her head in midline, separately from shoulders, with a good chin tuck. She brought open hands together in space and to knees.

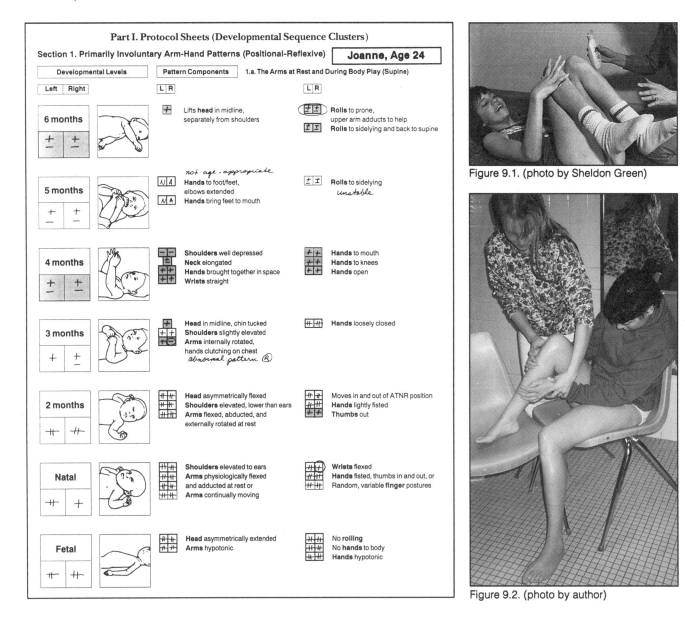

Figure 9.1. (photo by Sheldon Green)

Figure 9.2. (photo by author)

Delayed patterns (primary developmentally inappropriate): Joanne's shoulders were elevated at rest, increasing upon head lifting, and her neck was not fully elongated. Rolling was done with increased effort and was not a smooth transition.

Atypical patterns (secondary developmentally inappropriate): Hands together on the chest produced an atypical pattern in the right hand, with arm adducted instead of abducted, resulting in a flexed wrist.

Implications for function: Elevated shoulders interfere with fine grading of neck muscles for head control and with full range of arm movement. Without the variability of arm and hand positions learned in the supine position, Joanne often demonstrates atypical hand positions which interfere with dexterity for functional tasks. Trunk muscles developed during early rolling patterns prepare for necessary trunk control in sitting, standing, and walking. Muscles in Joanne's entire body, however, lack the ability to grade movement (midrange control), one of the reasons she moves quickly and bumps into people and objects. Inadequate automatic balance reactions are also a contributing factor to postural control problems. Some of these missing patterns may be remediated in sitting and standing, positions more age-appropriate than supine.

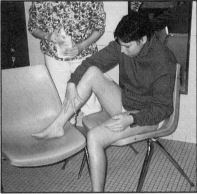

Figure 9.3. (photo by author)

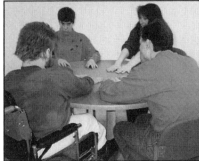

Figure 9.4. (photo by author)

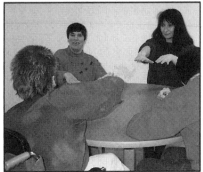

Figure 9.5. (photo by author)

Treatment Program

Joanne at 13

- In supine, Joanne should spread lotion on her legs to improve head lifting, extension of all arm joints, and improved use of trunk muscles for stability (figure 9.1).

Joanne at 24

- Rubbing lotion on all parts of her body after each bath and after swimming will improve Joanne's hand patterns as well as her dry skin. With assistance at first from her adult foster care supervisor, emphasis should be on using both hands, with slow, firm movements, wrist extension, and total contact of palm, fingers, and thumb on skin surface (figures 9.2, 9.3).

- T'ai Chi Chih, a series of slow, graceful, controlled movements involving full arm movements and the whole body, can be adapted as a group exercise at Joanne's day program, done in sitting and/or standing to slow, rhythmical music. To learn proper alignment of arms and hands for certain movements, table surfaces can be used as guides at first; then the same movements can be done in space (figures 9.4, 9.5).

- Graded structured activities can include:

  - rolling to improve trunk stability, needed for arm/hand mobility

  - rocker board to improve automatic balance reactions in sitting and standing, with support gradually decreased

  - wide walking board to improve balance in walking

  - ball skills such as bowling to improve eye-hand coordination

Evaluation Report

1.b. The Arms at Rest and during Head Raising (Prone)

Joanne at 13

When weight bearing on forearms, Joanne's shoulders were elevated, her arms were internally rotated and adducted, and her elbows were flexed and behind her shoulders. She did not have good head control with neck elongation. She rested her head back on her neck and supported herself on the bones of her arms rather than using appropriate shoulder girdle muscles. Rolling to the right was still accomplished with head hyperextension. In the hands-and-knees position, her elbows were only partly extended, head control was imperfect, and her balance was unstable. She pushed back to sitting from hands and knees to the W position rather than rotating to side-sitting. Her crawling pattern showed remnants of the Symmetrical Tonic Neck Reflex (STNR).

Joanne at 24

Normal patterns (developmentally appropriate): Joanne showed good balance and controlled rocking movements in the hands-and-knees position, with weight bearing on the open left hand, both wrists extended.

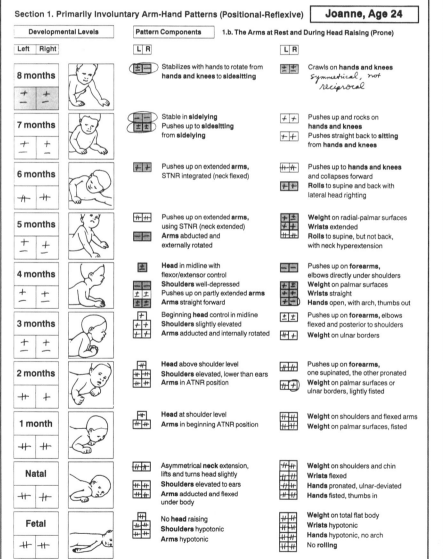

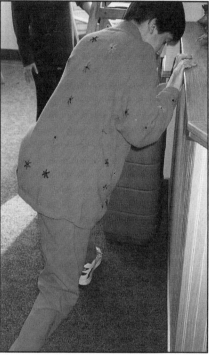

Figure 9.6. (photo by author)

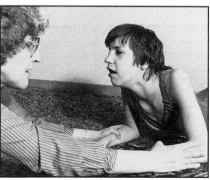

Figure 9.7. (photo by Sheldon Green)

Developmental Hand Dysfunction

Delayed patterns (primary developmentally inappropriate): Weight bearing was on the palmar surface of the lightly fisted right hand. When prone on forearms, Joanne demonstrated elevated shoulders and cervical, not capital, flexion, preventing fine grading of flexor/extensor head movement. Forearms were adducted and internally rotated instead of straight forward, and elbows were posterior to shoulders. The sidelying position (both left and right sides) was unstable. Transitions from sidelying to side-sitting and between side-sitting and hands and knees was very difficult toward the left, impossible toward the right. Crawling on hands and knees was done symmetrically, not reciprocally.

Atypical patterns (secondary developmentally inappropriate): Ankles were dorsiflexed in the hands-and-knees position, providing less stability than the normal plantar-flexed position.

Implications for function: Weight bearing on the upper extremities prepares for arm/hand strength and coordination, in addition to the use of the hands to stabilize during transitions. Because some of the janitorial tasks at her place of employment are done in kneeling positions, Joanne needs to have as much stability as possible as well as safe, efficient transitions from one position to another. She also has difficulty rising from the floor after falling (figure 9.6).

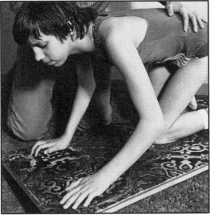

Figure 9.8. (photo by Sheldon Green)

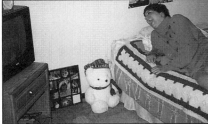

Figure 9.9. (photo by author)

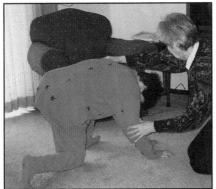

Figure 9.10. (photo by author)

Treatment Program

Joanne at 13

- In prone on forearms on rocker board, Joanne should be assisted in keeping arms abducted and externally rotated while developing true head control during weight shifting. Rocker board may have to be placed on an elevated surface to encourage neck flexion (capital flexion) and elongation (cervical extension) as Joanne looks downward at adult (figure 9.7).

- In the hands-and-knees position on rocker board, Joanne should develop balance shifting weight forward and backward as well as sideward, with elbows extended (figure 9.8).

Joanne at 24

- The sidelying position (both right and left), which develops important neck and trunk muscles, can provide variety when resting, sleeping, and watching television (figure 9.9).

- Postural control and transitions can be improved by working with a therapist who uses the NDT (Neuro-Developmental Treatment) approach (figure 9.10).

Evaluation Report

1.c. Asymmetrical Tonic Neck Reflex (ATNR)

Joanne at 13
This reflex was normally integrated: rotation of the head toward the side did not result in extension of the face limb and flexion of the skull limb.

Joanne at 24
Normal patterns (developmentally appropriate):
This reflex was fully integrated.

Implications for function: Joanne's voluntary movements are not contaminated by this reflex, which, when active, results in obligatory linked head/arm movements.

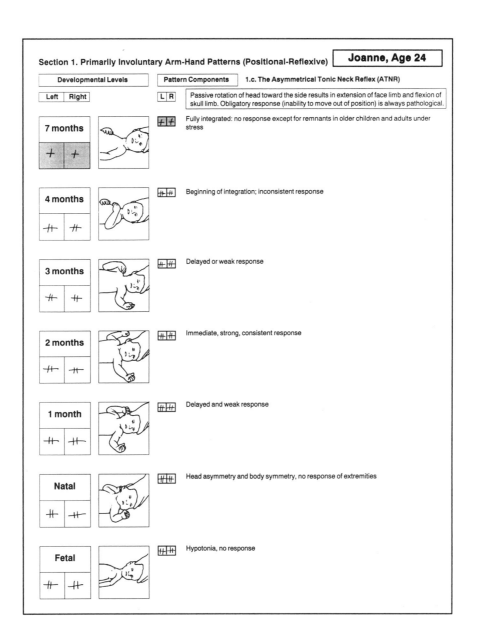

Evaluation Report

1.d. Grasping Reactions

Joanne at 13

The Grasp Reflex was normally integrated: stimulus in the palm did not result in involuntary grasp. Instinctive Grasp Reactions were also normally integrated: stimulus withdrawn from palm did not result in involuntary hand movement.

Joanne at 24

Normal patterns (developmentally appropriate): The Grasp Reflex was fully integrated. The Instinctive Grasp Reaction was integrated in the left hand.

Delayed patterns (primary developmentally inappropriate): The Instinctive Grasp Reaction was present in the right hand as Joanne responded to light touch on various parts of her hand when her vision was occluded by involuntarily orienting (turning hand over), groping (moving toward the stimulus), and sometimes trapping (grasping the stimulus).

Implications for function: Joanne's voluntary movements are not contaminated by the Grasp Reflex, which interferes with precise release when active. The Instinctive Grasp Reaction, which can interfere with the timing of voluntary release and precise manipulation if not integrated, is activated by light touch on various parts of the hand. Its reappearance in the right hand after integration at an earlier age may be due to sensory deficits and decreased hand use.

Section 1. Primarily Involuntary Arm-Hand Patterns (Positional-Reflexive)   **Joanne, Age 24**

1.d. Grasping Reactions
Note: Test in supine or with vision occluded to prevent contamination by voluntary movements.

Developmental Levels   Pattern Components

Left | Right   L | R
Instinctive Grasp Reaction: Light distally moving stimulus
Grasp Reflex: Firmly inserted stimulus

10 months
Instinctive Grasp Reaction: Integrated, stimulus withdrawn from **radial** side of palm results in voluntary, not involuntary movement

9 months
Grasp Reflex: Integrated, stimulus in **radial** side of palm results in voluntary, not involuntary grasp

8 months
Instinctive Grasp Reaction, trapping stage: Stimulus withdrawn from **radial** side of palm results in involuntary orienting, groping, and finally grasping

7 months
Instinctive Grasp Reaction, groping stage: Stimulus on **ulnar** border of hand results in involuntary pronation and movement toward stimulus

6 months
Instinctive Grasp Reaction, groping stage: Stimulus on **radial** border of hand results in involuntary supination and movement toward stimulus
Grasp Reflex: Beginning integration, weakening involuntary response to stimulus in **radial** side of palm

5 months
Instinctive Grasp Reaction, orienting stage: stimulus on **ulnar** border of hand results in involuntary pronation

Instinctive Grasp Reaction, orienting stage: Stimulus on **radial** border of hand results in involuntary supination

4 months

3 months
Grasp Reflex: Fully developed, stimulus in **radial** side of palm results in the **Catching phase:** Sudden finger flexion followed by the **Holding phase:** Sustained flexion when resisted

2 months
Grasp Reflex: Stimulus in **radial** side of palm results in thumb and all fingers flexion and adduction, followed by synergistic flexion of entire extremity

1 month
Grasp Reflex: Stimulus in **radial** side of palm results in thumb and index finger flexion and adduction, followed by synergistic flexion of entire extremity

Natal
Grasp Reflex: Stimulus in **ulnar** side of palm combined with traction results in involuntary grasp of middle, ring, little, and index fingers, and thumb in sequence, and synergistic flexion of entire extremity (lifting body weight)

Fetal
Grasp Reflex: Stimulus in **ulnar** side of palm results in slight or no involuntary grasp
Instinctive Grasp Reaction: No response to stimulus

Treatment Program

Joanne at 24

- Since improvement in voluntary skills helps decrease involuntary movements, treatment will be addressed in Section 2.

Evaluation Report

1.e. Placing Responses

Joanne at 13

Proprioceptive Placing was normally integrated: brushing the back of the hand against the table edge did not result in involuntary hand movement. Protective Extensor Thrust, stimulated from the sitting position, was normally present forward, sideward, and backward on elbows but was not well developed backward with arms extended, especially on the right.

Joanne at 24

Normal patterns (developmentally appropriate): Proprioceptive Placing (brushing back of hand against table edge with vision occluded) was integrated (no involuntary placing of hand on surface). Protective Extensor Thrust forward in standing was strong, consistent, and immediate.

Delayed patterns (primary developmentally inappropriate): Protective Extensor Thrust, stimulated from standing, was delayed sideward and backward, more so on the right side.

Implications for function: Proprioceptive Placing also prepares the wrist and hand for graceful voluntary movements but needs to be integrated or it will interfere with voluntary manipulation. Protective responses, which emerge developmentally at the same time as independent sitting and weight bearing on extended arms, protect the head during falls and reinforce the reaching pattern. As standing and walking become perfected, the responses become activated in those positions as well.

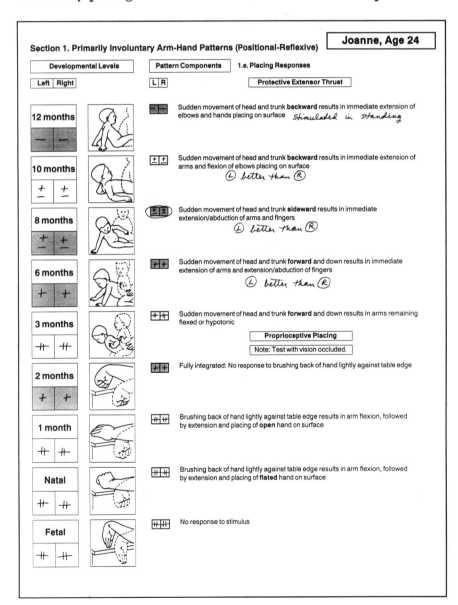

Treatment Program

Joanne at 24

- Because Joanne falls frequently, protective extension of the arms (to protect her head) can be facilitated by day program staff trained by Joanne's therapist. This can be done first against walls and furniture in standing, her primary functional position, right side twice as often as left (figure 9.11).

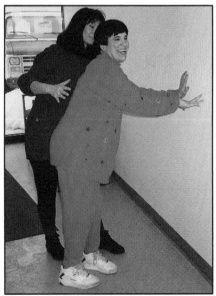

Figure 9.11. (photo by author)

Developmental Hand Dysfunction

Evaluation Report

1.f. Avoiding Responses

Joanne at 13
This response was normally integrated: stimulus to any part of the hand did not result in reflexive withdrawal.

Joanne at 24
Delayed patterns (primary developmentally inappropriate): With vision occluded, Joanne's left hand showed a slight involuntary response (spreading of fingers) to a distally moving light stimulus on the back of her hand or on the palmar surface of her fingertips. Her right hand showed an even stronger response.

Implications for function: This automatic response helps reduce the Grasp Reflex and open the hand during normal development. It decreases as voluntary control increases. If not eventually integrated, however, it interferes with sustained voluntary grasp and precise manipulation. Its reappearance after integration at an earlier age may be due to sensory deficits and decreased hand use.

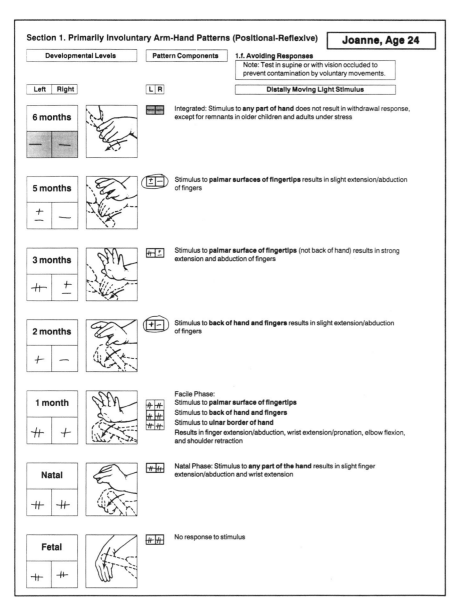

Section 1. Primarily Involuntary Arm-Hand Patterns (Positional-Reflexive) — **Joanne, Age 24**

Developmental Levels | Pattern Components | 1.f. Avoiding Responses
Note: Test in supine or with vision occluded to prevent contamination by voluntary movements.

Left | Right — L | R — **Distally Moving Light Stimulus**

6 months — Integrated: Stimulus to **any part of hand** does not result in withdrawal response, except for remnants in older children and adults under stress

5 months — Stimulus to **palmar surfaces of fingertips** results in slight extension/abduction of fingers

3 months — Stimulus to **palmar surface of fingertips** (not back of hand) results in strong extension and abduction of fingers

2 months — Stimulus to **back of hand and fingers** results in slight extension/abduction of fingers

1 month — Facile Phase:
Stimulus to **palmar surface of fingertips**
Stimulus to **back of hand and fingers**
Stimulus to **ulnar border of hand**
Results in finger extension/abduction, wrist extension/pronation, elbow flexion, and shoulder retraction

Natal — Natal Phase: Stimulus to **any part of the hand** results in slight finger extension/abduction and wrist extension

Fetal — No response to stimulus

Treatment Program

Joanne at 24
- The use of firm pressure with brush or washcloth to briskly rub all parts of the nails and hands on a daily basis will help reduce avoiding responses (especially in the right hand), stimulate healthy tissue, and activate sensory receptors. As Joanne gains more voluntary control of her hands, she can become more independent in grooming skills such as using an oversized emery board for nail care (figures 9.12, 9.13).

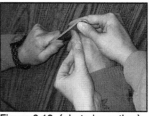

Figure 9.12. (photo by author)

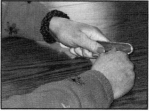

Figure 9.13. (photo by author)

Section 2. Primarily Voluntary Movements (Cognitively Directed)

Evaluation Report

2.a. The Arms on Approach (Supine)

Joanne at 13
Joanne used a direct unilateral approach with her left hand and a circular approach with her right. Her hands were open, and she was able to grasp with one hand, other joining. Her right elbow and wrist were not fully extended, and excessive extension was seen in the MCP (knuckle) joints.

Joanne at 24
Normal patterns (developmentally appropriate): Unilateral approach was direct and accurate, with both elbows fully extended and both hands open. Bilateral reach was symmetrical.

Delayed patterns (primary developmentally inappropriate): The left wrist was straight during approach, and the right was flexed. Fingers in both hands showed excessive extension.

Implications for function: Wrist extension and appropriate finger extension are necessary to prepare for accurate and stable grasp of differently sized objects.

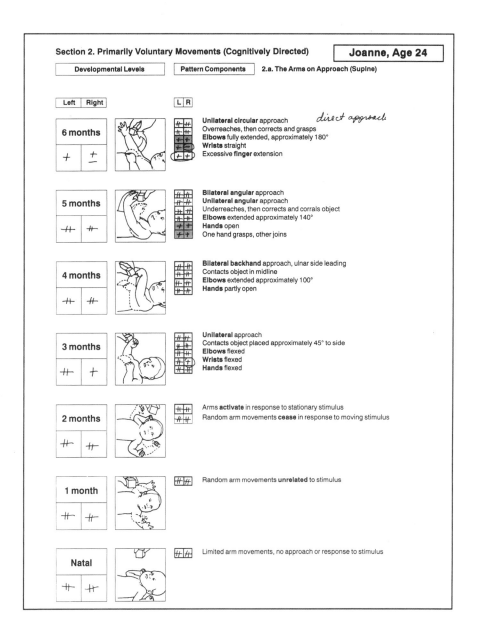

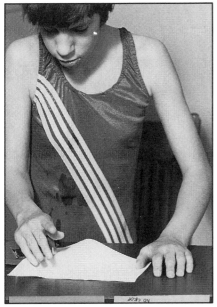

Figure 9.14. (photo by Sheldon Green)

Treatment Program

Joanne at 13

- Elbow and wrist extension in the right arm can be improved by pressing down on a stapler while standing (figure 9.14).

Joanne at 24

- To increase active wrist extension, Joanne should reach for objects above her head on grocery shelves and in her kitchen (figure 9.15).

- Learning to shape her hands around a variety of objects such as fruit and vegetables as she shops for food will improve Joanne's ability to use appropriate finger extension (figure 9.16). Activities which require identification of objects by touch, without vision, will increase sensitivity for this shaping, or accommodation (see 2.g.).

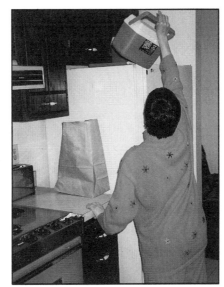

Figure 9.15. (photo by author)

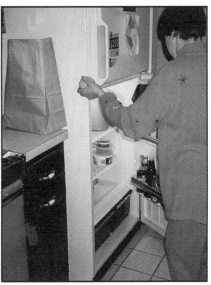

Figure 9.16. (photo by author)

Evaluation Report

2.b. The Arms on Approach (Prone)

Joanne at 13

In prone, Joanne avoided shifting weight to her right arm and chest when reaching with her left arm. She was not able to reach with one arm while bearing weight on the other forearm or extended arm, and her right hand was not open.

Joanne at 24

Normal patterns (developmentally appropriate): Reaching from hands and knees was fairly accurate, with left hand open and flat when weight bearing.

Delayed patterns (primary developmentally inappropriate): The weight-bearing right hand was lightly fisted in the hands-and-knees position. Lateral weight shifts were not as smooth when reaching from prone on forearms.

Implications for function: Head and arm function in prone positions are components of cleaning tasks at work and at home. Joanne does not always choose efficient movement patterns during these tasks.

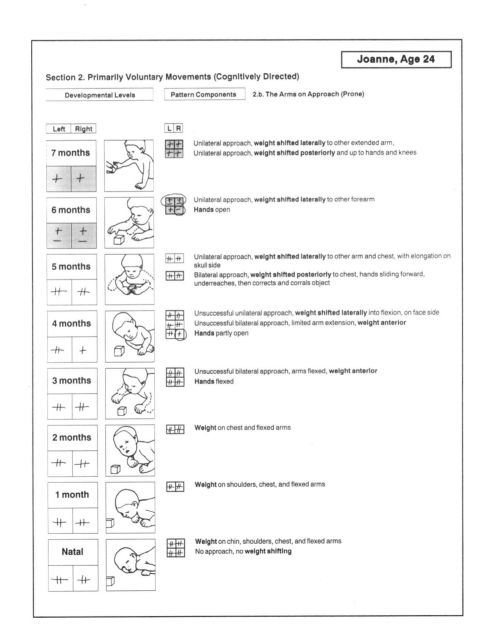

Developmental Hand Dysfunction

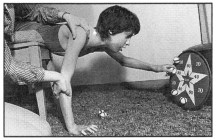

Figure 9.17. (photo by Sheldon Green)

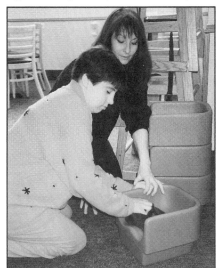

Figure 9.18. (photo by author)

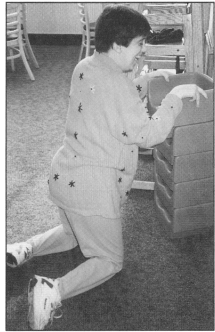

Figure 9.19. (photo by author)

Treatment Program

Joanne at 13

- Prone over a padded bench, Joanne should be assisted in bearing weight on her extended right arm while reaching with her left. Fingers of the right hand should be extended (figure 9.17).

Joanne at 24

- Joanne needs assistance in motor planning for proximal stability during distal mobility. Her job coach can help with adjustments in posture to encourage appropriate bilateral hand use (for example, during reaching to wash and stack booster chairs, figures 9.18, 9.19).

- Swimming with a life jacket which allows free arm movements in both prone and supine will improve strength, coordination, and symmetry as Joanne is required to make independent weight shifts and balance adjustments without a supporting surface or assistance from her adult foster care supervisor (figures 9.20, 9.21).

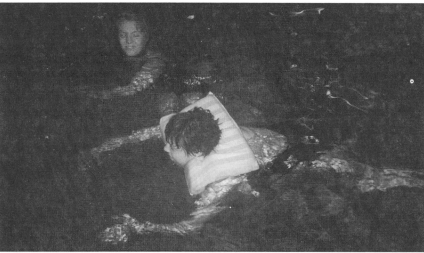

Figure 9.20. (photo by author)

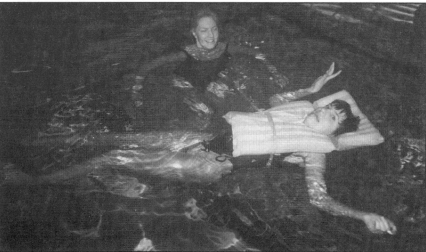

Figure 9.21. (photo by author)

Evaluation Report

2.c. The Arms on Approach (Sitting)

Joanne at 13

Joanne used a unilateral direct approach with her left hand, elbow and wrist straight, hand open, with appropriate finger extension. Voluntary supination was used to facilitate grasp. Joanne's right hand used a unilateral circular approach, with elbow not fully extended and wrist not extended. Voluntary supination (palm up) was limited.

Joanne at 24

Normal patterns (developmentally appropriate): Unilateral and bilateral approaches were fairly accurate, with elbows fully extended and appropriate finger extension in the left hand.

Delayed patterns (primary developmentally inappropriate): The left forearm had slight limitation of supination, and the left wrist was straight, not extended. Right-hand fingers showed excessive extension, especially at the MCP joints.

Atypical patterns (secondary developmentally inappropriate): Because she was unable to supinate her right forearm more than midposition, Joanne substituted trunk movement. The right wrist was flexed and forearm was pronated (palm down).

Implications for function: Atypical stereotypic patterns are used to compensate for lack of certain components of normal sequences. Additionally, Joanne's rapid, impulsive movements indicate lack of mid-range control and motor planning. Thus, precise reaching without knocking objects over is difficult.

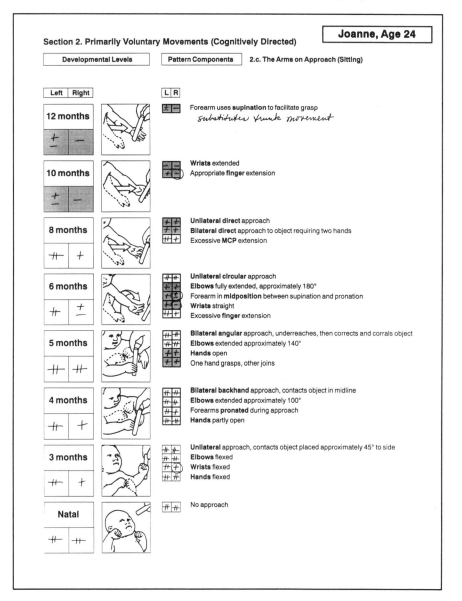

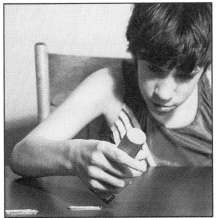

Figure 9.22. (photo by Sheldon Green)

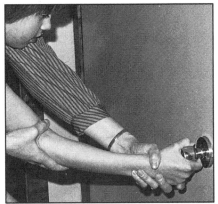

Figure 9.23. (photo by Sheldon Green)

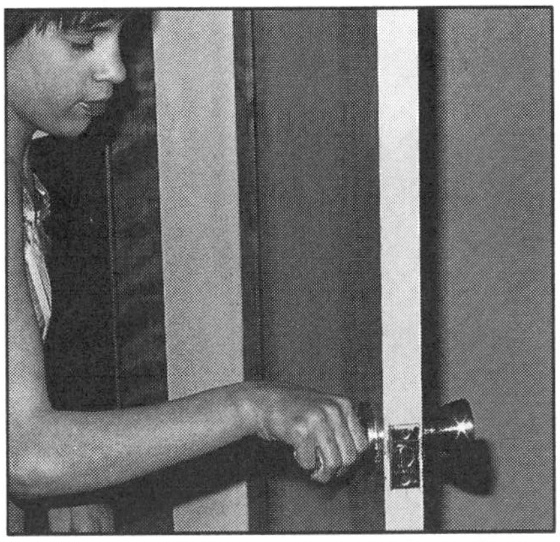

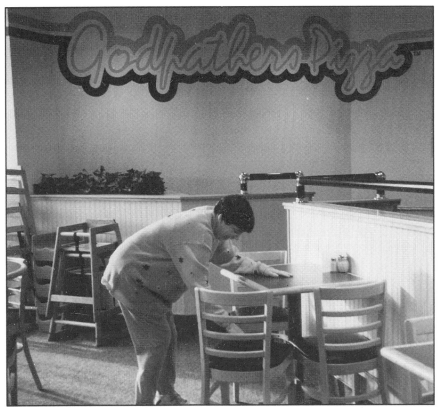

Figure 9.24. (photo by Sheldon Green)

Treatment Program

Joanne at 13

- Sitting at a desk, Joanne should grasp a magnetized dowel with her right hand to reach directly toward a series of paper clips placed at a distance—this requires complete elbow extension (figure 9.22).

- Joanne should be assisted in supinating her right forearm while turning a doorknob, then achieve the task independently (figures 9.23, 9.24).

Joanne at 24

- Arm movements on sticky or other resistive surfaces (such as sanding wood projects) will help Joanne slow down and be more aware of her position in space.

- While cleaning tables and chairs at work, Joanne's other hand should be stabilized flat on the surface for support and good alignment of wrist and finger joints (figure 9.25).

Figure 9.25. (photo by author)

Evaluation Report

2.d. Grasp of the Dowel and 2.e. Grasp of the Cube

Joanne at 13
Joanne used radial-palmar and radial-digital grasps in both hands, with wrist straight in right hand, extended in left.

Joanne at 24
Normal patterns (developmentally appropriate): Joanne had mature three-jawed chuck and radial-digital grasps (delicate grips) in both hands.

Delayed patterns (primary developmentally inappropriate): Radial-palmar grasps (power grip) were somewhat unstable because all surfaces of her palm and fingers were not in contact with the objects. Her left wrist was straight, not extended, and her right wrist was usually flexed during grasp.

Atypical patterns (secondary developmentally inappropriate): The right hand PIP joint was stiffly extended instead of slightly flexed, indicating inadequate midrange control.

Implications for function: Heavy or large objects require maximum hand surface to be in contact for efficient power grasp. Lighter, smaller objects require more mature, precise grasps, except during power tasks (knife and fork).

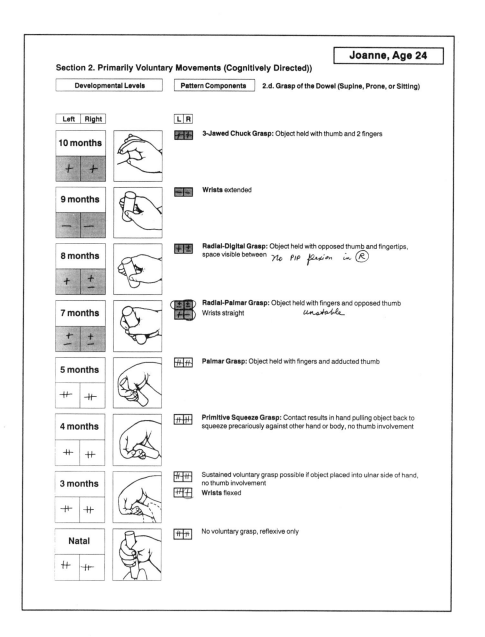

Developmental Hand Dysfunction

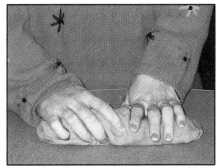

Figure 9.26. (photo by author)

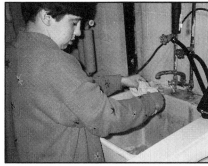

Figure 9.27. (photo by author)

Treatment Program

Joanne at 24

- Occupational therapy using graded structured exercises with clay can be individualized for Joanne to improve strength and control of her hand and finger joints. Kneading bread dough could be a functional application (figure 9.26).

- Power grasps can be improved during certain domestic tasks such as making the bed and wringing wet cloths, with positioning to facilitate supination (figure 9.27).

- Although Joanne prefers to use the same utensils as her peers, adapted handles would provide more efficient grips for tasks such as cutting food with a knife or brushing teeth. Many of these adaptations are simple variations used by people with normal abilities. They include sport water bottles with straws, large-handled kitchen utensils, and battery-operated toothbrushes (see 2.g.).

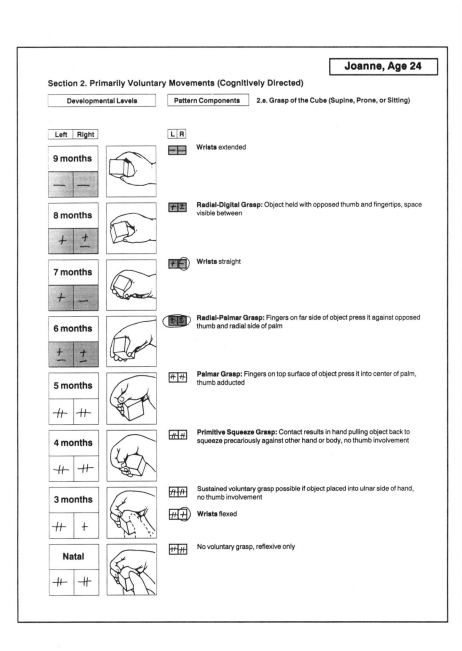

Joanne, Age 24

Section 2. Primarily Voluntary Movements (Cognitively Directed)

Developmental Levels | Pattern Components | 2.e. Grasp of the Cube (Supine, Prone, or Sitting)

Left | Right | L | R

9 months — Wrists extended

8 months — **Radial-Digital Grasp:** Object held with opposed thumb and fingertips, space visible between

7 months — **Wrists** straight

6 months — **Radial-Palmar Grasp:** Fingers on far side of object press it against opposed thumb and radial side of palm

5 months — **Palmar Grasp:** Fingers on top surface of object press it into center of palm, thumb adducted

4 months — **Primitive Squeeze Grasp:** Contact results in hand pulling object back to squeeze precariously against other hand or body, no thumb involvement

3 months — Sustained voluntary grasp possible if object placed into ulnar side of hand, no thumb involvement

Wrists flexed

Natal — No voluntary grasp, reflexive only

Evaluation Report

2.f. Grasp of the Pellet (Prone or Sitting)

Joanne at 13

The scissors grasp was well established in the left hand but still emerging in the right hand. No inferior-pincer, pincer, or fine pincer grasps were observed because of inadequate thumb opposition.

Joanne at 24

Normal patterns (developmentally appropriate): Joanne picked up a pellet using the inferior-pincer grasp (between ventral surfaces) with her left hand, and a scissors grasp (between thumb and side of curled index finger) with her right hand. She was unable to use a pincer grasp (between distal pads of thumb and index finger) or fine pincer grasp (between fingertips).

Implications for function: Although the scissors grasp is a developmentally earlier skill that remains throughout life for function (such as using a key), higher-level grasps such as the inferior-pincer and pincer are essential for a variety of independent activities. Dexterity is required for social activities such as playing cards with her niece and nephew (figure 9.28), health needs such as handling medications in pill form (figures 9.29, 9.30), and dressing components such as buttons, snaps, and zippers.

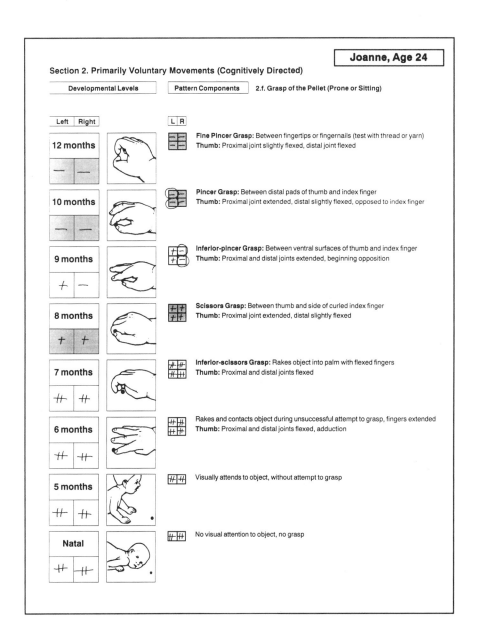

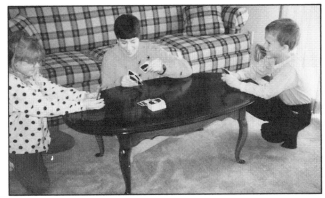

Figure 9.28. (photo by author)

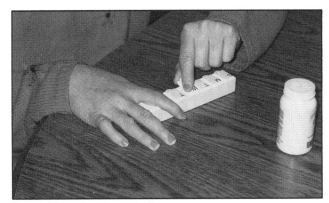

Figure 9.29. (photo by author)

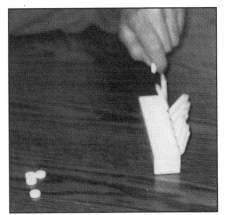

Figure 9.30. (photo by author)

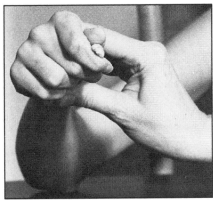

Figure 9.31. (photo by Sheldon Green)

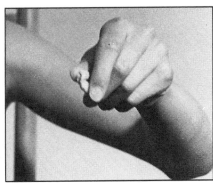

Figure 9.32. (photo by Sheldon Green)

Treatment Program

Joanne at 13

- Joanne should perfect the scissors grasp (pellet held between thumb and side of curled index finger) in the right hand with repeated practice (figure 9.31).

- The inferior-pincer grasp (pellet held between ventral surfaces of thumb and index finger) can begin with the left hand by presenting as large a pellet as needed, then gradually reducing size as skill improves (figure 9.32).

Joanne at 24

- Joanne's zippers can be adapted by inserting a large ring in the pull tab to help her be more independent.

- The pincer grasp can be facilitated in the left hand during therapy with structured activities such as pinching cotton balls from pegboard holes, or pinching clay while the entire arm rests on the surface for support. Pinching pie crust edging could be a functional application to achieve the pincer grasp in the left hand and to move from the scissors grasp to the inferior-pincer in the right (figures 9.33, 9.34).

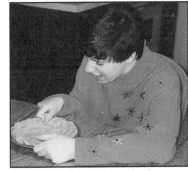

Figure 9.33. (photo by author)

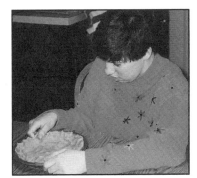

Figure 9.34. (photo by author)

Evaluation Report

2.g. Manipulation Skills (Prehension Schema)

Joanne at 13

Joanne was able to invert a container to reach contents, use both hands to combine objects, and build a tower of two block. When manipulating with one hand, she still demonstrated associated movements in the opposite hand. Reflexive-type movements of scratching and clutching were still present in the right hand, indicating that tactile recognition, repetition, and discrimination were not yet perfected. The right hand also did not accommodate well to new objects and positions. Coordination of hand, vision, and sucking schemata had not been fully developed, evidenced by Joanne's poor convergence, tracking, and alternating visual monitoring from one hand to the other. Reciprocal assimilation was limited as well, since she had lacked experience in watching the less functional right hand. Shaking movements were characterized by shoulder motion primarily in the right arm, and shoulder and elbow motion only in the left, with no wrist flexibility. Poking with index finger extended and others flexed was well established in the left hand but not in the right. Joanne still had difficulty holding an object with one hand while manipulating it with the other (right more than left).

Joanne at 24

Tactile Awareness

Normal patterns (developmentally appropriate): Joanne was able to discriminate among different textures and between objects and her own hand. Her left hand accommodated well to objects of different sizes and shapes.

Section 2. Primarily Voluntary Movements (Cognitively Directed)

Joanne, Age 24

Developmental Levels | Pattern Components | 2.g. Manipulation Skills (Prehension Schema)

Left | Right

15 months — Inverts container to reach contents / Intentional manipulation possible without hand and object within visual field | One hand manipulates object while other holds or assists

12 months — Both hands combine objects | **Tactile manipulation** (rotating, squeezing, transferring) replaces **oral exploration** (mouthing)

10 months — Isolates index finger to poke, others flexed / Tries unsuccessfully to reach into small container to remove object | One hand manipulates, other hand mirrors / **Shakes** object with arm, elbow, and wrist motion *wrist only on ⓛ*

9 months — Tries to poke, all fingers extended / Pokes with thumb | Increased **tactile manipulation**, **orally explores** new objects primarily

8 months — **Reciprocal Assimilation:** Watches hand and keeps it moving to make interesting sights last / Intentional manipulation possible when hand and object are within visual field | Drops object / Throws object / Pushes object / Pulls object

7 months — **Object Permanence:** Searches for lost or removed object, ignoring new stimulus / Drops object when grasping another | Retains object when grasping another / **Shakes** one or both objects, alternating visual monitoring back and forth

6 months — Beginning of **Object Permanence:** Searches for lost or removed object, but can be distracted by another | Alternately mouths, looks, shakes object, retaining grasp / **Shakes** object with arm and elbow motion

5 months — **Tactile Discrimination** between hand and object (bites object, not fingers) | Alternately mouths and shakes object / **Shakes** object with arm motion only

4 months — Mouths object or eats finger foods with insufficient **tactile discrimination** (may bite fingers by mistake) | Hand brings object to mouth, orally exploring both / Visually attends and swipes at object if within 1"

3 months — **Tactile Assimilation:** Hand movements extend to own face, body, clothing / **Tactile Accommodation:** Hands adapt to new objects, without visual attention | **Tactile Recognition** (eyes alert) leads to: Voluntary repetition of reflexive movements / Hand to mouth

1 month — **Reflexive Movements:** Scratching and clutching | Eyes watch moving hand

Natal — **Reflexive Grasp:** Involuntary, without tactile awareness (eyes do not alert) / No voluntary hand movements | Visually attends to object without reaching / No voluntary hand to mouth, head/mouth move to suck on hand

Atypical patterns (secondary developmentally inappropriate): Joanne's right hand did not accommodate completely to the shape of objects.

Implications for function: Joanne is able to eat finger foods without biting her fingers by mistake. She also identifies chairs she has cleaned at work by feeling the seats to see if they are wet or dry (figure 9.35). The abil-

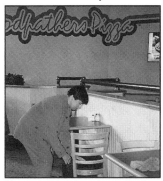

Figure 9.35. (photo by author)

ity to accommodate hands to the shape of objects is the precursor to complex manipulation skills. The tactile information derived from the total contact combines with the visual information to enhance motor planning and execution. Eventually, the tactile perception alone is necessary for certain tasks outside of the visual field (for example, fastening a bra in the back or a necklace at the back of the neck).

Prehension Schema
Normal patterns (developmentally appropriate): Joanne inverted a container to reach the contents with well-controlled graded movements with either hand. She was able to combine objects, with her left hand functioning better than the right. Her left hand was able to reach into a small container to remove an object. She could isolate both left and right index fingers as well as her thumbs to poke. Throwing was possible with the left arm.

Delayed patterns (primary developmentally inappropriate): Her right-hand fingers were unable to reach into a small container to remove an object. Throwing with the right arm was attempted but not successful.

Implications for function: Limited manipulative skills have interfered with Joanne's ability to open packages and remove food from wrappings. She needs dexterity to be more nearly equal in both hands as she folds laundry, makes her bed, and combines objects (such as putting a cap on a pen). Video games have helped maintain excellent thumb isolation in both hands. Using a calculator requires the ability to isolate each index finger. When bowling with her adapted ball (which has a retractable handle), Joanne needs full range of shoulder and elbow motion (figures 9.36, 9.37).

Hand/Mouth/Vision Schema
Normal patterns (developmentally appropriate): Hand-to-mouth patterns were observed during independent eating.

Delayed patterns (primary developmentally inappropriate): Joanne was aware that she needed to watch her hands with her eyes to achieve optimal function. Shaking objects was done with wrist movement primarily, with limited shoulder and elbow range, and without visual monitoring, left arm only.

Implications for function: Unless Joanne concentrated continuously, food sometimes dropped from the spoon or fell from her mouth to the table and floor. These problems are related to inadequate motor control of hands and arms and her inability to keep lips closed during chewing (total movement patterns, rather than dissociation of lips and jaw). Arm/elbow/wrist movements while shaking objects such as bottles of nail polish will loosen up the shoulder for larger arm movements needed for sports such as bowling and other recreational activities.

Unilaterality and Bilaterality (Hand Preference)
Normal patterns (developmentally appropriate): Joanne used both hands together spontaneously and appropriately but usually manipulated objects with her left hand while her right hand assisted or stabilized.

Delayed patterns (primary developmentally inappropriate): Her right hand rarely initiated manipulation and sometimes involuntarily dropped an object, especially when her left hand grasped another.

Implications for function: Although Joanne's left hand was fairly efficient using the spoon, she was unable to use both hands together to cut food with a knife and fork because of right hand limitations. Although pushing the grocery cart helps Joanne maintain balance, she needs steering guidance because of unequal strength in both hands. For this reason, she prefers to pull the garbage cart with one hand when moving it to the curb.

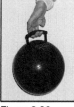

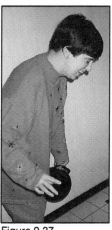

Figure 9.36. (photo by author)

Figure 9.37. (photo by author)

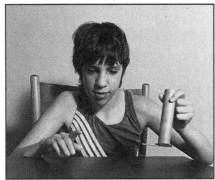

Figure 9.38. (photo by Sheldon Green)

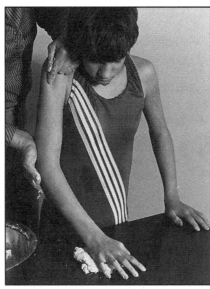

Figure 9.42. (photo by Sheldon Green)

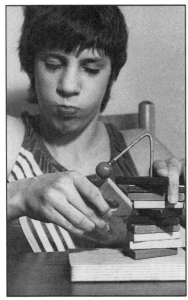

Figure 9.39. (photo by Sheldon Green)

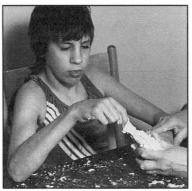

Figure 9.43. (photo by Sheldon Green)

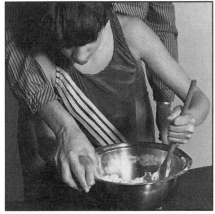

Figure 9.40. (photo by Sheldon Green)

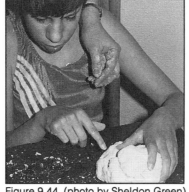

Figure 9.44. (photo by Sheldon Green)

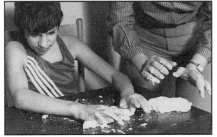

Figure 9.41. (photo by Sheldon Green)

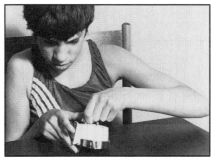

Figure 9.45. (photo by Sheldon Green)

Treatment Program

Joanne at 13

- Sitting at a desk, Joanne should grasp a magnetized dowel with each hand to reach and pick up a series of paper clips, alternating her visual gaze from her hand holding the dowel to each paper clip (figure 9.38).

- The threading toy can be used to improve coordination of hand and vision schemata, accommodation, elbow and wrist flexibility, and manipulation with one hand while holding with the other (figure 9.39).

- Bread dough can be used to improve manipulation with one hand while holding with the other (stirring ingredients together), experimental manipulation (rolling, pressing, pinching), and the poking index finger (figures 9.40 to 9.44).

- Winding a clock with one hand while holding with the other can improve manipulation as well as supination (figure 9.45).

Developmental Hand Dysfunction

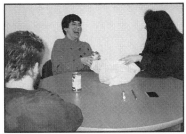

Figure 9.46. (photo by author)

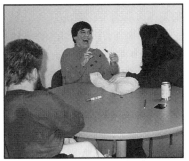

Figure 9.47. (photo by author)

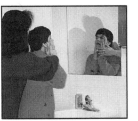

Figure 9.48. (photo by author)

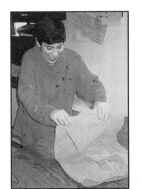

Figure 9.49. (photo by author)

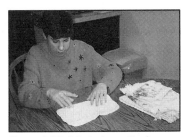

Figure 9.50. (photo by author)

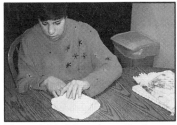

Figure 9.51. (photo by author)

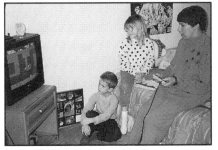

Figure 9.52. (photo by author)

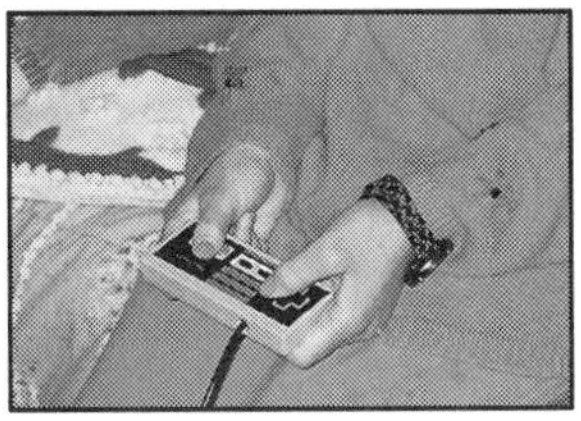

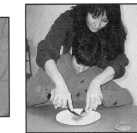

Figure 9.53. (photo by author)

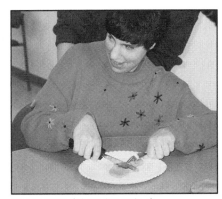

Figure 9.54. (photo by author)

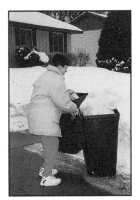

Figure 9.55. (photo by author)

Figure 9.56. (photo by author)

Treatment Program
Joanne at 24

- To improve tactile awareness and accommodation, Joanne can participate in group activities which require identifying or matching everyday articles such as beverage cans or marker pens with vision occluded (stereognosis) (figures 9.46, 9.47).
- Manipulation can be improved with graded activities (from large to small), such as folding laundry (figures 9.48 to 9.50).
- Joanne can be reminded and assisted by day program staff to rub lotion on her hands and face after every meal, emphasizing total contact of palms, fingers, and thumbs on skin surface (figure 9.51).
- Using the right hand as well as the left to wash table surfaces (push/pull motions) would improve finger alignment, equalize arm strength, and increase eye-hand coordination.
- Hand/mouth/vision interaction could be improved with further evaluation of oral-motor and visual-motor components.
- Video and computer games played with family members will continue to improve Joanne's ability to isolate finger and thumb function as well as eye-hand coordination (figures 9.52, 9.53).
- Shaking maracas or other instruments to music will increase freedom of shoulder and arm movement resulting in more range for sports such as bowling.
- Bilateral tasks such as cutting soft foods with a knife and fork may be possible with hand-over-hand assistance and adapted handles, which provide more stable power grasps (figures 9.54, 9.55).
- Joanne can be encouraged to use both hands to steer grocery and garbage carts as her eye-hand coordination improves (figure 9.56).

Evaluation Report

2.h. Release of the Dowel or Cube

Joanne at 13
All skills were present except for adept one-stage transfer and wrist extension in right hand. Joanne demonstrated a precise release into both large and small containers.

Joanne at 24
Normal patterns (developmentally appropriate): Joanne showed precise release with the left hand into both small and large containers, and with her right hand into large containers. Her left wrist was straight during release, especially the assistive release (against a surface). She showed an adept transfer from one hand to the other.

Delayed patterns (primary developmentally inappropriate): Precise release into small containers was more difficult with the right hand because the arm joints did not have the flexibility to orient the objects. The right wrist was flexed during release, especially against a surface (assistive release).

Implications for function: Joanne needs accurate release for many home and work tasks: placing food into the refrigerator (figure 9.16, page 115), putting paper trash into garbage when clearing after meals, sorting bottles and cans for recycling (figure 9.57), and releasing her time card into the slot (figure 9.58).

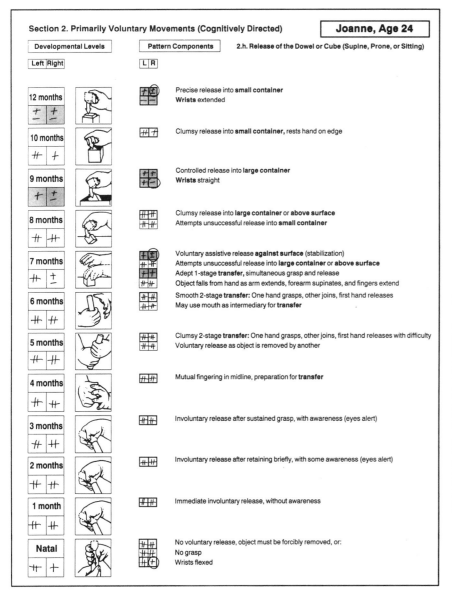

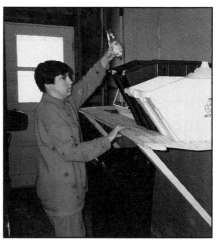

Figure 9.57. (photo by author)

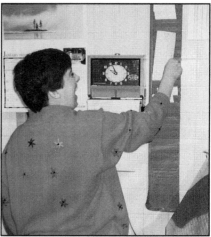

Figure 9.58. (photo by author)

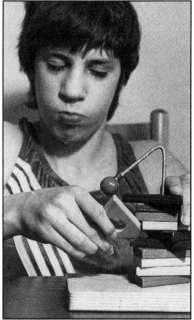

Figure 9.59. (photo by Sheldon Green)

Treatment Program

Joanne at 13

- Transfer of objects should be encouraged; for example, grasping shapes with one hand, transferring to the other, then placing them on the threading toy, which provides assistive release as well (figure 9.59).

Joanne at 24

- Wrist positioning can be improved (more extension and supination) during release activities if the trunk is stabilized against an appropriate surface and the opposite arm is either assisting or supporting.

- Releasing large objects with the right hand into a variety of gradually smaller containers will help Joanne improve her skill (figures 9.60, 9.61).

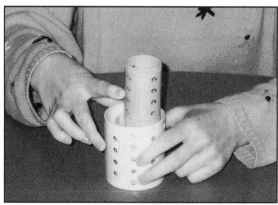

Figure 9.61. (photo by author)

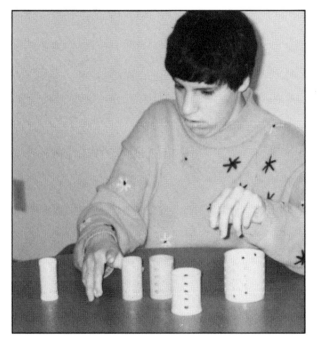

Figure 9.60. (photo by author)

Evaluation Report

2.l. Release of the Pellet

Joanne at 13

Joanne could not transfer a pellet from one hand to the other. Her right wrist was flexed rather than straight. She released the pellet clumsily from her right hand into a large container but not a small one. The left hand was able to release precisely into a small container with wrist straight rather than extended.

Joanne at 24

Normal patterns (developmentally appropriate): Precise release into a small container was done easily with the left hand. Release into a large container was done easily by both hands, with wrists straight.

Delayed patterns (primary developmentally inappropriate): Release into a small container was impossible for the right hand. Attempts to transfer the pellet from one hand to the other were unsuccessful.

Implications for function: Joanne needs precise fingertip release of pellet-sized objects such as pills for bilateral manipulative skills such as buttoning.

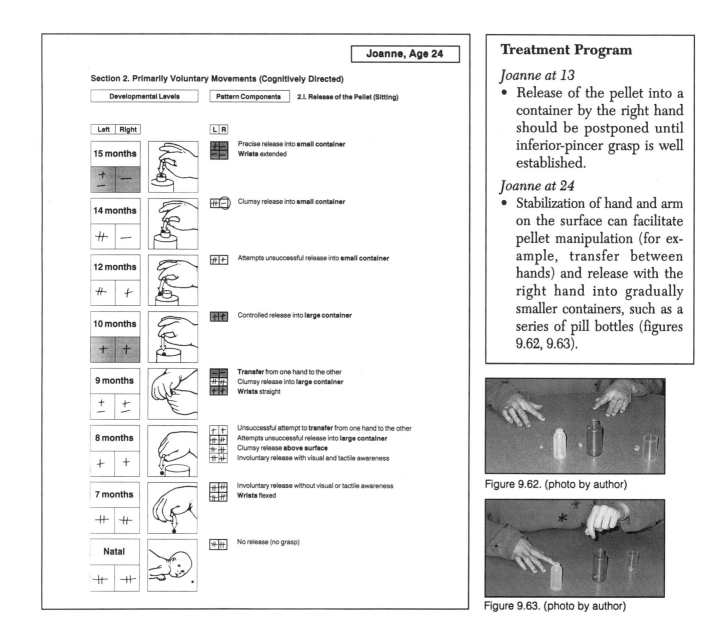

Joanne, Age 24

Section 2. Primarily Voluntary Movements (Cognitively Directed)

Developmental Levels | Pattern Components | 2.l. Release of the Pellet (Sitting)

15 months — Precise release into **small container** / **Wrists** extended

14 months — Clumsy release into **small container**

12 months — Attempts unsuccessful release into **small container**

10 months — Controlled release into **large container**

9 months — **Transfer** from one hand to the other / Clumsy release into **large container** / **Wrists** straight

8 months — Unsuccessful attempt to **transfer** from one hand to the other / Attempts unsuccessful release into **large container** / Clumsy release **above surface** / Involuntary release with visual and tactile awareness

7 months — Involuntary release without visual or tactile awareness / **Wrists** flexed

Natal — No release (no grasp)

Treatment Program

Joanne at 13

- Release of the pellet into a container by the right hand should be postponed until inferior-pincer grasp is well established.

Joanne at 24

- Stabilization of hand and arm on the surface can facilitate pellet manipulation (for example, transfer between hands) and release with the right hand into gradually smaller containers, such as a series of pill bottles (figures 9.62, 9.63).

Figure 9.62. (photo by author)

Figure 9.63. (photo by author)

Section 3. Prewriting Skills (Left Hand)

Evaluation Report

3.a. Crayon or Pencil Grasp

Joanne at 13

Joanne's left hand grasped the pencil with a static tripod posture (held proximally with crude approximation of thumb, index, and middle fingers, but MCP joints were not stabilized for fine, localized movements of PIP joints). Several components of the dynamic tripod posture were emerging: the wrist was slightly extended, and the ring and little fingers were flexed to form a stable arch, but Joanne was not able to draw tiny circles.

Joanne at 24

Delayed patterns (primary developmentally inappropriate): Joanne used a static tripod grasp of the pencil, with continual adjustments by the other hand.

Implications for function: The static tripod grasp, while not as mature as the dynamic tripod, is extremely functional and used by many adults without disabilities.

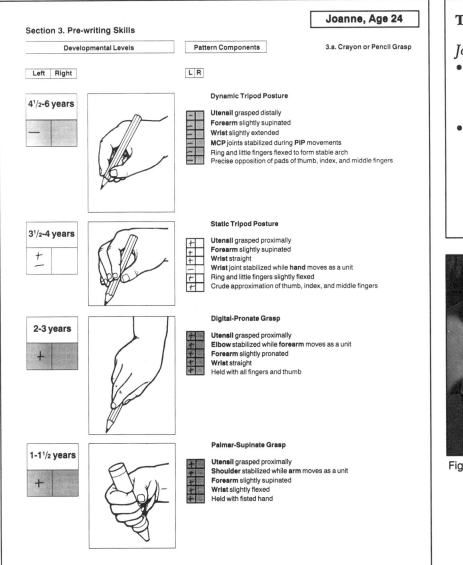

Treatment Program

Joanne at 13

- A triangular rubber pencil gripper can be used to encourage distal grasp.

- Joanne can trace circles of gradually smaller size to increase localized movements of digit components as MCP joints are stabilized (figure 9.64).

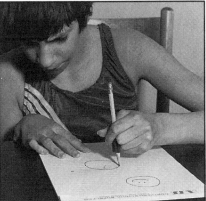

Figure 9.64. (photo by Sheldon Green)

Evaluation Report

3.b. Drawings

Joanne at 13

Joanne's drawings were at an approximate 4-year level. She copied a circle and a cross and an imperfect square, but she was not able to trace a cross or a diamond accurately. Without perceptual concepts of diagonal lines, she was unable to copy a triangle or a diamond.

Joanne at 24

Normal patterns (developmentally appropriate): Joanne was able to copy a circle.

Delayed patterns (primary developmentally inappropriate): She could imitate a horizontal line, a vertical line, a square, and a cross, and could trace a diamond, with corners rounded. She could not copy a square, a triangle, or a diamond.

Implications for function: Joanne is able to write her name and read some signs and some functional words. She signs cards and letters that she sends to friends and family, as well as her paychecks (figure 9.65). Perceptual-motor concepts form the foundation for these reading and writing skills.

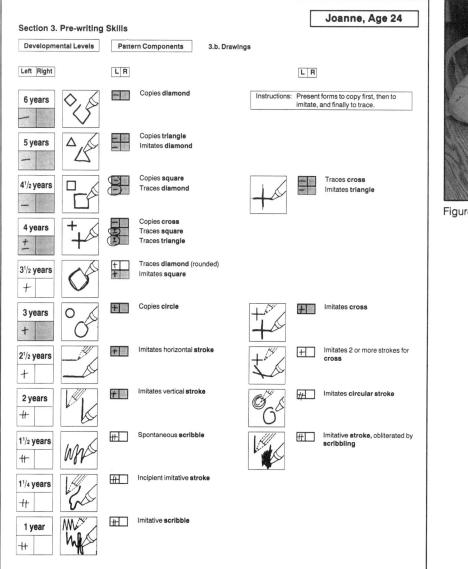

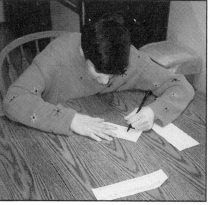

Figure 9.65. (photo by author)

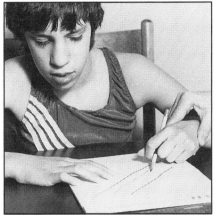

Figure 9.66. (photo by Sheldon Green)

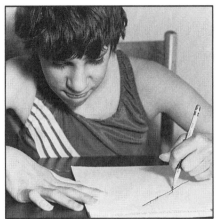

Figure 9.67. (photo by Sheldon Green)

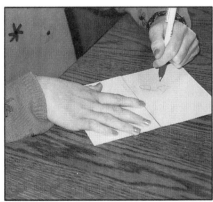

Figure 9.68. (photo by author)

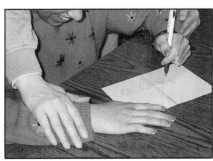

Figure 9.69. (photo by author)

Treatment Program

Joanne at 13
- Diagonal line activities can include:

  - assistive followed by independent drawing between two parallel diagonal lines, with sets gradually narrowing (figure 9.66)

  - independent tracing on a single line (figure 9.67)

  - independent drawing between two dots

  - independent drawing without guidelines

Joanne at 24
- Paper for writing, sketching, and painting should always be oriented for the left hand, to allow Joanne visual access to her work. Her forearms should rest on the table fully, with her right hand flat, stabilizing the paper. Her left hand should rest on the surface, grasping the pen close to the point for better control (figures 9.68, 9.69). Joanne's writing utensil could be chosen from the wide assortment now available to provide a larger handle for stability without requiring special adaptation.

- Structured graded drawing exercises of lines and shapes during occupational therapy will improve Joanne's perceptual concepts of letters and words for reading as well as writing. These activities could be designed to contain dates and times, which are Joanne's areas of strengths and highly motivating (for example, car on the road, railroad, ladder, hills, templates [guide, trace, copy, memorize]).

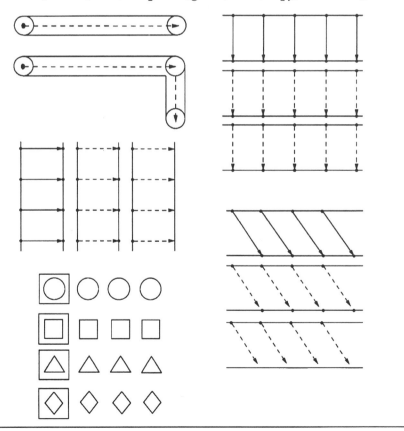

Summary and Conclusions

Joanne demonstrated certain important gaps in her early development, atypical distribution of muscle tone, delayed visual control, limited mobility, and resultant decreased environmental exploration. Her left hand was more functional than her right.

Recommendations

Joanne's occupational therapy program should include remediation of gaps in prehension development to maximize skill competence in self-help (independent living), functional academics (survival), and recreational and prevocational activities.

Sample IEP
(Individual Educational Plan)
Occupational Therapy Components

Present Level of Function

Joanne's prehension skills showed a scatter of missing skills throughout the first 15 months of development, interfering with independence in educational, recreational, self-help, and prevocational activities. Joanne's writing skills, including pencil grasp and drawing, were at a 3- to 4-year developmental level.

Goals and Objectives
Goal #1
To improve prehension skills to increase independence in the school environment

Objective 1.1
Joanne will use the inferior-pincer grasp with her left hand and the scissors grasp with her right to pick up and sort 25 mixed coins into five piles (pennies, nickels, dimes, quarters, and half dollars) with 80% accuracy by using tactile channels (feeling size and thickness) as well as visual, without a speed component.

Objective 1.2
Joanne will press down on a stapler with her right hand, using total elbow and wrist extension, holding the papers with her left hand, to staple ten sets of papers together in 20 seconds, to improve clerical skills for prevocational exploration.

Objective 1.3
Joanne will be able to read a series of seven telephone numbers and use her right index finger either to dial or to push buttons with 100% accuracy after first whispering the numbers aloud to herself.

Goal #2
To improve pencil grasp and drawing skills related to writing

Objective 2.1
Joanne will use the dynamic tripod posture to grasp a pencil while drawing circles of 1" diameter.

Objective 2.2
Joanne will be able to draw a triangle with 90% accuracy in preparation for writing letters such as V and W, which incorporate diagonal lines.

Joanne at 24

Summary and Conclusions

Although Joanne's hands are functional for many tasks, and she is independent in most activities in home, school, and community environments, she has difficulty with certain skills because of developmental motor delays and lack of automatic movement patterns. In other words, she has to concentrate on the motor components, compromising the cognitive components. Persistent involuntary reflexes sometimes interfere with voluntary movements. Most patterns are delayed, but normal rather than atypical.

Her left hand is significantly more adept than her right, but she does use both hands spontaneously for bilateral tasks. Joanne's type of spastic cerebral palsy causes movements throughout her body to be awkward and less refined because of her difficulty in grading movement (midrange control). This spasticity also affects oral-motor function (eating) and visual-motor function, primarily eye-hand coordination.

Recommendations

- Occupational therapy and/or physical therapy is recommended to improve postural control during transitions, fine motor function, and visual-perceptual-motor skills. Automatic movement patterns can be achieved with repetition if tasks are carefully structured for success each time.

- Because Joanne's social skills are one of her strengths, and sharing meals is an important social activity, the improvement of her eating skills should be a priority. A feeding evaluation of both oral-motor (chewing) and fine-motor (utensil use) functions would identify components for treatment, including prefeeding sensory stimulation of mouth, cheeks, jaw, lips, and tongue, and use of adapted utensils.

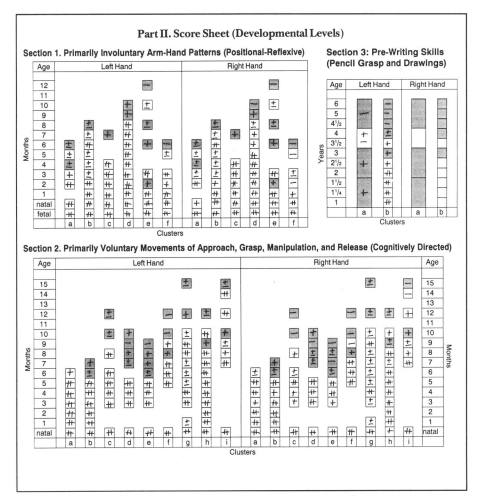

Sample ISP (Individual Service Plan) Occupational Therapy Components

Present Level of Function

Joanne is able to participate *independently* or with verbal reminders in the following activities: washing hair with hand-held shower while sitting in tub, toileting, bathing, eating (glass, spoon), dressing (except for buttons, snaps, zippers, and shoelaces), making her bed, dusting, setting and clearing the table, and laundry.

With *minimal assistance and/or adaptations,* she also participates in printing her name, brushing her hair, cooking, washing her face, sports (bowling with adapted handle), swimming, shopping for food, and cleaning tables and chairs.

She needs *maximal assistance* for cutting food (which needs to be small because of chewing problems) and certain dressing skills (buttons, snaps, zippers, shoelaces).

Goal and Objectives

Goal #1

To increase money management skills in the home and community environments

Objective 1.1

Joanne will budget and plan a well-balanced meal by choosing illustrated food cards from a card file box.

Objective 1.2

Joanne will identify the foods on her cards in the store and place them in her cart, using a stable accommodative grasp and precise release (to avoid bruising fruit or breaking glass containers).

Objective 1.3

Joanne will purchase her groceries with the correct amount of money, selecting appropriate bills and coins from her purse.

Objective 1.4

Joanne will push the cart with both hands through the entire store without hitting obstacles.

To Joey at age 8

from her sister Jacki at age 14

What can you say about a little girl?
A small child, filled with love.
A child whose smile
Never stops,
Always lingers
With that extra bit of love.
There's so much to say,
For she's unique in every way.
She gives,
With every day that she lives.
Never knowing,
That with each smile she bestows,
She shows
What it's like to be always growing.
To know her,
Is to know what love is,
For all you have to do,
Is look in the eyes
That always seem to say,
I love you!

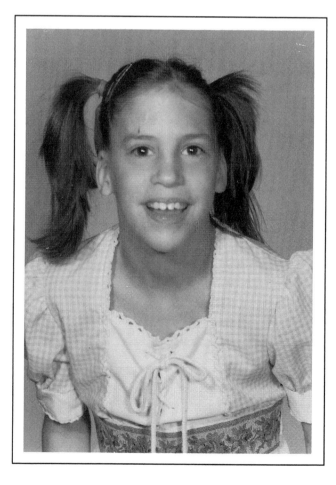

Chapter Ten
Patrick
Evaluation and Treatment
Transition from Childhood to Adulthood

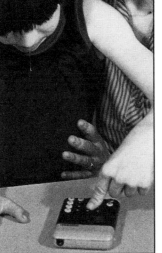

Date: 12-30-81

To: Whom it may concern

Re: Occupational therapy evaluation for Patrick M.

This 6-year-old male with a diagnosis of athetoid quadriplegia with spasticity was re-evaluated today in his home because of suspected regression in fine motor skills due to side effects of unregulated seizure medications. Patrick is presently mainstreamed into a kindergarten classroom. The Erhardt Developmental Prehension Assessment (EDPA) was used to measure arm as well as hand patterns, with his mother present and assisting in administration and observation.

The EDPA measures arm-hand patterns from the fetal and natal periods to 15 months, when the essential components of prehension are developed and functional. Because further refinement, increased skill, and the use of tools are the result of learned experiences, the 15-month level can be considered the maturity of prehension and thus an approximate norm for assessing older children. Pencil grasp and drawings are also measured from 1 to 6 years. Gaps in early developmental sequences, especially in primitive reflexes, often interfere with fine motor coordination later in life.

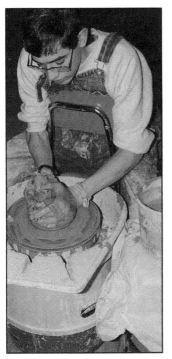

Date: 3-21-92

To: Whom it may concern

Re: Occupational therapy evaluation for Patrick M.

This 16-year-old male with a diagnosis of athetoid quadriplegia with spasticity was re-evaluated today in his home with the Erhardt Developmental Prehension Assessment (EDPA) to determine hand skills relating to educational performance now, and future function in transition areas of:

- home and independent living: cooking, cleaning, laundry, dressing, bathing, grooming, and eating
- recreation/leisure activities: art (pottery, painting), exercise and sports (badminton, basketball, biking, bowling, golf, horseback riding, cross-country skiing, weight lifting)
- community participation: mobility (transportation) and social access to people, public places, and activities (restaurants, shopping malls)
- career/vocational opportunities: clerical skills, gardening, and computer operation (manipulation of trackball, keyboard, and disks)

Patrick resides with his parents and younger brother and attends regular classes and resource rooms in a public high school. He has participated in a summer employment program involving clerical skills and lawn care.

Patrick was evaluated for head, arm, and hand function in various positions: supine (on his back), prone (on his stomach), and sitting. His physical therapist and his mother assisted in administration, observations, and interpretations.

Section 1. Primarily Involuntary Arm-Hand Patterns (Positional-Reflexive)

Evaluation Report

1.a. The Arms at Rest and during Body Play (Supine)

Patrick at 6

Patrick's shoulders were elevated (right more than left) rather than depressed, with neck elongation, and he did not tuck his chin well during head lifting. Rolling to sidelying and back while grasping knees was unstable, and rolling over to prone was accomplished with excess hip flexion rather than head lifting and adduction of upper arm.

Patrick at 16

Normal patterns (developmentally appropriate): In supine Patrick was able to lift his head in midline, separately from shoulders, with good neck elongation. He brought open hands together in space and to knees. Rolling was accomplished with upper arm leading and lateral head righting.

Delayed patterns (primary developmentally inappropriate): Patrick's shoulders were elevated at rest, increasing upon head lifting, right more than left. He hyperextended his head during effort (reaching for knees).

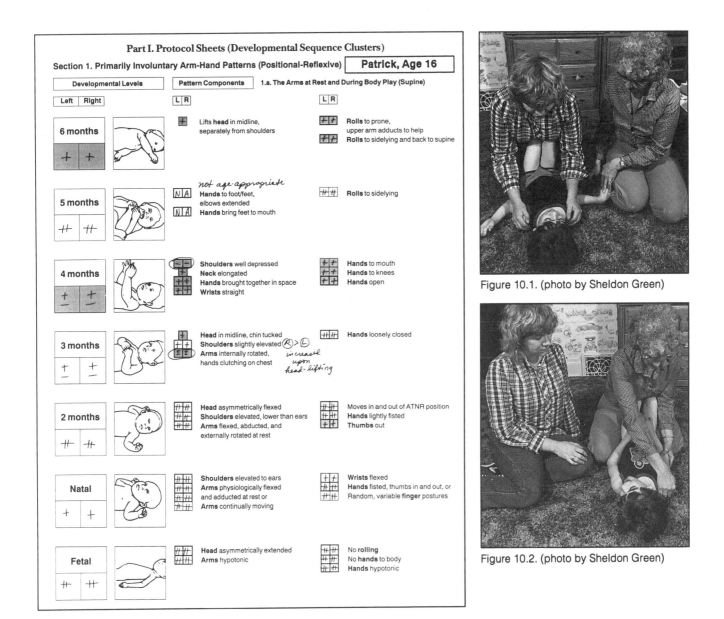

Figure 10.1. (photo by Sheldon Green)

Figure 10.2. (photo by Sheldon Green)

Atypical patterns (secondary developmentally inappropriate): Hands together on the chest produced an atypical pattern, with arms adducted instead of abducted, resulting in flexed wrists.

Implications for function: Elevated shoulders interfere with fine grading of neck muscles for head control and limit range of arm movement. Neck elongation and chin tuck are necessary for optimal visual function, especially at near point for downward gaze in reading. Rolling is important for repositioning in bed.

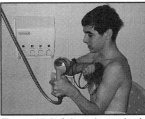

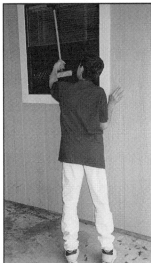

Figure 10.3. (photo by author)

Figure 10.4. (photo by author)

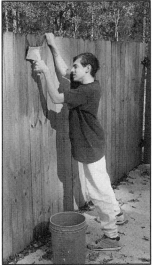

Figure 10.5. (photo by author)

Treatment Program

Patrick at 6

- Patrick's mother should be taught how to inhibit and depress his shoulders by rapid shaking and rotation. This should be followed by compression of his arm into the shoulder joint, which is stabilized by adult's hand, to provide normal co-contraction and prepare for true arm control without artificial stabilization by shoulder elevation (figures 10.1, 10.2).

Patrick at 16

- When sitting in the shower, Patrick should hold the hand-held shower head in his left hand and use his right hand to wash all body parts, especially his chest, with a large sponge in a net bag providing maximal hand contact (figure 10.3).

- Range of motion in shoulders and arms can be increased by washing windows (figure 10.4) or painting large areas (figure 10.5). The opposite hand should be used for stabilization when appropriate.

Evaluation Report

1.b. The Arms at Rest and during Head Raising (Prone)

Patrick at 6

When Patrick was weight bearing on forearms, his right elbow was further behind the shoulder than the left due to poor separation between the arm and scapula. The arms were not well abducted and externally rotated during head raising, and shoulders were elevated, the right barely lower than Patrick's ears. He was missing good neck elongation, and his hands were lightly fisted rather than open, with right thumb inside the palm, not outside. The Symmetrical Tonic Neck Reflex (STNR) was not fully integrated,

resulting in excess head extension, leg flexion in the hands-and-knees position, and poor balance rocking forward and crawling. Patrick could not push up to side-sitting from the sidelying position and could rotate from hands and knees to sitting toward the left but not toward the right.

Patrick at 16

Normal patterns (developmentally appropriate): Patrick was stable in sidelying. Excellent control was seen in transition from sidelying to side-sitting, transition between side-sitting and hands and knees (to the left better than to the right), and rolling. Abdominal muscles were very active.

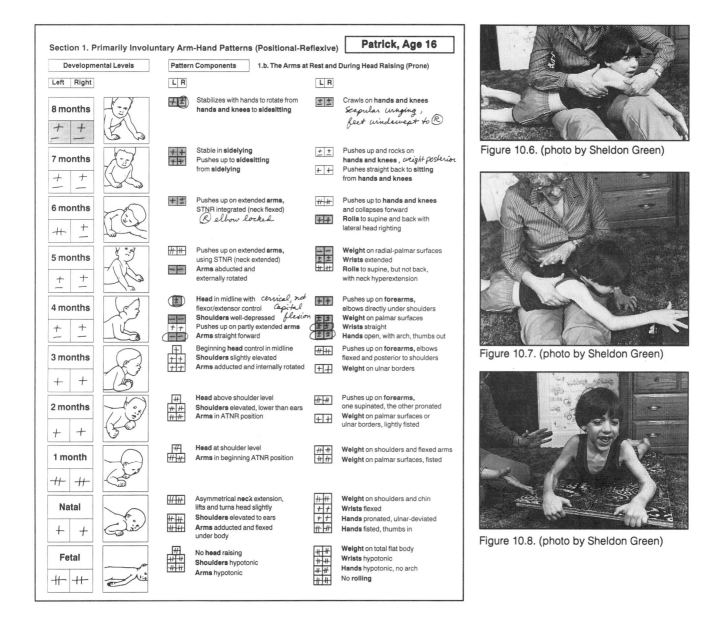

Figure 10.6. (photo by Sheldon Green)

Figure 10.7. (photo by Sheldon Green)

Figure 10.8. (photo by Sheldon Green)

Developmental Hand Dysfunction

Delayed patterns (primary developmentally inappropriate): Patrick demonstrated limited head control in the forearm position, with elevated shoulders and cervical, not capital, flexion. Forearms were adducted and internally rotated instead of straight forward. Hands were not completely open. In the hands-and-knees position, weight bearing on hands was sometimes on the ulnar surface, not consistently palmar, and weight was kept posterior.

Atypical patterns (secondary developmentally inappropriate): On forearms and in the hands-and-knees position, wrists were flexed and ulnar deviated instead of straight or extended, which interfered with integrity of the arches of the hands. Feet were windswept to the right in the hands-and-knees position, and the right elbow was locked. Scapular winging was observed during crawling, indicating shoulder instability.

Implications for function: Sidelying is an appropriate position for watching television or doing leg raises in physical education class. Weight bearing on the upper extremities prepares for arm/hand strength and coordination, as well as the use of the hands to stabilize during transitions. It is also functional in cleaning and gardening tasks.

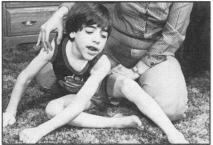

Figure 10.9. (photo by Sheldon Green)

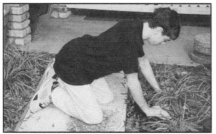

Figure 10.10. (photo by Sheldon Green)

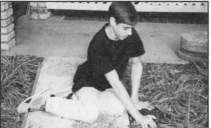

Figure 10.11. (photo by author)

Figure 10.12. (photo by author)

Treatment Program

Patrick at 6

- When Patrick is prone over adult's lap, his arm should be dissociated from his scapula (shoulder blade) by inhibition while entire scapula is stabilized by adult's hand. This should be followed by active reaching forward (figures 10.6, 10.7).

- Prone on forearms on rocker board, Patrick should improve balance and weight shifting sideward. Hands should be flat rather than grasping edge to decrease total flexion pattern. The board may need to be placed on an elevated surface to encourage neck flexion (capital flexion) and elongation (cervical extension) as he looks downward at adult (figure 10.8).

- Pushing up to side-sitting from sidelying should be done with adult assistance at shoulders and hips, gradually reducing control (figures 10.9, 10.10).

Patrick at 16

- Gardening on hands and knees will improve head control and shoulder stability. Normal hand posture and arch integrity will be preserved as his hands bear weight on soft soil. Although Patrick prefers to transition from hands and knees to side-sitting toward the left, he should make a conscious effort to transition to the right as well (figures 10.11, 10.12).

Evaluation Report

1.c. Asymmetrical Tonic Neck Reflex (ATNR)

Patrick at 6
This reflex was fully integrated to the left and beginning to be integrated toward the right. Rotation of the head toward the side resulted in inconsistent extension of the face limb and flexion of the skull limb.

Patrick at 16
Normal patterns (developmentally appropriate): This reflex was fully integrated.

Implications for function: Patrick's voluntary movements are not contaminated by this reflex, which results in obligatory linked head/arm movements when active.

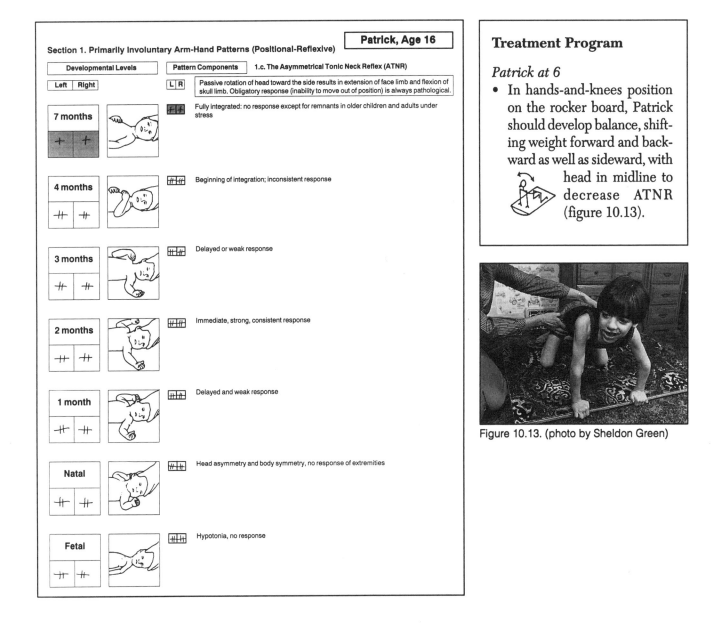

Figure 10.13. (photo by Sheldon Green)

Treatment Program

Patrick at 6
- In hands-and-knees position on the rocker board, Patrick should develop balance, shifting weight forward and backward as well as sideward, with head in midline to decrease ATNR (figure 10.13).

Evaluation Report

1.d. Grasping Reactions

Patrick at 6

The Grasp Reflex was normally integrated. A stimulus in the palm did not result in involuntary grasp. Instinctive Grasp Reactions were also normally integrated. A stimulus withdrawn from the palm did not result in involuntary hand movements of orienting, groping, and trapping.

Patrick at 16

Normal patterns (developmentally appropriate): The Grasp Reflex was fully integrated.

Delayed patterns (primary developmentally inappropriate): The Instinctive Grasp Reaction was present. Patrick involuntarily oriented, groped, and sometimes grasped the stimulus with vision occluded.

Atypical patterns (secondary developmentally inappropriate): Intermittent involuntary athetoid movements were also observed, right more than left.

Implications for function: The Instinctive Grasp Reaction, which is meant to prepare wrist and hand for graceful voluntary movements, can interfere with voluntary release and precise manipulation if not integrated. It is activated by light touch on various parts of the hand, which is not processing sensory input normally. Its reappearance after integration at an earlier age may be due to decreased right hand use compared with the left. Improvement in voluntary skills helps decrease involuntary movements.

Section 1. Primarily Involuntary Arm-Hand Patterns (Positional-Reflexive)

Patrick, Age 16

1.d. Grasping Reactions

Note: Test in supine or with vision occluded to prevent contamination by voluntary movements.

Evaluation Report

1.e. Placing Responses

Patrick at 6

Proprioceptive Placing was normally integrated. Brushing the back of the hand stimulated from sitting against the table edge did not result in involuntary hand movements. Protective Extensor Thrust forward was normally present sideward to the left but not well developed to the right, forward, or backward.

Patrick at 16

Normal patterns (developmentally appropriate): Protective Extensor Thrust stimulated from kneeling was strong, consistent, and immediate in the left arm. Proprioceptive Placing (brushing back of hand against table edge with vision occluded) was integrated (no involuntary placing of hand on surface).

Delayed patterns (primary developmentally inappropriate): Protective Extensor Thrust stimulated from kneeling was slightly delayed forward in the right arm, sideward to the left, and backward on both elbows. It was absent sideward to the right and backward on extended arms. Patrick compensated on his right side by deliberately falling forward instead of sideward.

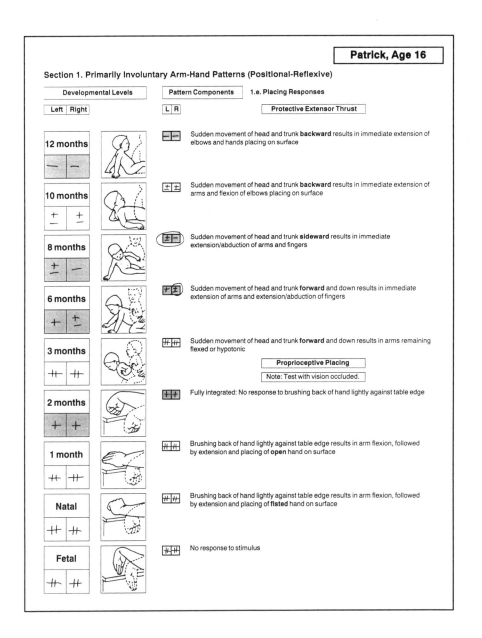

Implications for function: Protective responses, which emerge developmentally at the same time as independent sitting and weight bearing on extended arms, protect the head during falls and reinforce the reaching pattern. As kneeling and standing become perfected, the responses become activated in those positions as well. Proprioceptive Placing also prepares wrist and hand for graceful voluntary movements but needs to be integrated or it will interfere with voluntary manipulation.

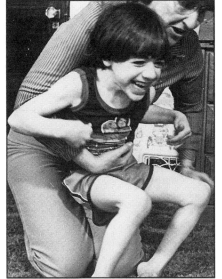

Figure 10.14. (photo by Sheldon Green)

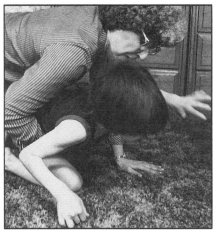

Figure 10.15. (photo by Sheldon Green)

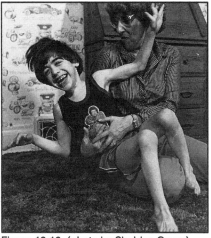

Figure 10.16. (photo by Sheldon Green)

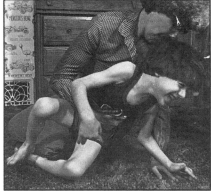

Figure 10.17. (photo by Sheldon Green)

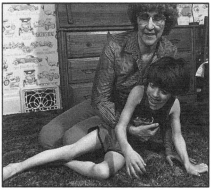

Figure 10.18. (photo by Sheldon Green)

Treatment Program

Patrick at 6
- Patrick can be tossed from adult's lap either forward, sideward, or diagonally backward, without knowing which way, in order to eliminate any voluntary spastic postures and movements and allow automatic reactions. When landing sideward on the right arm, his elbow should be flexed so he bears weight on the forearm, but the left arm can take his weight sideward with the elbow straight. After he lands, he should be helped to stay in position and rock slowly to feel the compression (figures 10.14 to 10.18).

Patrick at 16
- Patrick can practice catching himself against walls and furniture from standing, a primary functional position, with emphasis on his right arm, singly as well as together with his left.

Evaluation Report

1.f. Avoiding Responses

Patrick at 6
This response was normally integrated. A stimulus to any part of the hand did not result in reflexive withdrawal.

Patrick at 16
Delayed patterns (primary developmentally inappropriate): With vision occluded, Patrick showed a slight involuntary response (spreading of fingers) to a distally moving light stimulus on the back of his hand or on the palmar surface of his fingertips, right more than left.

Atypical patterns (secondary developmentally inappropriate): Athetoid movements in the right hand were again observed, especially when the arm was held in space. Patrick also exhibited avoiding reactions to associated auditory stimuli (verbal preparation), in anticipation of the tactile stimulus.

Implications for function: This automatic response helps reduce the Grasp Reflex and open the hand during normal development. It decreases as voluntary control increases. If not eventually integrated, however, it interferes with sustained voluntary grasp and precise manipulation. Its reappearance after integration at an earlier age may be due to incomplete sensory integration.

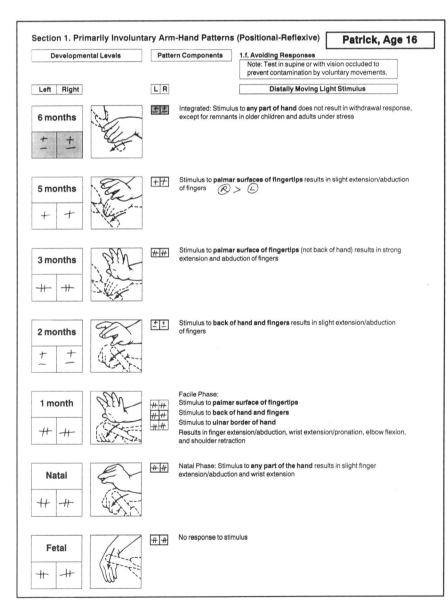

Section 1. Primarily Involuntary Arm-Hand Patterns (Positional-Reflexive) — **Patrick, Age 16**

1.f. Avoiding Responses
Note: Test in supine or with vision occluded to prevent contamination by voluntary movements.

Distally Moving Light Stimulus

6 months — Integrated: Stimulus to **any part of hand** does not result in withdrawal response, except for remnants in older children and adults under stress

5 months — Stimulus to **palmar surfaces of fingertips** results in slight extension/abduction of fingers (R) > (L)

3 months — Stimulus to **palmar surface of fingertips** (not back of hand) results in strong extension and abduction of fingers

2 months — Stimulus to **back of hand and fingers** results in slight extension/abduction of fingers

1 month — Facile Phase:
Stimulus to **palmar surface of fingertips**
Stimulus to **back of hand and fingers**
Stimulus to **ulnar border of hand**
Results in finger extension/abduction, wrist extension/pronation, elbow flexion, and shoulder retraction

Natal — Natal Phase: Stimulus to **any part of the hand** results in slight finger extension/abduction and wrist extension

Fetal — No response to stimulus

Treatment Program

Patrick at 16
- Recreational arts and crafts activities such as pottery provide rich tactile information (texture, temperature, shape, size), to help Patrick increase sensory discrimination and decrease avoiding responses (see 2.g.).

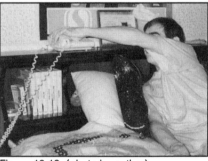

Figure 10.19. (photo by author)

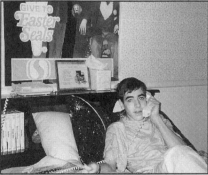

Figure 10.20. (photo by author)

Developmental Hand Dysfunction

Section 2. Primarily Voluntary Movements (Cognitively Directed)

Evaluation Report

2.a. The Arms on Approach (Supine)

Patrick at 6
Patrick used a direct unilateral approach with his left hand and a circular approach with the right. His wrists were straight, hands open.

Patrick at 16
Normal patterns (developmentally appropriate): Left-hand approach was direct and fairly accurate, with appropriate finger extension. The right hand spontaneously joined the left, which usually initiated reaching. Bilateral reach was fairly symmetrical.

Delayed patterns (primary developmentally inappropriate): The right arm did not reach accurately.

Although both wrists were extended during approach, they usually flexed upon grasping, and right fingers showed excessive extension.

Atypical patterns (secondary developmentally inappropriate): Elbows were somewhat hyperextended, locked for stability, because of inadequate midrange control.

Implications for function: The challenge of new or difficult tasks may produce reversion to earlier or atypical patterns such as wrist flexion or excessive finger extension. These patterns interfere with accurate and stable grasp of various objects. Patrick needs skill in both hands to reach for a lamp switch, alarm clock, or telephone on either side of his bed.

Section 2. Primarily Voluntary Movements (Cognitively Directed) — **Patrick, Age 16**

| Developmental Levels | Pattern Components | 2.a. The Arms on Approach (Supine) |

Left | Right   **L | R**

6 months
Unilateral circular approach *Unilateral approach is direct on L, slightly inaccurate on R*
Overreaches, then corrects and grasps
Elbows fully extended, approximately 180°
Wrists straight
Excessive **finger** extension *L has inconsistent appropriate extension*

5 months
Bilateral angular approach *bilateral is fairly symmetrical, less accuracy on R*
Unilateral angular approach
Underreaches, then corrects and corrals object
Elbows extended approximately 140°
Hands open
One hand grasps, other joins

4 months
Bilateral backhand approach, ulnar side leading
Contacts object in midline
Elbows extended approximately 100°
Hands partly open

3 months
Unilateral approach
Contacts object placed approximately 45° to side
Elbows flexed
Wrists flexed *upon grasp*
Hands flexed

2 months
Arms **activate** in response to stationary stimulus
Random arm movements **cease** in response to moving stimulus

1 month
Random arm movements **unrelated** to stimulus

Natal
Limited arm movements, no approach or response to stimulus

Treatment Program

Patrick at 16

- Reaching for the telephone should be done with the right arm as well as the left (figures 10.19, 10.20).

- With his father as a spotter, Patrick lifts weights in supine to improve right-arm strength and control as it is paired with his more skillful left (figure 10.21).

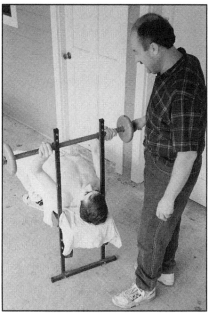

Figure 10.21. (photo by author)

Evaluation Report

2.b. The Arms on Approach (Prone)

Patrick at 6
All skills were present except for bilateral approach and right hand open. Patrick sought stability with hip abduction-flexion. He reached with each arm while bearing weight on the other forearm or extended arm. His left hand was open.

Patrick at 16
Normal patterns (developmentally appropriate): Reaching from hands and knees with one arm was accurate, with symmetrical body positioning and open left hand. Bilateral reaching (sliding with the floor as a guide) was symmetrical.

Delayed patterns (primary developmentally inappropriate): Patrick had difficulty with his lateral weight shifts when reaching from prone on forearms. His neck extended, he overshifted, and flexed into the weight-bearing side instead of elongating it. His right arm was internally rotated with wrist flexed. Reaching into space from flat on the floor was asymmetrical and was done with an inappropriate weight shift (leaning into same side).

Implications for function: Head and arm function in various prone positions are components of swimming, cleaning, and gardening.

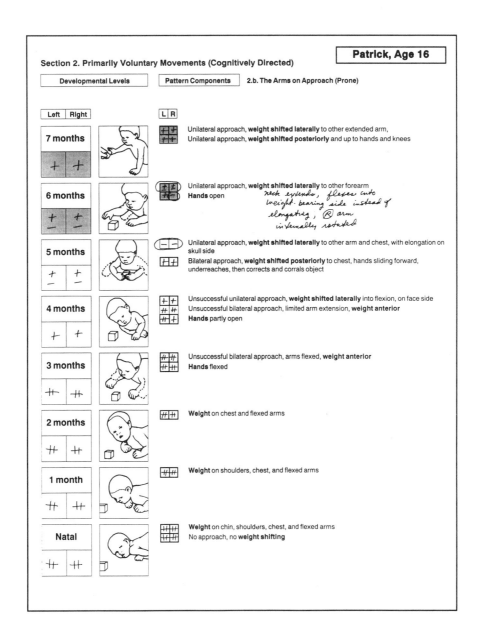

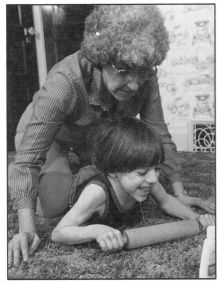

Figure 10.22. (photo by Sheldon Green)

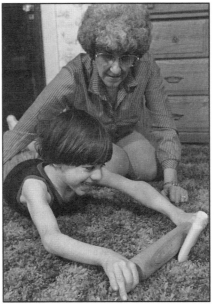

Figure 10.23. (photo by Sheldon Green)

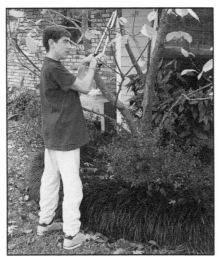

Figure 10.24. (photo by author)

Treatment Program

Patrick at 6

- Prone on floor, Patrick can use a rolling pin to knock over an object to improve bilateral approach and right elbow extension. His pelvis should be stabilized to prevent him from "fixing" with his hips (figures 10.22, 10.23).

Patrick at 16

- Swimming with flotation devices on upper arms will increase strength, coordination, symmetry, and balance. Full arm extension forward with each arm stroke should be emphasized.

- Bilateral activities such as using pruning shears (figure 10.24) require arm control forward at various heights.

Evaluation Report

2.c. The Arms on Approach (Sitting)

Patrick at 6

All skills were present in the left hand but not in the right, where Patrick used a circular rather than direct approach with flexed wrist and excessive MCP (knuckle) joint extension. He could supinate (turn palm up) his right hand only with the elbow flexed, not extended. His left hand used a unilateral direct approach, with elbow and wrist extended, appropriate finger extension, and voluntary supination to facilitate grasp, with elbow either flexed or extended.

Patrick at 16

Normal patterns (developmentally appropriate):
Unilateral and bilateral approaches were accurate and controlled, with appropriate finger extension in the left hand and inconsistent wrist extension (easier if object was placed high, further away, or if elbow rested on surface for support), left better than right. Supination was used to facilitate grasp on the left. When grasping a dowel, Patrick brought his left hand into midposition and then joined his right in a pronated (palm down) position.

Delayed patterns (primary developmentally inappropriate): Shoulders elevated upon effort, and upper extremities showed either increased flexion or elbow locking into extension. Right hand was not always open, fingers showed excessive MCP extension, and stabilization on the surface was needed in order to supinate enough to grasp an object with straight wrist in midposition.

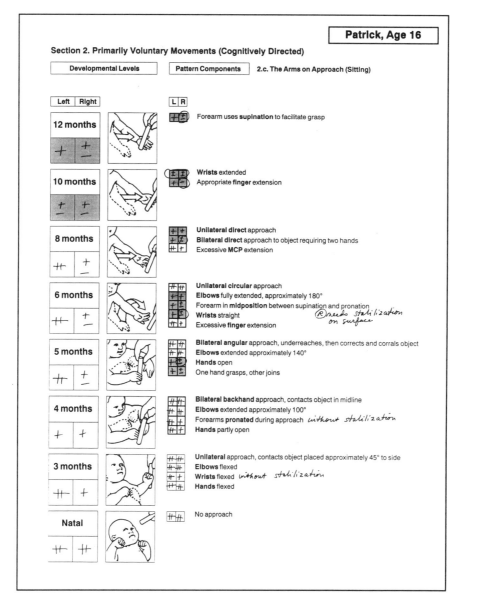

Atypical patterns (secondary developmentally inappropriate): Without a surface for stabilization, the right wrist was flexed and forearm pronated.

Implications for function: To use a rake or golf club, one hand first grasps and the other joins, with forearm flexibility needed for proper positioning, and shoulder/elbow control for function. Grasping a glass or beverage can requires a straight wrist in midposition to avoid spilling.

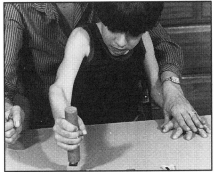

Figure 10.25. (photo by Sheldon Green)

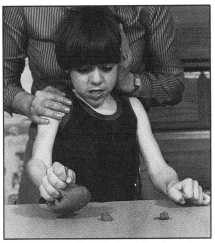

Figure 10.26. (photo by Sheldon Green)

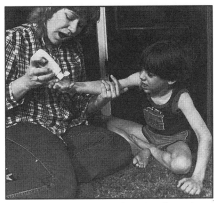

Figure 10.27. (photo by Sheldon Green)

Treatment Program

Patrick at 6

- Sitting at a desk, Patrick can grasp a magnetized dowel with his right hand to reach directly toward a series of magnetized alphabet letters. His left hand should be stabilized on the surface (figure 10.25).

- Sitting at a desk, Patrick can grasp a ball of clay with his right hand to reach directly toward a series of clay bits, pressing down on each to "clean" the table, to improve approach, wrist extension, and hand position. The ball of clay could be formed to fit his hand appropriately; his opposite hand should be stabilized flat on the surface, and he should be assisted in keeping his head in midline and his right shoulder down (figure 10.26).

- Patrick should be assisted in keeping his elbow extended while actively supinating his hand to receive lotion, with assistance gradually reduced (figure 10.27).

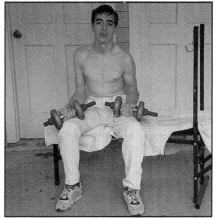

Figure 10.28. (photo by author)

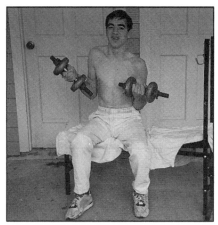

Figure 10.29. (photo by author)

Treatment Program

Patrick at 16

- Lifting weights in sitting can improve forearm supination but symmetry may be jeopardized (figures 10.28, 10.29). Weight machines can help get good alignment of trunk as well as arms. The therapist observes hyperextension of Patrick's lower back, corrects it with her hands, and places a belt in the same place so he can continue independently (figures 10.30 to 10.32).

- Operating oars in rowing machine or boat will equalize bilateral function.

- In a lead-up activity for basketball, Patrick and his brother throw the ball into the trash can. After eye-hand coordination improves, Patrick is ready to achieve more bilateral arm extension as he throws the ball overhead into the regular basket (figures 10.33, 10.34).

- Patrick should reach and grasp a rake with right hand first (in midposition), then left joining (figure 10.35).

- Cleaning kitchen counters and dusting can be done by sliding the right hand on the surface for support and good alignment of wrist and finger joints (figure 10.36).

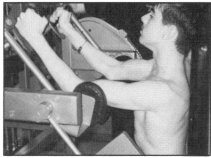

Figure 10.30. (photo by author)

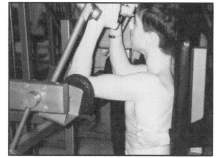

Figure 10.31. (photo by author)

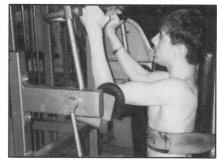

Figure 10.32. (photo by author)

Developmental Hand Dysfunction

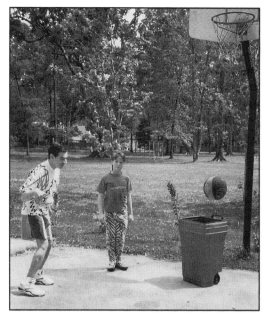

Figure 10.33. (photo by author)

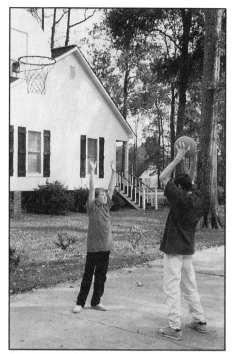

Figure 10.34. (photo by author)

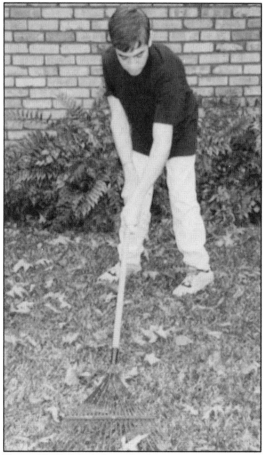

Figure 10.35. (photo by author)

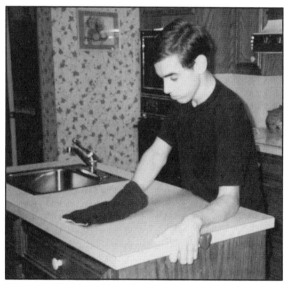

Figure 10.36. (photo by author)

Chapter Ten/Patrick

Evaluation Report

2.d. Grasp of the Dowel (Supine, Prone, or Sitting)

Patrick at 6

The left hand used a radial-palmar grasp, with the radial-digital grasp emerging. The right hand used a palmar grasp, thumb adducted, with a radial-palmar grasp emerging.

Patrick at 16

Normal patterns (developmentally appropriate): Patrick used his opposite hand to place the dowel correctly into each hand for a mature three-jawed chuck grasp. Radial-palmar grasp (power grip) of a dowel with both one-hand and two-hand grasps was excellent. He often rested his elbows on the surface for better control of his hands.

Delayed patterns (primary developmentally inappropriate): Although wrists were straight upon approach, they often flexed upon grasp. Patrick grasped objects having smaller handles with a more unstable, primitive palmar grasp, thumb adducted, not opposed, with associated shoulder elevation and wrist flexion.

Atypical patterns (secondary developmentally inappropriate): Although his radial-digital grasp (thumb and all fingertips) was functional, inadequate midrange control of finger joints caused inadequate control and poor alignment, especially of the PIP joints and the left little finger. When stabilizing his right hand on the surface, Patrick's flexed wrist caused MCP hyperextension.

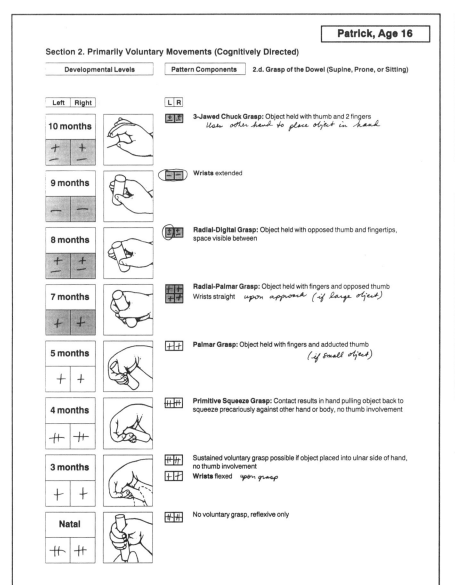

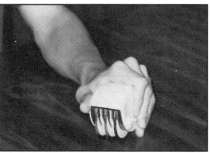

Figure 10.37. (photo by author)

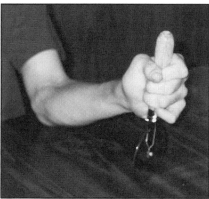

Figure 10.38. (photo by author)

Developmental Hand Dysfunction

Implications for function: Heavy or large objects such as a tennis or badminton racket require maximum hand surface to be in contact for efficient power grasp. Lighter, smaller objects such as a toothbrush or eating utensils usually require more mature, precise grasps, except during power tasks such as cutting with a knife and fork, rolling knife, or pizza cutter (figures 10.37, 10.38).

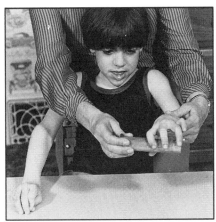

Figure 10.39. (photo by Sheldon Green)

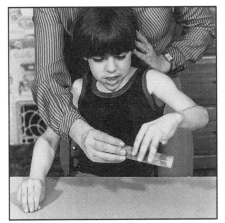

Figure 10.40. (photo by Sheldon Green)

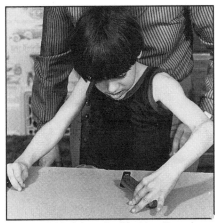

Figure 10.41. (photo by Sheldon Green)

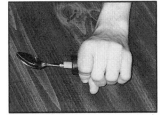

Figure 10.42. (photo by author)

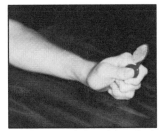

Figure 10.43. (photo by author)

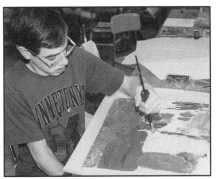

Figure 10.44. (photo by author)

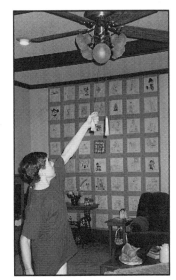

Figure 10.45. (photo by author)

Treatment Program

Patrick at 6
- Radial-digital grasp can be improved by first placing the dowel in Patrick's hand appropriately, then having him reach for it in space and finally grasp it from the surface (figures 10.39 to 10.41).

Patrick at 16
- Various adapted utensil handles for eating, tooth brushing, and painting can be explored to improve grip and finger alignment (figures 10.42 to 10.44).

- Grasping with extended wrists can be facilitated when reaching upward for a ceiling fan cord (figure 10.45).

Evaluation Report

2.e. Grasp of the Cube (Supine, Prone, or Sitting)

Patrick at 6

The left hand used both radial-palmar and radial-digital grasps with wrist extension, but the right used an atypical pattern of flexed wrist, adducted thumb, and components of both the radial-palmar and radial-digital grasp (figure 5.3, page 48).

Patrick at 16

Normal patterns (developmentally appropriate): Patrick used a radial-digital grasp of the small cube and a radial-palmar grasp of the larger one with his left hand. He used modified radial-digital grasps (middle finger and thumb with left hand, index finger and thumb with his right hand).

Delayed patterns (primary developmentally inappropriate): Although he was able to use his opposite hand to place the smaller object correctly into his hand, he could not pick the objects up from the table easily. Patrick compensates appropriately by using his other hand to place the object correctly in his hand or by sliding the object off the surface to grasp it.

Atypical patterns (secondary developmentally inappropriate): The right-hand radial-digital and

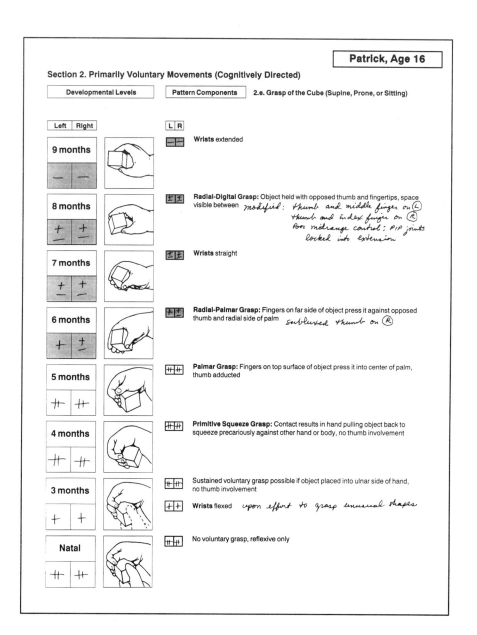

radial-palmar grasps were characterized by poor midrange finger control (PIP joints locked into extension) and a subluxed right thumb (proximal joint with distal joint hyperextended).

Implications for function: Good thumb alignment and control are necessary for Patrick to grasp cube-shaped objects such as the box holding his computer disks, individual floppy disks, and audiocassettes.

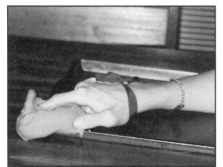

Figure 10.46. (photo by author)

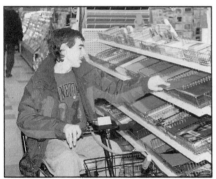

Figure 10.47. (photo by author)

Treatment Program

Patrick at 6
- The emerging radial-palmar grasp of the cube in the right hand can be improved by placing, then reaching in space, and finally grasping from the surface, as with the dowel.

Patrick at 16
- Specific exercises with therapy putty or clay will improve manipulation, midrange strength, and control of finger joints. For example, Patrick exercised with clay while wearing a pincher mitt to isolate index finger for appropriate thumb opposition (figure 10.46). This pattern helped improve his radial-digital grasp of a notebook selected for purchase from a store in the mall (figure 10.47).

- A large mass of therapy putty, providing total contact with Patrick's entire hand, can facilitate the radial-palmar grasp with thumb opposition to each of his fingers (figure 10.48).

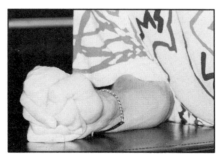

Figure 10.48. (photo by author)

Evaluation Report

2.f. Grasp of the Pellet (Prone or Sitting)

Patrick at 6

The left hand used the pincer grasp with thumb opposed. The right hand usually raked the pellet into the palm with adducted thumb and flexed fingers. The scissors grasp was emerging in the right hand, but with subluxation of the proximal thumb joint. As Patrick tried to grasp the pellet, he first adducted the thumb. As he pressed it against the side of the index finger, the distal thumb joint flexed and the proximal thumb joint hyperextended or subluxed (figure 5.4, page 49).

Patrick at 16

Normal patterns (developmentally appropriate): Fine pincer grasp was accomplished with good control of all finger joints in the left hand but some hyperextension of the distal thumb joint. The scissors grasp (lateral pinch) was excellent in the left hand.

Delayed patterns (primary developmentally inappropriate): Scissors grasp with the right hand was not possible.

Atypical patterns (secondary developmentally inappropriate): Fine pincer grasp by the right hand required some compensatory stabilization of fingers against each other, since PIP and thumb control were inadequate. Without perfect control of arm, elbow, and wrist joints, Patrick needed to slide his fingers on the surface to use pincer grasp. Wrist flexion,

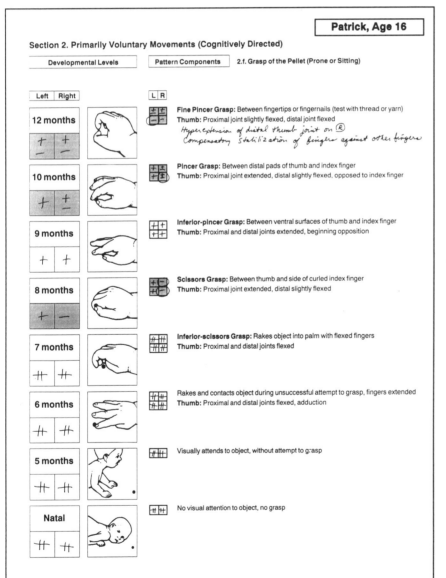

Patrick, Age 16

Section 2. Primarily Voluntary Movements (Cognitively Directed)

Developmental Levels | Pattern Components | 2.f. Grasp of the Pellet (Prone or Sitting)

Fine Pincer Grasp: Between fingertips or fingernails (test with thread or yarn)
Thumb: Proximal joint slightly flexed, distal joint flexed

Hyperextension of distal thumb joint on Ⓡ
Compensatory stabilization of fingers against other fingers

Pincer Grasp: Between distal pads of thumb and index finger
Thumb: Proximal joint extended, distal slightly flexed, opposed to index finger

Inferior-pincer Grasp: Between ventral surfaces of thumb and index finger
Thumb: Proximal and distal joints extended, beginning opposition

Scissors Grasp: Between thumb and side of curled index finger
Thumb: Proximal joint extended, distal slightly flexed

Inferior-scissors Grasp: Rakes object into palm with flexed fingers
Thumb: Proximal and distal joints flexed

Rakes and contacts object during unsuccessful attempt to grasp, fingers extended
Thumb: Proximal and distal joints flexed, adduction

Visually attends to object, without attempt to grasp

No visual attention to object, no grasp

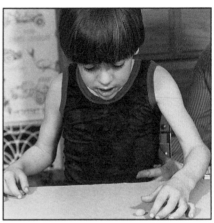

Figure 10.49. (photo by Sheldon Green)

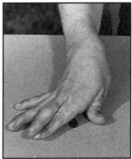

Figure 10.50. (photo by Sheldon Green)

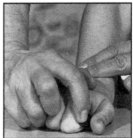

Figure 10.51. (photo by Sheldon Green)

Developmental Hand Dysfunction

however, caused only the tips of his extended fingers and hyperextended thumb to be in contact.

Implications for function: Managing money requires a high level of skill for grasping and manipulating coins and bills within the hand. Precise grasp of tiny objects such as raisins or thread depends on appropriate points of stability as well as midrange control in all finger joints. The scissors grasp of an object such as a key is an example of developmentally earlier skills that remain throughout life for functional use. Peeling address labels and placing them on envelopes requires sustained fine pinch against the resistance of adhesive as well as precise release.

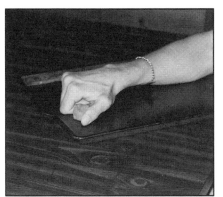

Figure 10.52. (photo by author)

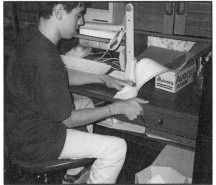

Figure 10.53. (photo by author)

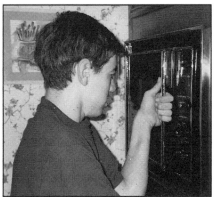

Figure 10.54. (photo by author)

Treatment Program

Patrick at 6

- Patrick should work toward the fine pincer grasp in the left hand by grasping gradually smaller pellets. His right hand should be stabilized on the surface to prevent associated reactions (figure 10.49).

- To move from the inferior-scissors grasp to the scissors grasp, Patrick's right hand should be placed on the surface with thumb extended, the pellet should be placed against the side of the curled index finger, and he should actively slide his thumb along the surface to grasp without subluxation of the proximal thumb joint (figures 10.50, 10.51) and hyperextension of the distal thumb joint.

Patrick at 16

- Pincer grasp of coins can begin with the largest coins (50¢), gradually reducing to quarters, nickels, and dimes. A large pellet of therapy putty, gradually reduced in size, can be used to achieve the scissors grasp, with isolated thumb movement in the right hand. The forearm and fist should rest on the surface (figure 10.52).

- Peeling labels should also be done with entire forearm resting on the surface to provide as much stability as possible (figure 10.53).

- Patrick must monitor his thumb alignment during functions such as opening the microwave door to avoid subluxation and distal hyperextension (figure 10.54).

Evaluation Report

2.g. Manipulation Skills (Prehension Schema)

Patrick at 6

All skills were present in the left hand except shaking objects with shoulder, elbow, and wrist motion. Patrick used shoulder and elbow only. The poking index finger was emerging. He could manipulate objects without visual monitoring. Eye, hand, and mouth coordination were also emerging well. The left hand could drop, throw, push, and pull objects, build a tower of two blocks, and perform manipulative skills such as rotating.

Patrick's right hand did not accommodate to the form of new objects and new positions well, did not bring objects to mouth easily, did not shake objects well even with merely shoulder motion, had not coordinated hand, vision, and sucking schemata, and had difficulty pushing, pulling, dropping, and throwing objects. Patrick tried to poke with his right index finger, but all fingers extended. Manipulation was limited, not possible unless hand and object were in the same visual field and other hand performed associated movements rather than holding.

Patrick at 16

Tactile Awareness
Atypical patterns (secondary developmentally inappropriate): Patrick's hands did not accommodate completely to the shape of objects (for example, when petting his dog). Fingertips of the left hand and all fingers of the right hand lacked contact.

Section 2. Primarily Voluntary Movements (Cognitively Directed) **Patrick, Age 16**

Developmental Levels   **Pattern Components**   **2.g. Manipulation Skills (Prehension Schema)**

Left | Right

For difficult tasks, RUE flexed and shoulders elevated during excessive effort

15 months
- Inverts container to reach contents
- Intentional manipulation possible without hand and object within visual field
- One hand manipulates object while other holds or assists

12 months
- Both hands combine objects *wrists flexed*
- **Tactile manipulation** (rotating, squeezing, transferring) replaces **oral exploration** (mouthing)

10 months
- Isolates index finger to poke, others flexed
- Tries unsuccessfully to reach into small container to remove object
- One hand manipulates, other hand mirrors
- **Shakes** object with arm, elbow, and wrist motion

9 months
- Tries to poke, all fingers extended
- Pokes with thumb *Hyperextended on (R)*
- *Needs to stabilize hand on surface*
- Increased **tactile manipulation, orally explores** new objects primarily

8 months
- **Reciprocal Assimilation:**
  - Watches hand and keeps it moving to make interesting sights last
  - Intentional manipulation possible when hand and object are within visual field
- Drops object *wrist flexed on both (R) > (L)*
- Throws object
- Pushes object
- Pulls object

7 months
- **Object Permanence:**
  - Searches for lost or removed object, ignoring new stimulus
  - Drops object when grasping another
- Retains object when grasping another
- **Shakes** one or both objects, alternating visual monitoring back and forth

6 months
- Beginning of **Object Permanence:**
  - Searches for lost or removed object, but can be distracted by another
- Alternately mouths, looks, shakes object, retaining grasp
- **Shakes** object with arm and elbow motion

5 months
- **Tactile Discrimination** between hand and object (bites object, not fingers)
- Alternately mouths and shakes object
- **Shakes** object with arm motion only

4 months
- Mouths object or eats finger foods with insufficient **tactile discrimination** (may bite fingers by mistake)
- Hand brings object to mouth, orally exploring both
- Visually attends and swipes at object if within 1"

3 months
- **Tactile Assimilation:** Hand movements extend to own face, body, clothing
- **Tactile Accommodation:** Hands adapt to new objects, without visual attention *(L) > (R)*
- **Reflexive Movements:**
  - Scratching and clutching
- **Tactile Recognition** (eyes alert) leads to: Voluntary repetition of reflexive movements
- Hand to mouth
- Eyes watch moving hand

1 month

Natal
- **Reflexive Grasp:** Involuntary, without tactile awareness (eyes do not alert)
- No voluntary hand movements
- Visually attends to object without reaching
- No voluntary hand to mouth, head/mouth move to suck on hand

Implications for function: The ability to accommodate hands to the shape of objects is the precursor to complex manipulation skills. The tactile information derived from the total contact combines with the visual information to enhance motor planning and execution. Eventually, the tactile perception alone is necessary for certain tasks outside of the visual field (such as buttoning at the back of the neck).

Prehension Schema
Normal patterns (developmentally appropriate): Patrick inverted a container to reach the contents with well-controlled, graded movements with his left hand. He could isolate his left index finger to poke. Throwing was possible with the left arm. He used his hands together for a variety of bilateral functions: combining objects, doing the same thing with both hands, and holding with one hand while manipulating with the other. His left hand rotated an object held by his right.

Delayed patterns (primary developmentally inappropriate): When combining objects, his wrists were flexed. He could not isolate his right index finger for poking. Throwing with the right arm alone was attempted, but because shoulder and elbow movement were limited, release (dropping) could be accomplished with wrist flexion only. He dropped an object using the primitive wrist flexion pattern in both left and right hands. Insufficient arm movement and no elbow movement also prevented free shaking movements. The left arm moved only through internal and external rotation at the shoulder, while the right arm moved appropriately up and down but in small ranges.

Atypical patterns (secondary developmentally inappropriate): All joints of the right upper extremity became totally flexed and shoulders elevated as he tried more difficult skills such as inverting a container to reach the contents, pushing and pulling, and poking with finger or thumb. During poking with the right index finger, he needed to stabilize on the surface with his thumb; his wrist was flexed, MCP joints hyperextended, and DP flexed. Poking with thumbs could be accomplished only by stabilizing other fingers on the surface. His fingers were abducted and extended when dropping objects with his right hand.

Implications for function: Patrick needs to invert the paintbrush container carefully to select a brush without spilling all of them. Isolated finger and thumb function, better in the left hand than the right, is needed in both hands for faster and more efficient use of keyboards, calculators, and the potter's wheel. Bilateral hand use includes combining objects (cap on pen), doing the same thing with both hands (carrying two beverage cans), holding with one hand while manipulating with the other (paper and pencil), and rotating with one hand to screw or unscrew the top of a jar held by the other hand. Dropping objects (a biscuit into his dog's mouth) is more accurate if wrist is in proper alignment. Shaking objects such as spraypaint cans requires free shoulder, elbow, and wrist movements. Some bilateral tasks, such as carrying a tray in the school lunchroom, will be difficult because of the added motor component of walking.

Hand/Vision Schema
Normal patterns (developmentally appropriate): Eye-hand coordination was generally consistent as Patrick maintained visual monitoring of each hand.

Delayed patterns (primary developmentally inappropriate): Patrick still needed to watch his hands with his eyes to achieve optimal function. He alternated visual monitoring from one hand to the other during bilateral activities.

Implications for function: Patrick needs to keep his eyes on his left hand when drawing and painting, and on his right hand when using the chalkboard eraser.

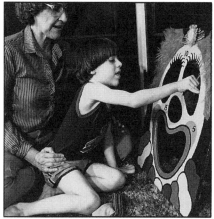

Figure 10.55. (photo by Sheldon Green)

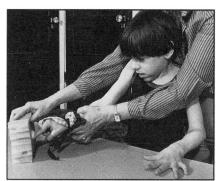

Figure 10.56. (photo by Sheldon Green)

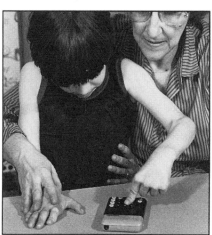

Figure 10.57. (photo by Sheldon Green)

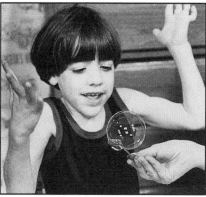

Figure 10.58. (photo by Sheldon Green)

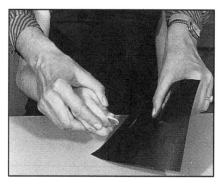

Figure 10.59. (photo by Sheldon Green)

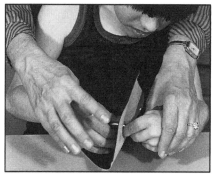

Figure 10.60. (photo by author)

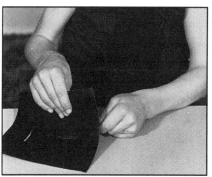

Figure 10.61. (photo by Sheldon Green)

Treatment Program

Patrick at 6

- Coordination of hand, sucking, and vision schemata can be remediated by encouraging Patrick to finger feed appropriate foods with the right hand while continuing spoon feeding with the left.

- Shaking of objects such as rhythm band instruments can be improved by preceding active movements with inhibition (rapid shaking) of entire arm. Patrick should visually monitor each hand alternately.

- Dropping and throwing objects with the right hand can be improved with a beanbag game. Patrick should side-sit, with pelvic stabilization if necessary (figure 10.55).

- Poking with the right index finger can be improved by using a pincher mitt, which keeps other fingers flexed (figure 10.56).

- Extension of the distal joint of the left poking finger while using a calculator can be improved with manual assistance, gradually reduced (figure 10.57).

- Active experimental manipulation within the visual field can include creative activities with soap bubbles (figure 10.58).

- The ability to manipulate an object with one hand while holding with the other can be improved by as much assistance as necessary in lead-up button activities using a large button and a leather square (figures 10.59 to 10.61).

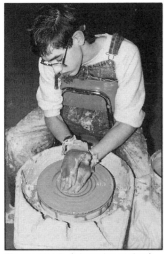

Figure 10.62. (photo by author)

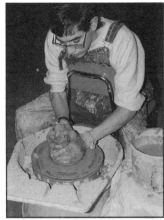

Figure 10.63. (photo by author)

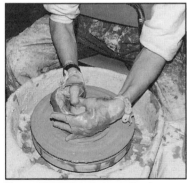

Figure 10.64. (photo by author)

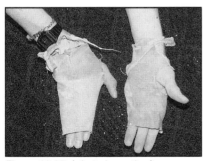

Figure 10.65. (photo by author)

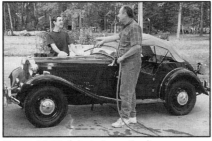

Figure 10.66. (photo by author)

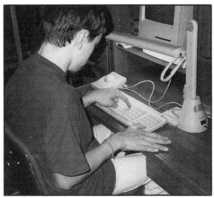

Figure 10.67. (photo by author)

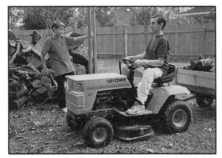

Figure 10.68. (photo by author)

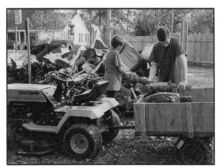

Figure 10.69. (photo by author)

Patrick at 16

- Pottery activities will improve accommodation, bilateral coordination, and hand/finger strength. Adapted leather gloves can help keep fingers in good alignment and as much hand surface as possible in contact with the material (figures 10.62 to 10.65).

- When helping his father wash the car, Patrick can use a large sponge fitting into the right hand for push/pull motions to increase range of motion and eye-hand coordination (figure 10.66).

- Poking (finger isolation) can be improved in the right hand, using a pincher mitt, so that both index fingers can be used for the computer keyboard, increasing speed (figure 10.67).

- Shaking spray-paint cans will increase shoulder and arm range of motion.

- Patrick develops upper extremity symmetry and bilaterality as he uses both hands on the steering wheel to drive the tractor and to help his brother load firewood (figures 10.68, 10.69).

2.h. Release of the Dowel or Cube (Supine, Prone, or Sitting)

Patrick at 6

The left hand demonstrated precise release into large or small containers, with wrist extension. Assistive release against a surface was functional, and transfer from left to right was adept. Patrick did not transfer objects smoothly from right to left, and released clumsily with his right wrist flexed above a surface or into a container. Assistive release was emerging in the right hand.

Patrick at 16

Normal patterns (developmentally appropriate): Patrick showed precise release with the left hand into a small container. Forearms were in midposition and wrists were straight during assistive release on a surface.

Delayed patterns (primary developmentally inappropriate): Precise release into both small and large containers was more difficult with the right hand because upper extremity joints did not have the flexibility to orient the objects. Both wrists were flexed when releasing against a surface (assistive release) in the pronated position. Transferring objects from one hand to the other was much better from left to right than from right to left.

Implications for function: Assistive release with wrist straight and forearm in midposition is used to place a cup on the table. Patrick needs precise release to place his books into the wire basket on his three-wheeled power scooter. Flexed wrists when the forearm is pronated (palm down) interfere with insertion of floppy disks into disk drives and envelopes into mail slots.

Section 2. Primarily Voluntary Movements (Cognitively Directed) **Patrick, Age 16**

Developmental Levels | Pattern Components | 2.h. Release of the Dowel or Cube (Supine, Prone, or Sitting)

Left | Right | L | R

Level		Description
12 months (+ / −)		Precise release into **small container** Wrists extended
10 months		Clumsy release into **small container**, rests hand on edge
9 months (+ / +)		Controlled release into **large container** Wrists straight
8 months		Clumsy release into **large container** or **above surface** Attempts unsuccessful release into **small container**
7 months		Voluntary assistive release **against surface** (stabilization) Attempts unsuccessful release into **large container** or **above surface** Adept 1-stage **transfer**, simultaneous grasp and release Object falls from hand as arm extends, forearm supinates, and fingers extend
6 months		Smooth 2-stage **transfer**: One hand grasps, other joins, first hand releases May use mouth as intermediary for **transfer**
5 months		Clumsy 2-stage **transfer**: One hand grasps, other joins, first hand releases with difficulty Voluntary release as object is removed by another
4 months		Mutual fingering in midline, preparation for **transfer**
3 months		Involuntary release after sustained grasp, with awareness (eyes alert)
2 months		Involuntary release after retaining briefly, with some awareness (eyes alert)
1 month		Immediate involuntary release, without awareness
Natal		No voluntary release, object must be forcibly removed, or: No grasp Wrists flexed *for certain tasks*

Developmental Hand Dysfunction

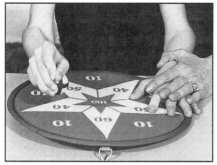

Figure 10.70. (photo by Sheldon Green)

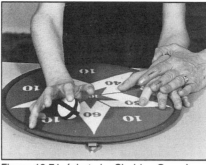

Figure 10.71. (photo by Sheldon Green)

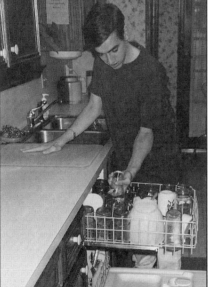

Figure 10.72. (photo by author)

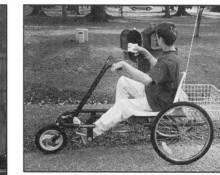

Figure 10.73. (photo by author)

Treatment Program

Patrick at 6

• Transfer of objects from right to left should be encouraged as much as possible.

• Assistive release with right hand should be continued to increase wrist extension and prepare for normal patterns during release above a surface and into a container (figures 10.70, 10.71.)

Patrick at 16

• If Patrick's trunk is stabilized against an appropriate surface and his opposite arm is either assisting or supporting, more forearm supination (palm up) and wrist extension are possible during release activities such as placing a glass into the dishwasher (figure 10.72) or a letter into the mailbox (figure 10.73).

Evaluation Report

2.i. Release of the Pellet (Sitting)

Patrick at 6
The left hand used a controlled release into a large container and a clumsy release into a small container, without wrist extension. Patrick was unable to transfer the pellet in either direction. His right hand released clumsily with flexed wrist into a large container but unsuccessfully into a small container.

Patrick at 16
Normal patterns (developmentally appropriate): Release into a large container was done easily by both hands.

Delayed patterns (primary developmentally inappropriate): Release into a small container was difficult for the left hand, with fingers resting on the edge for support; right-hand release was even more difficult, with index finger entering the container. Wrists were flexed.

Implications for function: Precise release is needed for putting pills into a small bottle or medication sorter.

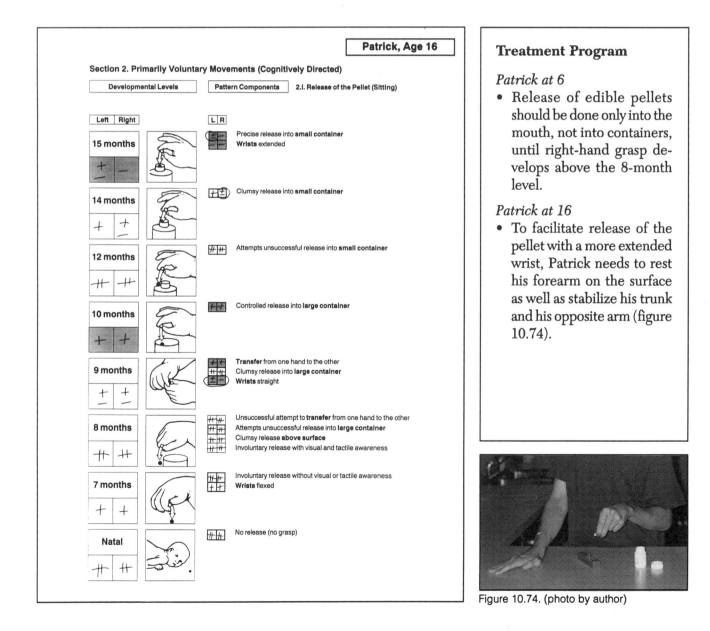

Patrick, Age 16

Section 2. Primarily Voluntary Movements (Cognitively Directed)

Developmental Levels   Pattern Components   2.i. Release of the Pellet (Sitting)

Left | Right   L | R

15 months — Precise release into **small container** / **Wrists** extended

14 months — Clumsy release into **small container**

12 months — Attempts unsuccessful release into **small container**

10 months — Controlled release into **large container**

9 months — **Transfer** from one hand to the other / Clumsy release into **large container** / **Wrists** straight

8 months — Unsuccessful attempt to **transfer** from one hand to the other / Attempts unsuccessful release into **large container** / Clumsy release **above surface** / Involuntary release with visual and tactile awareness

7 months — Involuntary release without visual or tactile awareness / **Wrists** flexed

No release (no grasp)

Natal

Treatment Program

Patrick at 6
- Release of edible pellets should be done only into the mouth, not into containers, until right-hand grasp develops above the 8-month level.

Patrick at 16
- To facilitate release of the pellet with a more extended wrist, Patrick needs to rest his forearm on the surface as well as stabilize his trunk and his opposite arm (figure 10.74).

Figure 10.74. (photo by author)

Section 3. Prewriting Skills (Left Hand)

Evaluation Report

3.a. Crayon or Pencil Grasp

Patrick at 6

Patrick's left hand used either a palmar-supinate or digital-pronate grasp of the pencil. Normal patterns were seen with the former, but the latter resulted in excessive pronation and ulnar deviation of the wrist (figure 5.5, page 50).

Patrick at 16

Normal patterns (developmentally appropriate): Patrick used a functionally appropriate, adapted grasp of the marker, held between index and middle finger and captured in the web space of the left hand. Normal adults and children use a variety of pencil grasps. Patrick's adaptation, which provides excellent stability of the utensil in the hand, is similar to the grip used for tiny drawings by the well-known artist of the *Where's Waldo?* books.

Delayed patterns (primary developmentally inappropriate): Patrick stabilized at his shoulder to move his left arm as a unit. He held an adapted paintbrush with a palmar-supinate grasp (fisted hand, with wrist slightly flexed and supinated away from midposition). He did not keep his arm on the surface to avoid smearing the paint, which provided freedom of mobility at the expense of stability (figure 10.75).

Implications for function: Writing, drawing, and painting utensils can be held with different grasps or have adapted handles to provide effective stability and mobility for function.

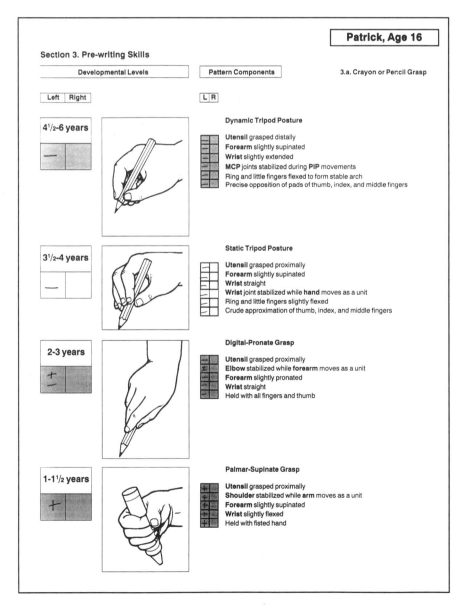

Section 3. Pre-writing Skills

Developmental Levels

| Left | Right |

Pattern Components

| L | R |

3.a. Crayon or Pencil Grasp

4½-6 years

Dynamic Tripod Posture
Utensil grasped distally
Forearm slightly supinated
Wrist slightly extended
MCP joints stabilized during **PIP** movements
Ring and little fingers flexed to form stable arch
Precise opposition of pads of thumb, index, and middle fingers

3½-4 years

Static Tripod Posture
Utensil grasped proximally
Forearm slightly supinated
Wrist straight
Wrist joint stabilized while **hand** moves as a unit
Ring and little fingers slightly flexed
Crude approximation of thumb, index, and middle fingers

2-3 years

Digital-Pronate Grasp
Utensil grasped proximally
Elbow stabilized while **forearm** moves as a unit
Forearm slightly pronated
Wrist straight
Held with all fingers and thumb

1-1½ years

Palmar-Supinate Grasp
Utensil grasped proximally
Shoulder stabilized while **arm** moves as a unit
Forearm slightly supinated
Wrist slightly flexed
Held with fisted hand

Patrick, Age 16

Treatment Program

Patrick at 6

- The palmar-supinate grasp should be used by the left hand for all prewriting activities until developmentally equivalent drawings are perfected. Similar activities by the right hand, such as drawing in a sand tray, can improve arm control without leading to writing, which may confuse dominance (figures 10.76, 10.77).

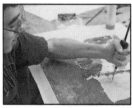

Figure 10.75. (photo by author)

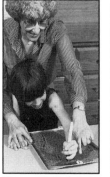

Figure 10.76. (photo by Sheldon Green)

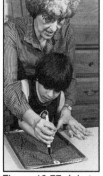

Figure 10.77. (photo by Sheldon Green)

Evaluation Report

3.b. Drawings

Patrick at 6

All skills were present at the 2½-year level with scatter to 4½ years. Patrick imitated vertical, horizontal, and circular strokes but had not perfected the circle, square, or cross. His tracing was not accurate.

Patrick at 16

Normal patterns (developmentally appropriate): Patrick produced perfect vertical and horizontal lines, a circle, cross, square, and triangle from memory, as well as copying and imitating examiner's productions. Patrick was able to trace a circle and diamond perfectly.

Delayed patterns (primary developmentally inappropriate): He could not draw a diamond from memory, and his imitation of a diamond drawing was imperfect.

Implications for function: Patrick's ability to trace well indicates excellent motor control. Reproduction of more difficult forms by imitation and from memory indicates some perceptual delays.

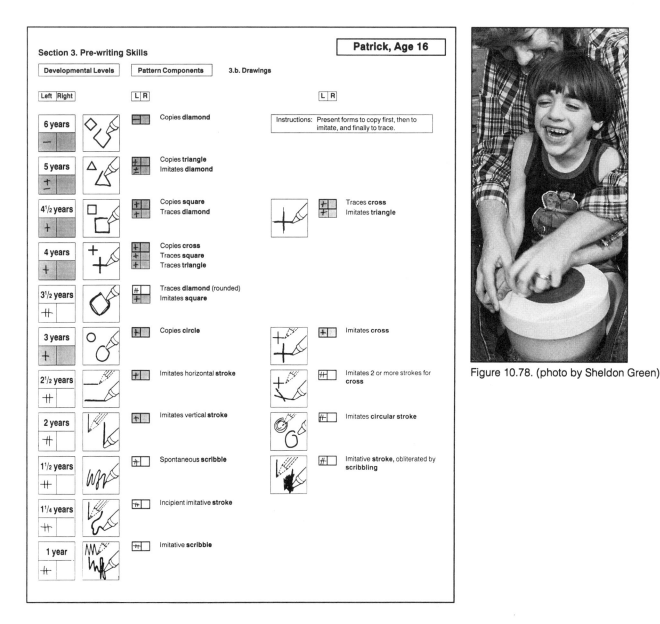

Figure 10.78. (photo by Sheldon Green)

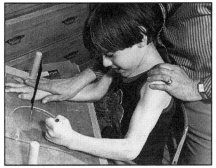

Figure 10.79. (photo by Sheldon Green; desk courtesy of Courtney Rotzien)

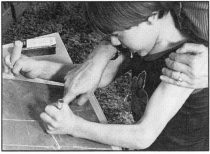

Figure 10.80. (photo by Sheldon Green; desk courtesy of Courtney Rotzien)

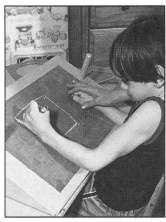

Figure 10.81. (photo by Sheldon Green; desk courtesy of Courtney Rotzien)

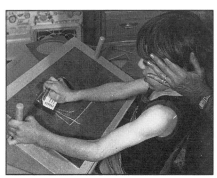

Figure 10.82. (photo by Sheldon Green; desk courtesy of Courtney Rotzien)

Treatment Program

Patrick at 6

- The salad spinner can be used to develop rhythmical circular movements, followed by independent use of the circle template as a guide. Patrick should stabilize his opposite hand either by grasping a dowel or keeping the hand flat on the surface (figures 10.78, 10.79).

- The ladder drawing activity (see page 133) can prepare for the square. Patrick should connect two dots placed on parallel vertical lines, first with manual and verbal assistance ("go" and "stop"), then verbal only (figure 10.80).

- The square can first be drawn with the template (page 133) as a guide, then traced, copied, and finally drawn from memory. Patrick's nondominant hand should do all the erasing, and his head should be in midline (figures 10.81, 10.82).

Patrick at 16

- Paper for writing, sketching, and painting should always be oriented for the left hand to allow Patrick visual access to his work. An easel or other inclined surface is also visually helpful because the surface is parallel to his face and eyes. When possible, Patrick should stabilize on the surface with elbow or entire forearm.

- Drawing exercises to improve concepts of diagonal lines and shapes (page 133) will improve Patrick's perceptual concepts of letters and words for reading as well as writing.

- Unstructured, abstract art work should be encouraged to give Patrick the opportunity to be creative and to refine eye-hand skills as he experiments with line, shape, and texture (figure 10.83).

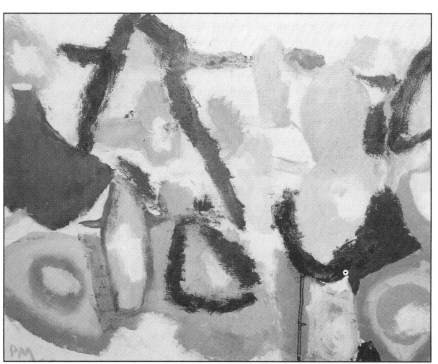

Figure 10.83. Original black and white painting by Patrick, age 16 (photo by author)

Summary and Conclusions

Patrick's difficulties with higher-level prehension skills can be traced to insufficient head control and shoulder stabilization. His compensatory patterns, such as shoulder elevation and retraction, became blocks to further development. Attempts to achieve skills out of sequence (developmentally inappropriate) resulted in atypical patterns such as grasping with flexed wrist, hyperextended MCP (knuckle) joints, and subluxed thumb.

Recommendations

Patrick's occupational therapy program should emphasize reduction of compensatory patterns of stabilization, improvement of midrange control, and facilitation of fine motor skills in developmental sequence.

Sample IEP (Individual Educational Plan) (Occupational Therapy Components)

Present Level of Function

Patrick's prehension skills showed a scatter of missing skills throughout the first 15 months of development, interfering with independence in educational, self-help, and play activities. Patrick's prewriting skills, including pencil grasp and drawing, were at a 2½- to 4½-year developmental level.

Goals and Objectives
Goal #1
To improve prehension skills to increase independence in the school environment

Objective 1.1
Patrick will be able to catch himself with his hands to protect his head from injury when losing his balance from a sitting position nine out of ten times.

Objective 1.2
Patrick will be able to shake a rhythm band instrument (such as maracas) with shoulder, elbow, and wrist motion ten times in ten seconds with the left hand, and with shoulder and elbow motion five times in ten seconds with the right hand.

Objective 1.3
Patrick will be able to throw a beanbag into a container at a 3-foot distance with 90% accuracy with his left hand and at a 1-foot distance with 75% accuracy with his right hand.

Objective 1.4
Patrick will be able to press number buttons on a calculator from 1 to 10 in sequence with 100% accuracy and with his left index finger straight.

Goal #2
To improve pencil grasp and drawing skills related to writing

Objective 2.1
Patrick will use the palmar-supinate grasp of the pencil with his left hand to trace a square within ¹/16″ accuracy.

Objective 2.2
Patrick will use the palmar-supinate grasp of the pencil to copy a circle with accurate closure nine out of ten times.

Summary and Conclusions

Patrick's hands are extremely functional, and he is independent in most activities in home, school, and community environments, but he has difficulty with certain tasks because of developmental motor delays and compensatory atypical patterns. Persistent involuntary reflexes sometimes interfere with voluntary movements. Patrick's type of athetoid cerebral palsy with spasticity causes slow, stiff movements throughout his body and occasional slight involuntary movements in his hands. Although Patrick uses both hands spontaneously for necessary bilateral tasks, much of his right-hand function is underdeveloped because of insufficient practice during his early years. During that time when he preferred his more efficient left hand, the gap between skill levels widened, causing even greater motivation to use his left more than his right. Many high-level skills, however, require equal skill in both hands. Asymmetries are still present throughout his body, but to a much lesser degree than formerly, because of ongoing therapy, with emphasis on the NDT (Neuro-Developmental Treatment) approach.

Recommendations

Occupational therapy and physical therapy with continued NDT emphasis is recommended to improve total body symmetry, fine motor function, and perceptual skills.

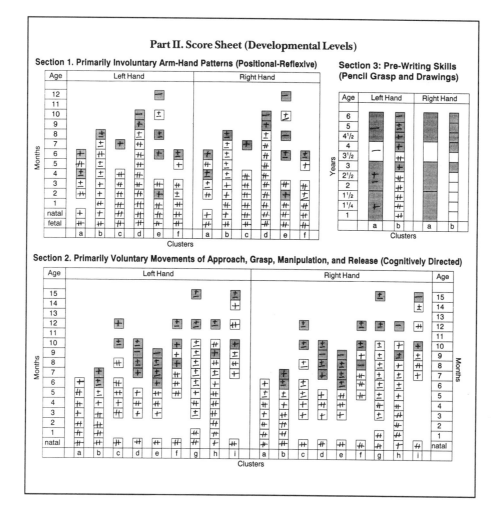

Sample ITP (Individual Transition Plan) Occupational Therapy Components

Present Level of Function: Patrick is able to participate *independently* in the following activities: walking short distances, driving a powered three-wheel scooter, pedaling a bicycle, dressing and eating, and operating a computer with keyboard and trackball.

With appropriate adaptations to compensate for physical limitations, he also participates in gardening, printing his name, oil painting and pottery, housekeeping and cooking, and sports (badminton, basketball, biking, bowling, cross-country skiing, golf, horseback riding, and weight lifting).

Area #1. Competitive employment

School Action: Teach vocational curriculum, with emphasis on computer data entry.

Family Action: Investigate possibilities of starting a family landscape business.

Objective 1.1
Patrick will use his right index finger equally as well as his left to type on the computer keyboard, doubling his speed, by the end of the school year.

Area #2. Independent living

School Action: Teach daily living skills, including balancing checkbook.

Family Action: Allocate increasing responsibilities to Patrick (for example, managing his own money).

Objective 2.1
Patrick will learn to take a handful of coins from his pocket with one hand and select the ones he needs with the other hand.

Chapter Eleven
Kristy
Evaluation and Treatment
Transition from Childhood to Adulthood

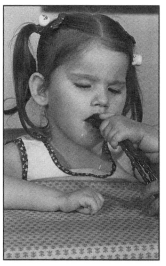

Date: 12-29-81

To: Whom it may concern

Re: Occupational therapy evaluation for Kristy C.

This 3½-year-old female with a diagnosis of hypotonia with spasticity was re-evaluated today in her home to update her occupational therapy program and pinpoint specific gaps in prehension development interfering with the progression of milestones. Kristy is presently attending a preschool program for children with special needs. Her mother assisted with administration, observation, and historical information.

The Erhardt Developmental Prehension Assessment (EDPA) was used to measure arm-hand patterns from the fetal and natal periods to 15 months, when the essential components of prehension are developed and functional. Because further refinement, increased skill, and the use of tools are the result of learned experiences, the 15-month level can be considered the maturity of prehension and thus an approximate norm for assessing older children.

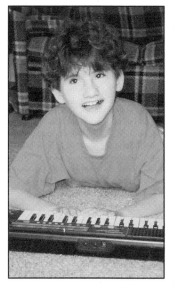

Date: 4-15-92

To: Whom it may concern

Re: Occupational therapy evaluation for Kristy C.

This 14-year-old female with a diagnosis of hypotonia with spasticity was re-evaluated today in her home with the Erhardt Developmental Prehension Assessment (EDPA) to determine hand function relating to educational performance now and future function in secondary transition areas of:

- home and independent living: self-care (feeding, dressing, bathing, grooming)
- recreation and leisure: music, television
- community participation: mobility through transitions (weight bearing, stabilizing)
- post-secondary learning opportunities: switch operation (indicating needs and choices, general communication)

Kristy resides with her parents and older sister and attends a class for individuals with severe and multiple handicaps in a public junior high school.

Kristy was evaluated for head, arm, and hand function in various positions: supine (on her back), prone (on her stomach), and sitting (in her wheelchair, which provided support up to midback). Her occupational therapist and her mother contributed historical and observational information.

Section 1. Primarily Involuntary Arm-Hand Patterns (Positional-Reflexive)

Evaluation Report

1.a. The Arms at Rest and during Body Play (Supine)

Kristy at 3¹/2

Missing skills were observed in both arms. Because of hypotonia originating at birth, Kristy had never experienced physiological flexion. Her arms had never been adducted and flexed nor her hands fisted. She had never brought hands to knees, hands to feet, or feet to mouth, patterns that elongate the neck and prepare for head lifting. Kristy was beginning to roll to prone, toward the left better than toward the right. She was beginning to lift her head in midline with chin tucked. She could bring both hands to mouth.

Kristy at 14

Normal patterns (developmentally appropriate): In supine Kristy was able to lift her head in midline, separately from shoulders, with good neck elongation. Intentional hands-to-face and body movements included rubbing face, eyes, behind ears, top of head. She was able to roll to her left side, especially when tired.

Delayed patterns (primary developmentally inappropriate): At rest, her arms were internally rotated, hands clutching on chest, with hands open and thumbs out. She did not lift her arms against gravity to bring hands together in space. Immature patterns

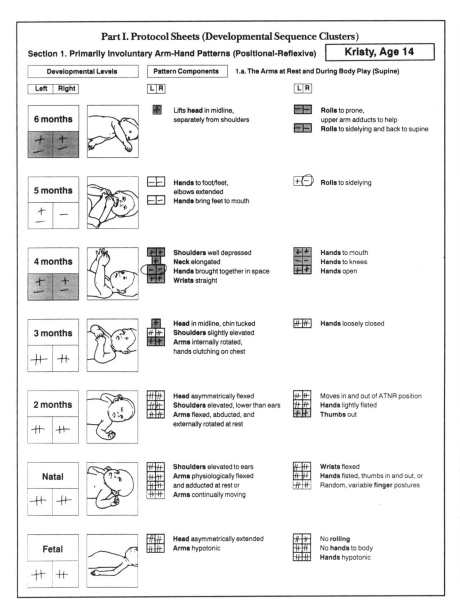

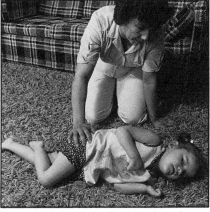

Figure 11.1. (photo by Sheldon Green)

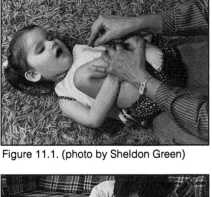

Figure 11.2. (photo by Sheldon Green)

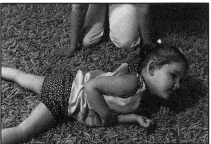

Figure 11.3. (photo by Sheldon Green)

included fingers in mouth (alternate hands) and repetitive wrist movements of patting chest (especially left hand).

Implications for function: Excellent head control in supine allows Kristy to cooperate in dressing and prevents injury when falling from sitting, especially backward. Interlocking of hands, resting arms on chest, and limited arm movements in space are signs of her need for stability and lack of strength against gravity. Movement of hands to face and body make possible a variety of grooming skills such as face washing, bathing, hair brushing, shampooing, and applying lotion or powder. Ability to roll means she can change position in bed independently. Difficulty lifting her arms prevents full participation in dressing, however; she presently cooperates by bending elbow only to insert her hand into the sleeve after a visual cue of caregiver's hand placed in sleeve. Immature, stereotypic hand patterns, observed during periods without structured activity, indicate Kristy's need for sensory input, which she fulfills in age-inappropriate ways.

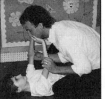
Figure 11.4. (photo by author)

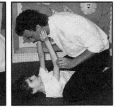
Figure 11.5. (photo by author)

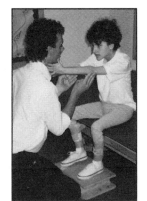
Figure 11.6. (photo by author)

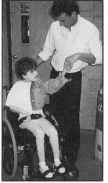
Figure 11.7. (photo by author)

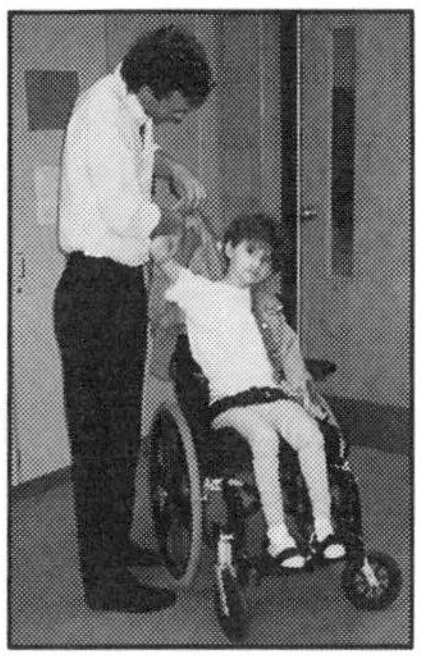

Figure 11.8. (photo by author)

Treatment Program

Kristy at 3½

- In supine, Kristy should be assisted in grasping her flexed knees while lifting her head to reach for food (figure 11.1).

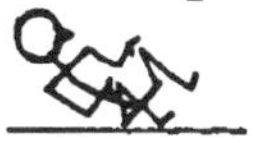

- Kristy's mother can assist her in rolling from supine to prone by rotating the hip of her flexed upper leg and by protracting her shoulder if necessary (figures 11.2, 11.3).

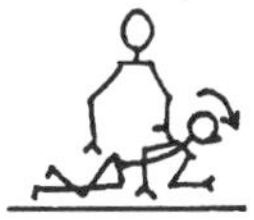

Kristy at 14

- Arm movements related to dressing skills

  - To improve arm extension against gravity, Kristy will be encouraged to reach for her therapist's face from supine (figures 11.4, 11.5) and sitting (figure 11.6). He can place his face in a variety of positions to stimulate increasing range of motion and strength for Kristy's forward, sideward, and upward arm movements as he reduces his manual assistance.

  - In sitting, because Kristy's left arm is tighter than her right, the left arm needs to be inserted into her jacket sleeve first, with her cooperation in extending it forward (figure 11.7). Her right arm is then moved upward and backward to insert into the other sleeve (figure 11.8). Removing the jacket is easiest when her right arm is removed first.

Evaluation Report

1.b. The Arms at Rest and during Head Raising (Prone)

Kristy at 3¹/2

Missing skills were observed in both arms. Kristy had never experienced natal physiological flexion, arms adducted and flexed under the body, which provides stability for beginning head control. She had rarely been placed in the prone position and was still most comfortable with her arms at her sides. She was able to maintain the forearm position with elbows flexed and behind the shoulders for a short time, but when raising her head, her shoulders and arms retracted, right more than left.

Rolling to supine independently was accomplished with a total extension pattern. When assisted in flexing her upper leg and keeping her arms forward, Kristy was able to use some lateral head righting but no neck flexion.

Kristy at 14

Kristy was observed first for independent positioning and movement, and then facilitated at higher antigravity levels.

Normal patterns (developmentally appropriate): In prone, without assistance, she could lift her head above shoulder level. When placed with her arms at her sides or forward, she could push up on forearms (elbows flexed and posterior to shoulders). Hands were open, with thumbs out, on ulnar or palmar surfaces, with good arch integrity. When a mirror was used to facilitate downward gaze, she showed improved head control.

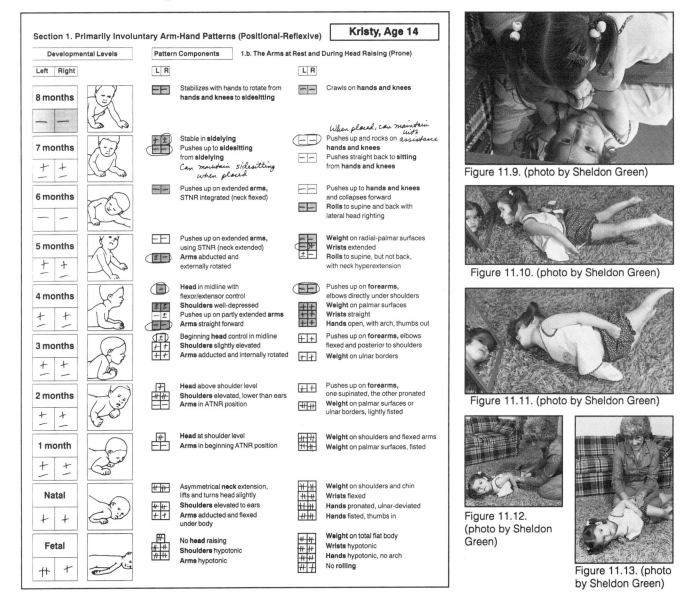

Figure 11.9. (photo by Sheldon Green)

Figure 11.10. (photo by Sheldon Green)

Figure 11.11. (photo by Sheldon Green)

Figure 11.12. (photo by Sheldon Green)

Figure 11.13. (photo by Sheldon Green)

Delayed patterns (primary developmentally inappropriate): In prone, without assistance, she was not able to move her arms from under her body. Less internal rotation of the arms was evident, but arms were not yet straight forward. She used neck hyperextension to push up on her left forearm and a partly extended right arm and, with manual assistance, roll to her left side, a stable resting position. She could not push up to hands and knees or to sitting but could maintain those positions with moderate assistance after being placed.

Atypical patterns (secondary developmentally inappropriate): Winging of shoulder blades due to shoulder girdle instability and inactive abdominal muscles was observed when weight bearing in prone without facilitation.

Implications for function: Although Kristy has limited function in the prone position, therapy emphasizing head control and weight bearing on the arms (forearms, extended arms, hands and knees) is very effective for development of shoulder and arm stability needed for all hand function.

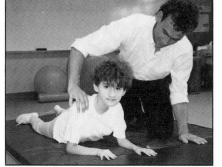

Figure 11.14. (photo by author)

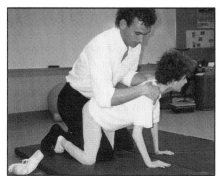

Figure 11.15. (photo by author)

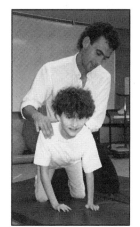

Figure 11.16. (photo by author)

Treatment Program

Kristy at 3¹/₂

- In prone on forearms over mother's lap, elbows internally rotated and adducted, hands lightly fisted, Kristy can improve flexor-extensor head control in midline and neck elongation by raising her head slowly to see herself in a mirror. Her pelvis should be stabilized to prevent excessive hip abduction and extension (figure 11.9).

- In prone on flexed arms or forearms, Kristy can be assisted in roll- ing without the total extension pattern by flexing her upper leg as she pushes off with forearm or hand, using lateral head righting (figures 11.10 to 11.13).

Kristy at 14

- Upper extremity weight bearing related to independent sitting

  - Shoulder, elbow, and wrist stability can be facilitated in a variety of prone positions (forearms [figure 11.14], hands and knees [figures 11.15, 11.16]), emphasizing good postural alignment, with minimal to maximal assistance, as needed, and combined with transitions to and from sitting, using Neuro-Developmental Treatment (NDT) techniques.

  - Independent side-sitting, important in community social settings (figure 11.17), can best be accomplished when Kristy is placed with both hands supporting on the surface and arms externally, not internally, rotated.

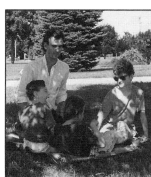

Figure 11.17. (photo by author)

Evaluation Report

1.c. Asymmetrical Tonic Neck Reflex (ATNR)

Kristy at 3¹/₂

Kristy had never experienced this primitive reflex, which provides the infant with beginning hand regard in supine and beginning stability during asymmetrical head raising in prone.

Kristy at 14

Normal patterns (developmentally appropriate): This reflex had never been experienced by Kristy because of persistent hypotonia in her early years.

Implications for function: Kristy's voluntary movements are not contaminated by this reflex, which results in obligatory head/arm movements when active.

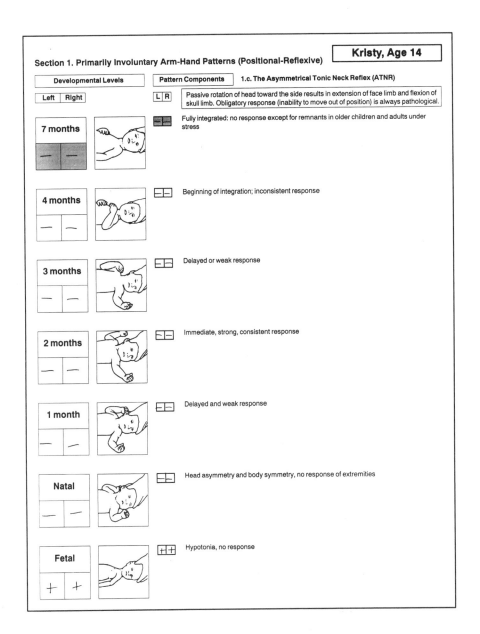

Evaluation Report

1.d. Grasping Reactions

Kristy at 3¹/₂

Because of hypotonia, Kristy had never experienced the Grasp Reflex, but through recent stimulation with therapeutic activities, she was beginning to respond to tug-of-war by catching and holding, phases of the fully developed Grasp Reflex, with synergistic (total) flexion. Instinctive Grasp Reactions were not observed.

Kristy at 14

Delayed patterns (primary developmentally inappropriate): The Grasp Reflex appears to be fully developed (firm stimulus in radial side of palm results in sudden finger flexion followed by sustained flexion when resisted), left hand stronger than right. The Instinctive Grasp Reaction was also present on the left as she involuntarily oriented (turned hand over) and groped (moved toward the stimulus) when her eyes were occluded. Without eyes occluded, she demonstrated an immediate eye/head turn toward the tactile stimulus on her left hand only.

Implications for function: The Grasp Reflex, which was not present at earlier ages, helps Kristy sustain grasp on objects for bringing to her mouth (spoon) and manipulating (shaking maracas). The Instinctive Grasp Reaction, also just emerging, can prepare wrist and hand for graceful voluntary movements. If not eventually integrated, however, these reflexive patterns can interfere with voluntary release and precise manipulation. Improvement in voluntary skills helps decrease involuntary movements.

Section 1. Primarily Involuntary Arm-Hand Patterns (Positional-Reflexive) — **Kristy, Age 14**

1.d. Grasping Reactions

Note: Test in supine or with vision occluded to prevent contamination by voluntary movements.

Developmental Levels | **Pattern Components**

| Left | Right |

| L | R | | Instinctive Grasp Reaction: Light distally moving stimulus / Grasp Reflex: Firmly inserted stimulus |

| 10 months | | **Instinctive Grasp Reaction:** Integrated, stimulus withdrawn from **radial** side of palm results in voluntary, not involuntary movement |

| 9 months | | **Grasp Reflex:** Integrated, stimulus in **radial** side of palm results in voluntary, not involuntary grasp |

| 8 months | | **Instinctive Grasp Reaction, trapping stage:** Stimulus withdrawn from **radial** side of palm results in involuntary orienting, groping, and finally grasping |

| 7 months | + / − | **Instinctive Grasp Reaction, groping stage:** Stimulus on **ulnar** border of hand results in involuntary pronation and movement toward stimulus |

| 6 months | + / − | **Instinctive Grasp Reaction, groping stage:** Stimulus on **radial** border of hand results in involuntary supination and movement toward stimulus / **Grasp Reflex:** Beginning integration, weakening involuntary response to stimulus in **radial** side of palm |

| 5 months | + / − | **Instinctive Grasp Reaction, orienting stage:** stimulus on **ulnar** border of hand results in involuntary pronation |

| 4 months | + / − | **Instinctive Grasp Reaction, orienting stage:** Stimulus on **radial** border of hand results in involuntary supination |

| 3 months | + / + | **Grasp Reflex:** Fully developed, stimulus in **radial** side of palm results in the **Catching phase:** Sudden finger flexion followed by the **Holding phase:** Sustained flexion when resisted |

| 2 months | ++ / ++ | **Grasp Reflex:** Stimulus in **radial** side of palm results in thumb and all fingers flexion and adduction, followed by synergistic flexion of entire extremity |

| 1 month | ++ / ++ | **Grasp Reflex:** Stimulus in **radial** side of palm results in thumb and index finger flexion and adduction, followed by synergistic flexion of entire extremity |

| Natal | ++ / ++ | **Grasp Reflex:** Stimulus in **ulnar** side of palm combined with traction results in involuntary grasp of middle, ring, little, and index fingers, and thumb in sequence, and synergistic flexion of entire extremity (lifting body weight) |

| Fetal | ++ / + | **Grasp Reflex:** Stimulus in **ulnar** side of palm results in slight or no involuntary grasp / **Instinctive Grasp Reaction:** No response to stimulus |

Treatment Program

Kristy at 3¹/₂

- Sitting in mother's lap, Kristy's wrist can be given joint compression before tug-of-war activities with the dowel, elbow flexed as well as extended (figures 11.18 to 11.20).

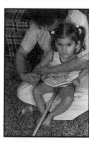

Figure 11.18. (photo by Sheldon Green)

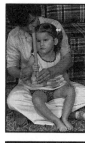

Figure 11.19. (photo by Sheldon Green)

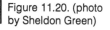

Figure 11.20. (photo by Sheldon Green)

Evaluation Report

1.e. Placing Responses

Kristy at 3¹/₂

Because of hypotonia, Kristy had never experienced the Proprioceptive Placing responses (brushing back of hand against table edge resulting in involuntary placing of hand on surface), which are normally present at birth and integrated at 2 months. Protective Extensor Thrust, stimulated from sitting, was beginning to emerge in the left arm but not in the right.

Kristy at 14

Normal patterns (developmentally appropriate): Proprioceptive Placing was not observed.

Delayed patterns (primary developmentally inappropriate): Protective Extensor Thrust stimulated from sitting was not present (arms remained flexed instead of extending) when Kristy was suddenly moved forward or sideward.

Implications for function: Protective responses, which emerge developmentally at the same time as independent sitting and weight bearing on extended arms, protect the head during falls.

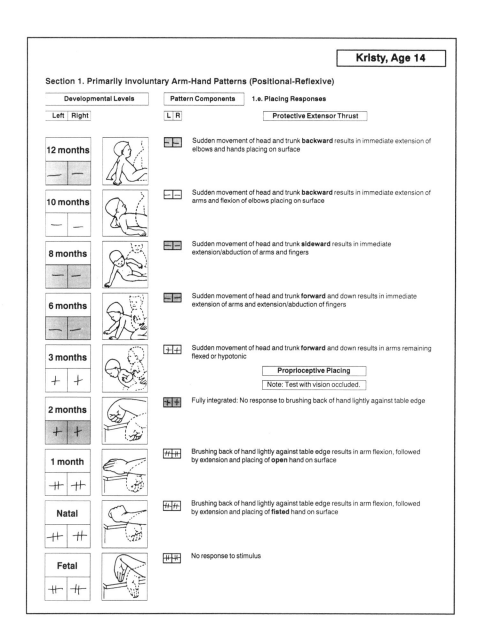

Evaluation Report

1.f. Avoiding Responses

Kristy at 3¹/₂

Kristy had not experienced these reactions in the early months of her life, probably because of a high threshold to tactile stimulation. However, a distally moving stimulus to the back of the hand and fingers now resulted in finger extension and abduction, wrist extension, and elbow flexion, stronger in the left. Automatic opening and closing of fingers was observed frequently.

Kristy at 14

Normal patterns (developmentally appropriate): Kristy showed a slight response (spreading of fingers) to a distally moving light stimulus on the back of her hand, left more than right.

Implications for function: This automatic response helps reduce the Grasp Reflex and open the hand during normal development. It decreases as voluntary control increases. If not eventually integrated, however, it interferes with sustained voluntary grasp and precise manipulation. Improvement in voluntary skills helps decrease involuntary movements.

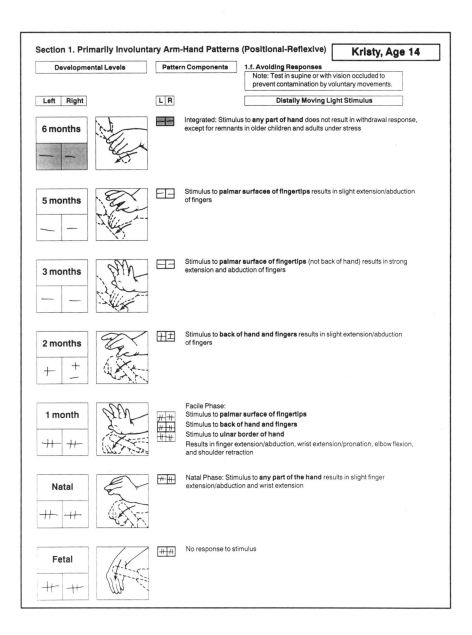

Section 2. Primarily Voluntary Movements (Cognitively Directed)

Evaluation Report

2.a. The Arms on Approach (Supine)

Kristy at 3¹/2
Kristy used a unilateral circular approach with elbows extended, wrists straight, and excessive finger extension. She contacted the object only, with open or partly open hands. Kristy had never used a consistent bilateral approach nor reached with one hand while the other joined.

Kristy at 14
Normal patterns (developmentally appropriate): Kristy demonstrated random hand movements unrelated to a stimulus and limited voluntary arm movements. However, her arms activated in response to a stimulus, or, less frequently, random arm movements ceased in response to a stimulus as she visually attended. Manual cuing (upper arm assistance) facilitated voluntary reaching toward her therapist's face, for example (figure 11.5, page 175). She used a unilateral circular approach, easier to the side. Her elbows usually stayed flexed, so contact was accomplished with objects no more than 8" to 10" away. Her hands were open or partly open, but wrists were flexed during approach, and she often underreached, then corrected to corral the object.

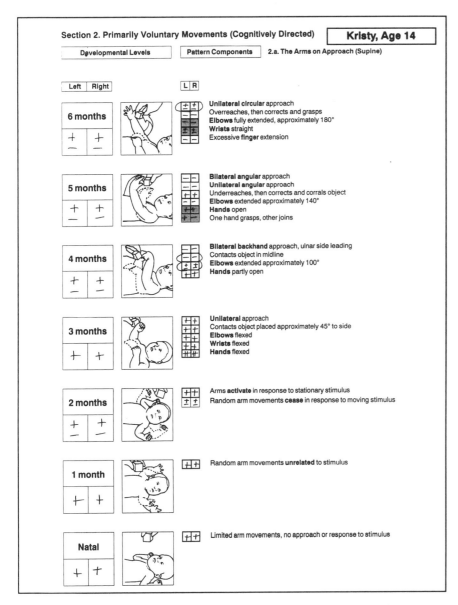

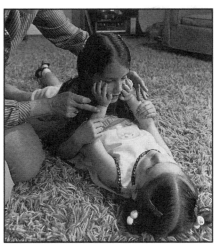

Figure 11.21. (photo by Sheldon Green)

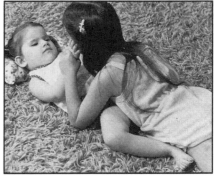

Figure 11.22. (photo by Sheldon Green)

Developmental Hand Dysfunction

Implications for function: Since Kristy's limited mobility and arm strength do not allow her to reach objects more than a few inches away, she has not had the opportunity to gain information through her hands as much as through her eyes and her ears. Yet the desire for movement is present in her arms and hands. She has demonstrated motivation and some ability to adjust arm/hand movement to contact an object, as well as interest in putting her hand into a sleeve (figure 11.7, page 175).

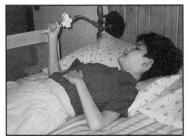

Figure 11.23. (photo by author)

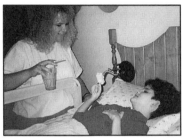

Figure 11.24. (photo by author)

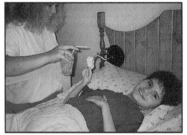

Figure 11.25. (photo by author)

Treatment Program

Kristy at 3¹/₂
- Supine with head on pillow to encourage chin tucking, Kristy should reach for her sister's face with both hands, an early infant-caregiver pattern she had missed (figures 11.21, 11.22).

Kristy at 14
- Reaching and pushing switches for communication and environmental control

  - An adapted switch alarm system can be used for Kristy to call her caregiver for help, a drink, or other attention. It can be mounted on the headboard of her bed, with a gooseneck connection for appropriate placement overhead as she lies supine (figures 11.23 to 11.25).

  - Adapted switches can also be used to operate a VCR or TV for music videos which Kristy enjoys. At home Kristy can be placed on her right side on the couch, with her left hand operating the switch (figure 11.26). If possible, sidelying on her left side should be attempted also, to encourage right-hand use.

  - As Kristy becomes aware of the cause-and-effect power of switch use, she can be introduced to appropriate computer programs which can lead to increased communication and learning (figure 11.27).

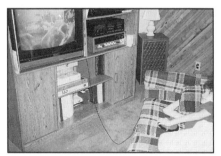

Figure 11.26. (photo by author)

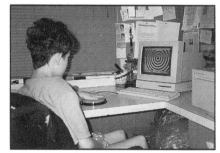

Figure 11.27. (photo by author)

Evaluation Report

2.b. The Arms on Approach (Prone)

Kristy at 3¹/₂
Kristy had had limited experience in prone and did not try to reach in this position, either bilaterally or unilaterally. Some weight shifting was seen with arms at side but not forward.

Kristy at 14
Delayed patterns (primary developmentally inappropriate): When placed with her weight on her right arm and side, Kristy was able to slide her left arm on the floor to contact an object with her open hand a few inches away. She was not able to use the right arm in the same manner.

Implications for function: Reaching in this position is easier than moving the arm against gravity, since the surface provides support and tactile input. This prone position could be used during therapy to improve accuracy and range of motion, especially in the right arm, for carryover into her more functional sitting position.

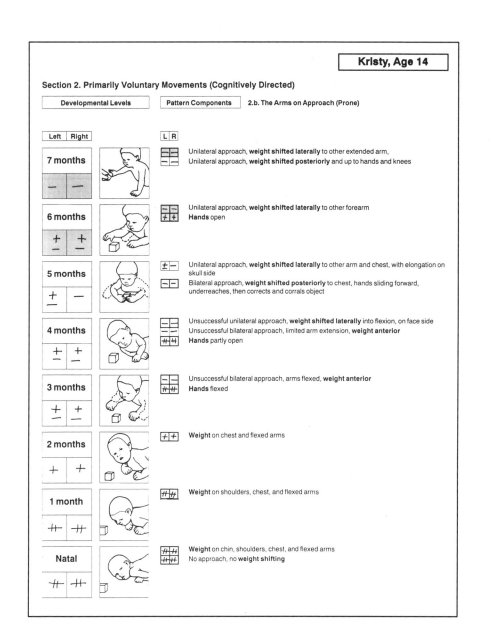

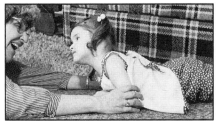

Figure 11.28. (photo by Sheldon Green)

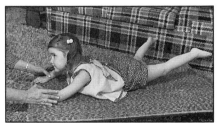

Figure 11.29. (photo by Sheldon Green)

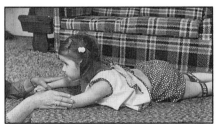

Figure 11.30. (photo by Sheldon Green)

Treatment Program

Kristy at 3¹/₂

- Weight shifting with arms adducted and flexed as well as forward should be done on a rocker board to prepare 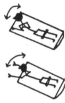 for reaching with one arm while bearing weight on other arm and chest. Kristy's legs may need to be strapped together at first to prevent the total extension-abduction pattern (figures 11.28 to 11.30).

Evaluation Report

2.c. The Arms on Approach (Sitting)

Kristy at 3^1/$_2$

Kristy used an emerging unilateral circular approach, with elbow extended, wrist straight, and excessive finger extension. She contacted and pushed an object only with open or partly open hand. Kristy had never used a bilateral approach and did not reach consistently with either hand.

Kristy at 14

Delayed patterns (primary developmentally inappropriate): Kristy used a unilateral approach to contact an object placed a few inches away at the side, with elbows flexed and wrists straight or very extended as she tried to grasp. Her forearms were pronated or in mid-position, and her hands open or partly open. She corralled her water bottle to bring it closer for her mouth to take the straw. She could lift her right arm easily, but not her left, and used some elbow and excessive wrist motion primarily with both left and right to adjust hand placement for grasp. She was also observed once reaching across midline to her right side with her left hand, but reaching for an object in midline was generally too difficult. Bilateral reaching was not observed, but Kristy could sustain bilateral grasp on an ice cream cup placed in her hands and bring it to her mouth if her elbows were provided with support.

Implications for function: Normally, the shoulder and elbow joints transport the hand to the precise place

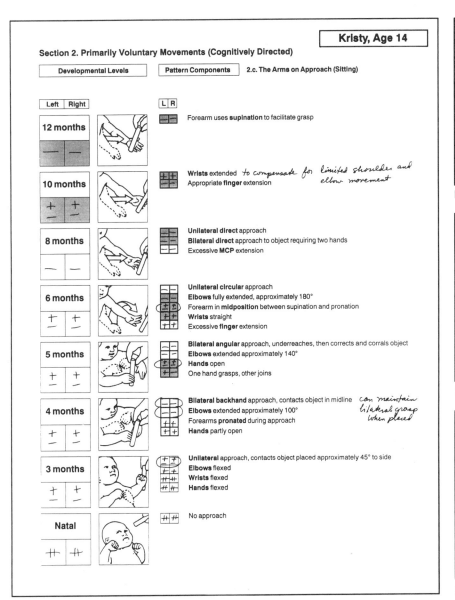

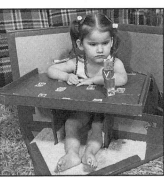

Figure 11.31. (photo by Sheldon Green)

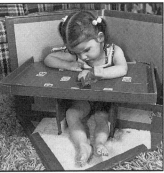

Figure 11.32. (photo by Sheldon Green)

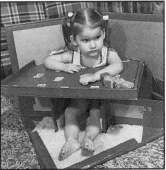

Figure 11.33. (photo by Sheldon Green)

necessary for grasp. Since limited shoulder movement and poorly graded elbow control interferes with the accuracy of Kristy's hand placement, she compensates with excessive wrist extension to achieve grasp. Increased shoulder and elbow movement and control are needed to allow more functional reaching and grasping for self-help skills such as feeding. Bilateral function is necessary for transitions such as stabilizing hands on caregiver's shoulders or chair arms during sit/stand/sit.

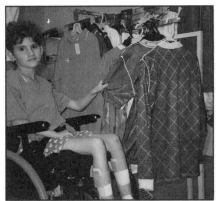

Figure 11.34. (photo by author)

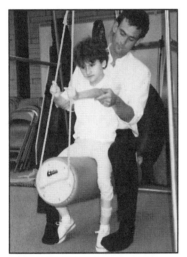

Figure 11.35. (photo by author)

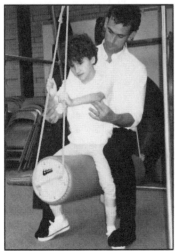

Figure 11.36. (photo by author)

Treatment Program

Kristy at 3¹/₂

Sitting at an adapted desk constructed of four-ply cardboard, consistent unilateral approach to the side can be improved by encouraging Kristy to knock down a tower of blocks (figures 11.31 to 11.33).

Kristy at 14

- Reaching to indicate choices and use of hands for transitions

    - Hand pointing as well as eye pointing could be encouraged for choices such as food or clothes (figure 11.34), since Kristy has demonstrated the ability to reach, grasp, and pull a tablecloth off a table.

    - While receiving vestibular stimulation sitting on the bolster swing during therapy, realistic fear of falling can motivate Kristy to grasp the ropes of the swing with both hands, after first being cued by her therapist (figures 11.35, 11.36).

    - Kristy should be encouraged to use both hands together for transitions, such as stabilizing her hands on caregiver's shoulders or on chair arms during sit/stand/sit (figures 11.37, 11.38).

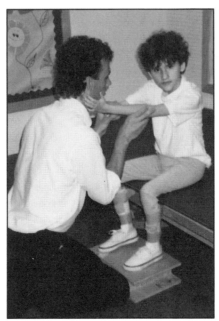

Figure 11.37. (photo by author)

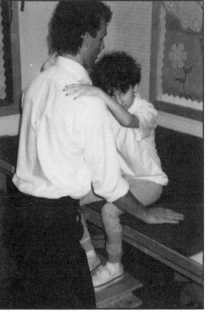

Figure 11.38. (photo by author)

Evaluation Report

2.d. Grasp of the Dowel (Supine, Prone, or Sitting)

Kristy at 3½

Kristy could sustain a voluntary grasp when an object was placed in the ulnar side of her hand, left better than right, and was beginning to develop the primitive squeeze grasp (contact results in hand pulling object back to squeeze precariously against other hand or body, minimal thumb involvement).

Kristy at 14

Delayed patterns (primary developmentally inappropriate): An important new skill is Kristy's ability to combine reach and grasp. She was formerly able only to reach and contact an object or maintain grasp if it was placed in her hand. She still needs facilitation (placement in space or in her hand) to use most efficient grasps: the radial-palmar grasp (object held with fingers and opposed thumb) or the palmar grasp (object held with fingers and adducted thumb). When reaching and grasping independently, however, her usual grasp was the primitive squeeze grasp.

Implications for function: Since correct hand placement in preparation for grasp is difficult for Kristy, her best dowel grasp for spoon or finger food (beef jerky, cookie biscuit, fruit or chocolate rolls) is achieved when the object is placed into her hand or oriented in space for her to grasp.

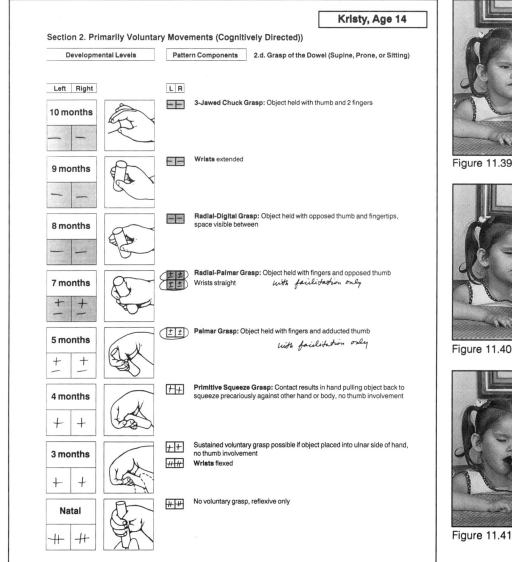

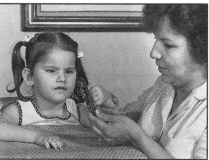

Figure 11.39. (photo by Sheldon Green)

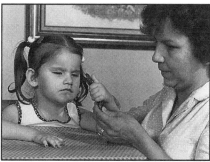

Figure 11.40. (photo by Sheldon Green)

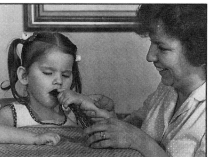

Figure 11.41. (photo by Sheldon Green)

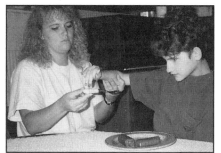

Figure 11.42. photo by author)

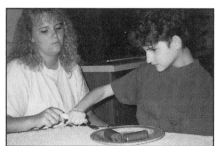

Figure 11.43. (photo by author)

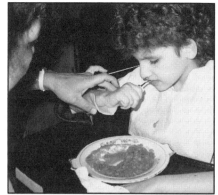

Figure 11.45. (photo by author)

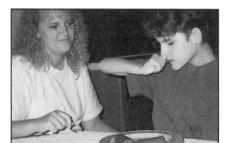

Figure 11.44. (photo by author)

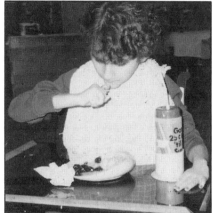

Figure 11.46. (photo by author)

Treatment Program

Kristy at 3¹/₂

- The primitive squeeze grasp can be improved by mother placing food 1" from Kristy's hand and waiting for her to reach, grasp, and pull it to her mouth (figures 11.39 to 11.41).

Kristy at 14

- Grasp of food and utensils while sitting in the wheelchair

  - To encourage the most functional hand position and independent grasp rather than totally passive placement, Kristy's caregiver can present the spoon or dowel-shaped finger food in the correct orientation (horizontally in space), rather than on the table. Support can be given at the elbow or the wrist as needed (figures 11.42 to 11.45).

  - The tall cup can be placed where Kristy can actively corral it with her left hand, bringing it close enough to drink independently from the straw (figure 11.46).

Evaluation Report

2.e. Grasp of the Cube (Supine, Prone, or Sitting)

Kristy at 3½

Kristy could sustain a voluntary grasp when an object was placed in the ulnar side of her hand, left better than right, and was beginning to develop the primitive squeeze grasp (contact results in hand pulling object back to squeeze precariously against other hand or body, no thumb involvement).

Kristy at 14

Delayed patterns (primary developmentally inappropriate): As in the dowel grasp, Kristy's most efficient cube grasps were the radial-palmar grasp (fingers on far side of object press it against opposed thumb and radial side of palm), or the palmar grasp (fingers on top surface of object press it into center of palm, thumb adducted), which were possible only if the object was placed into her hand. When reaching and grasping independently, however, her usual grasp was the primitive squeeze grasp.

Implications for function: Dowel shapes rather than cubes are easier for the caregiver to present and for Kristy to hold, and are usually more functionally common (spoon, food, hairbrush, hair spray bottle, maracas).

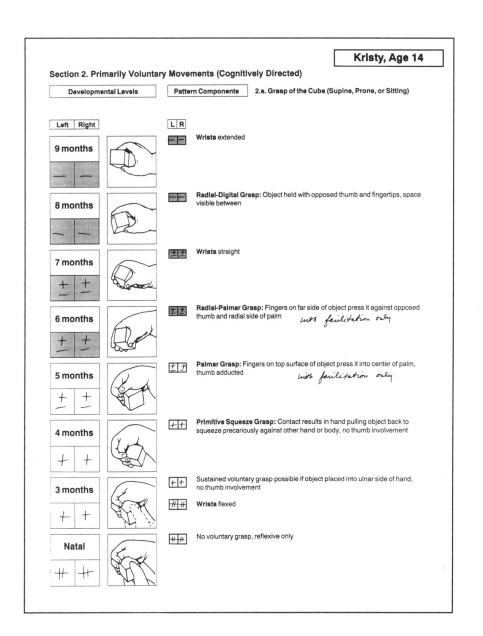

Evaluation Report

2.f. Grasp of the Pellet (Prone or Sitting)

Kristy at 3½
Kristy attempted to grasp the pellet but succeeded only in raking and contacting it.

Kristy at 14
Delayed patterns (primary developmentally inappropriate): Kristy did not demonstrate a pincer grasp, nor did she visually attend to a pellet.

Implications for function: Without the ability to grasp a pellet, Kristy's motivation to attend and reach for one was not stimulated. Finger feeding small edibles is not a realistic goal for Kristy because of concern for swallowing problems and choking, as well as limited digital manipulation.

Section 2. Primarily Voluntary Movements (Cognitively Directed)

Kristy, Age 14

Developmental Levels   Pattern Components   2.f. Grasp of the Pellet (Prone or Sitting)

Left | Right   L R

12 months
Fine Pincer Grasp: Between fingertips or fingernails (test with thread or yarn)
Thumb: Proximal joint slightly flexed, distal joint flexed

10 months
Pincer Grasp: Between distal pads of thumb and index finger
Thumb: Proximal joint extended, distal slightly flexed, opposed to index finger

9 months
Inferior-pincer Grasp: Between ventral surfaces of thumb and index finger
Thumb: Proximal and distal joints extended, beginning opposition

8 months
Scissors Grasp: Between thumb and side of curled index finger
Thumb: Proximal joint extended, distal slightly flexed

7 months
Inferior-scissors Grasp: Rakes object into palm with flexed fingers
Thumb: Proximal and distal joints flexed

6 months
Rakes and contacts object during unsuccessful attempt to grasp, fingers extended
Thumb: Proximal and distal joints flexed, adduction

5 months
Visually attends to object, without attempt to grasp

Natal
No visual attention to object, no grasp

2.g. Manipulation Skills (Prehension Schema)

Kristy at 3¹/₂

Repetitive scratching movements were frequent, and tactile discrimination was not well developed. Kristy demonstrated very little interaction of hand and sucking schemata and few exploratory movements, especially with objects. She was beginning reciprocal assimilation, watching her hand to prolong movement, and keeping her hand moving to make interesting sights last. Object permanence was beginning, but Kristy would not actively search for a removed object.

Kristy at 14

Kristy demonstrated developmental progression in a variety of new manipulation skills in several categories.

Tactile Awareness

Delayed patterns (primary developmentally inappropriate): She showed significant improvement in assimilation (hand movements extend to own face, body, clothing), accommodation (hand adapts to shape of new objects, especially the left), and tactile discrimination (can distinguish hand from object while finger feeding, although she still may accidentally bite her fingers or thumb while mouthing a toy). Nonpurposeful scratching and patting movements persisted in the left hand.

Implications for function: Kristy's hands appear to become more active when her vision is occluded. As tactile exploration skills increase, oral exploration (mouthing) should decrease. Increased tactile

Section 2. Primarily Voluntary Movements (Cognitively Directed)   Kristy, Age 14 awareness has led to hands to face and body more often, as well as shaping the hand around objects, important for grooming activities such as face washing, hair brushing, and applying lotion.

Prehension Schema

Delayed patterns (primary developmentally inappropriate): Emerging schemata included pushing, pulling, and dropping, but not throwing. Kristy intentionally and consistently pushed her adapted switch with either hand to receive a drink of water after initial prompting, and pressed on the electronic keyboard to hear sounds. She demonstrated intentional pulling by using her left hand to grasp and remove a towel placed over her head. She appeared to demonstrate intentional dropping by supinating (turning her hand over to let an object fall out) but did not visually monitor the act. She could not intentionally throw an object. She was sometimes able to retain grasp of an object when grasping another object with the other hand but often dropped the first object. Kristy appeared to possess more strength in her right arm, which could lift the spoon to her mouth with shoulder motion, than her left arm, which rested on or near the surface, using elbow and wrist motion only. However, her left hand had a stronger grasp, responded to touch with exploratory movements, and appeared to be more generally active and functional in all activities except feeding.

Implications for function: Kristy demonstrated increased awareness of cause and effect. Her emerging imitation skills could be utilized for training new hand schemata. Increased strength and mobility of arms would allow more participation in new activities.

Hand/Mouth Schema

Delayed patterns (primary developmentally inappropriate): Kristy has not yet replaced mouthing with tactile exploration, and often explores a new object orally.

Implications for function: Persistent mouthing satisfies the need for tactile information and delays development of manual exploration.

Hand/Vision Schema

Delayed patterns (primary developmentally inappropriate): Eye-hand coordination has improved and shows potential for further improvement. Excellent progress was seen in Kristy's ability to alternately look at and shake objects (maracas, hair spray bottles) in one or both hands, retaining grasp. Shaking movements involve primarily wrist and elbow, with slight motion in the right shoulder, more when excited. Kristy also alternately and repetitively imitated her therapist's shaking movements. She searched visually for lost or removed objects (object permanence) but could be distracted by another object. Eye-hand coordination was at several different developmental levels simultaneously: (a) she often visually attended to objects without reaching, (b) she sometimes explored tactually without visual attention, (c) her eyes watched her moving hand, and (d) she approached an object if it was within a few inches of her hand.

Implications for function: Intense eye gaze which is now used for food and clothes selection can be expanded to eye/hand pointing. The adapted switch, also used for choices, can be used for age-appropriate activities such as listening to music on the cassette player and operating computer programs with visual and auditory interest.

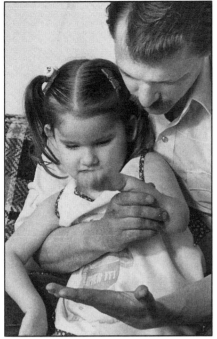

Figure 11.47. (photo by Sheldon Green)

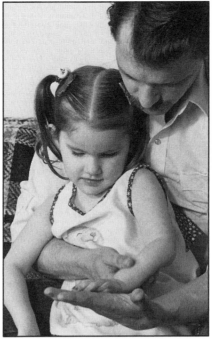

Figure 11.48. (photo by Sheldon Green)

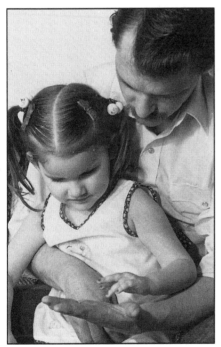

Figure 11.49. (photo by Sheldon Green)

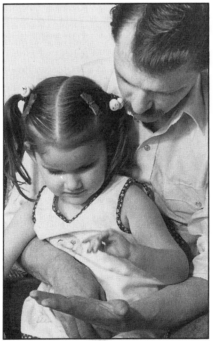

Figure 11.50. (photo by Sheldon Green)

Treatment Program

Kristy at 3¹/₂

- Passive, assistive, and active sensory stimulation can be done to Kristy's palms in particular to improve tactile awareness and discrimination. A variety of textures found in the home or neighborhood can include coarse and fine screen, cork, corduroy, suede, silk, rock, bark, coarse and fine sandpaper, shag carpet, terry cloth, velvet, foam sponge, chenille, animal fur, and fine steel wool.

- Finger feeding should be encouraged as much as possible (figures 11.39 to 11.41, page 188) to coordinate hand, sucking, and vision schemata.

- Kristy's father can improve reciprocal assimilation by first assisting her hand in "Give me five," then encouraging her to imitate the movement independently (figures 11.47 to 11.50).

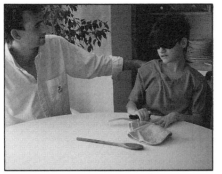

Figure 11.51. (photo by author)

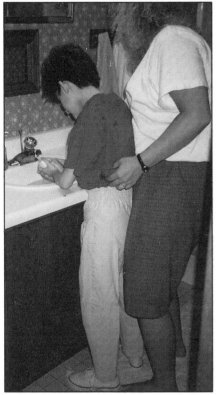

Figure 11.52. (photo by author)

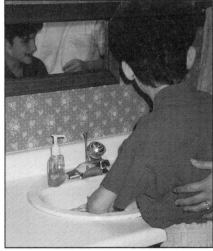

Figure 11.53. (photo by author)

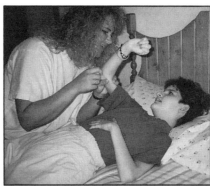

Figure 11.54. (photo by author)

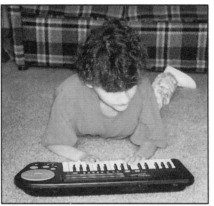

Figure 11.55. (photo by author)

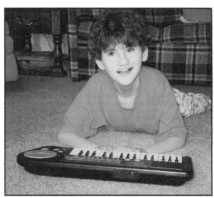

Figure 11.56. (photo by author)

Kristy at 14

- General manipulation and tactile awareness

  - Exploring familiar objects (comb, brush, spoon, cup) with vision occluded (dark goggles) can improve tactile awareness and reduce the need for oral exploration (figure 11.51).

  - While standing supported at the bathroom sink and using the mirror, Kristy can be helped to wash her face and both hands (figures 11.52, 11.53), pull the towel from the rack, and apply lotion.

- Eye-hand coordination

  - Bright nail polish and shiny bracelets can be used by Kristy's caregiver to cue visual attention to her hand in supine or sitting (figure 11.54).

  - The electronic keyboard can be used at home as well as school, with Kristy prone on forearms, using elbow and wrist motion, and monitoring her hand with downward gaze, which improves head control (figures 11.55, 11.56).

2.h. Release of the Dowel or Cube (Supine, Prone, or Sitting)

Kristy at 3¹/₂

Mutual fingering in midline (preparation for transfer) was observed, but no transfer was seen. Kristy had never experienced the strong reflexive grasp requiring forcible removal at the natal stage. She still released involuntarily without full awareness, left hand sustaining grasp longer than right. Voluntary release linked with adult removal of object was just emerging. No transfer was seen.

Kristy at 14

Delayed patterns (primary developmentally inappropriate): Kristy demonstrated most of the preparatory skills leading to intentional release: mutual fingering in midline to prepare for transferring, voluntary release as object is removed by another person, and two-stage transfer (one hand grasps, other joins, first hand releases after a period of time). She also appeared to release by supinating her hand and letting her wrist fall into extension, thus allowing the object to fall out. She did not show the

---

Section 2. Primarily Voluntary Movements (Cognitively Directed)

Kristy, Age 14

| Developmental Levels | | Pattern Components | 2.h. Release of the Dowel or Cube (Supine, Prone, or Sitting) |

Left | Right

L | R

12 months

Precise release into **small container**
Wrists extended *into gravity, not active*

10 months

Clumsy release into **small container**, rests hand on edge

9 months

Controlled release into **large container**
Wrists straight

8 months

Clumsy release into **large container** or **above surface**
Attempts unsuccessful release into **small container**

7 months

Voluntary assistive release **against surface** (stabilization)
Attempts unsuccessful release into **large container** or **above surface**
Adept 1-stage **transfer**, simultaneous grasp and release
Object falls from hand as arm extends, forearm supinates, and fingers extend

6 months

Smooth 2-stage **transfer:** One hand grasps, other joins, first hand releases
May use mouth as intermediary for **transfer**

5 months

Clumsy 2-stage **transfer:** One hand grasps, other joins, first hand releases with difficulty
Voluntary release as object is removed by another

4 months

Mutual fingering in midline, preparation for **transfer**

3 months

Involuntary release after sustained grasp, with awareness (eyes alert)

2 months

Involuntary release after retaining briefly, with some awareness (eyes alert)

1 month

Immediate involuntary release, without awareness

Natal

No voluntary release, object must be forcibly removed, or:
No grasp
Wrists flexed

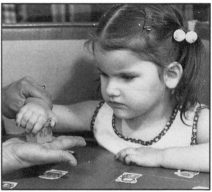

Figure 11.57. (photo by Sheldon Green)

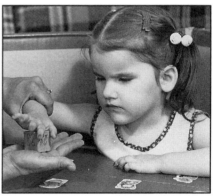

Figure 11.58. (photo by Sheldon Green)

assistive release of an object against the surface, such as placing a cup on her tray, nor release into a container. Kristy still showed evidence of involuntary release after brief or sustained grasp, with or without awareness.

Implications for function: Intentional release of objects on the surface or into containers can decrease dependence on caregivers, and can lead to more interesting manipulation activities for recreation and leisure and more opportunities for vocational potential.

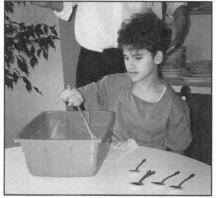

Figure 11.59. (photo by author)

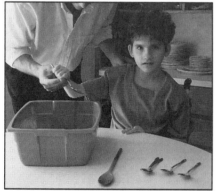

Figure 11.60. (photo by author)

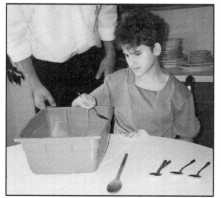

Figure 11.61. (photo by author)

Treatment Program

Kristy at 3¹/₂

- Voluntary release linked with adult removal of object should be continued until Kristy can consistently release on command.

- The two-stage transfer should be encouraged as Kristy's reach and grasp improve.

- Assistive release against a surface can be done with adult assistance (figures 11.57, 11.58).

Kristy at 14

- Sorting objects for prevocational tasks

  - To prepare for release into containers, Kristy can grasp large utensils such as wooden spoons and release them into her therapist's hand.

  - Sorting silverware into bins can also begin with large utensils and large bins, gradually reducing the sizes of both. Kristy may need her wrist stabilized (either manually or on the edge of the bin) to open her hand for release (figures 11.59 to 11.61).

Evaluation Report

2.i. Release of the Pellet (Sitting)

Kristy at 3¹/₂

Because Kristy had no grasp of the pellet, release was not measured.

Kristy at 14

Because Kristy had no grasp of the pellet, release was not possible.

Section 3. Prewriting Skills

Evaluation Report

3.a. Crayon or Pencil Grasp

3.b. Drawings

Kristy at 3¹/₂ and 14

Cognitive and motor levels preclude prewriting activities.

Kristy, Age 14

Section 2. Primarily Voluntary Movements (Cognitively Directed)

Developmental Levels | Pattern Components | 2.i. Release of the Pellet (Sitting)

Left	Right		L	R	
15 months					Precise release into **small container** / **Wrists** extended
14 months					Clumsy release into **small container**
12 months					Attempts unsuccessful release into **small container**
10 months					Controlled release into **large container**
9 months					**Transfer** from one hand to the other / Clumsy release into **large container** / **Wrists** straight
8 months					Unsuccessful attempt to **transfer** from one hand to the other / Attempts unsuccessful release into **large container** / Clumsy release **above surface** / Involuntary release with visual and tactile awareness
7 months					Involuntary release without visual or tactile awareness / **Wrists** flexed
Natal					No release (no grasp)

Developmental Hand Dysfunction

Summary and Conclusions

Kristy demonstrated significant gaps in development, particularly in the first two months, when physiological flexion and primitive reflexes provide a foundation for later skilled voluntary movements in the normal infant. Her hypotonia also resulted in a higher threshold of tactile awareness, decreasing her motivation to use her hands to explore her environment. Kristy used total extension patterns with intermittent rigidity or spasticity in her efforts to gain stability to move against gravity. However, these inappropriate patterns blocked further development and interfered with eye-hand coordination.

Recommendations

Kristy's occupational therapy program should emphasize development of head control, weight bearing on arms, and tactile awareness and discrimination.

Sample IEP (Individual Educational Plan) (Occupational Therapy Components)

Present Level of Function

Kristy's prehension skills ranged from the fetal stage to 6 months, preventing her from participating in age-appropriate educational, self-help, and play activities.

Goals and Objectives

Goal #1

To improve prehension skills to increase participation in school activities

Objective 1.1

Kristy will maintain head control and arms forward in the prone-on-forearms position for 60 seconds during classroom activities such as reading time.

Objective 1.2

Kristy will be able to roll independently across the classroom to reach a group of children, using lateral head righting and arm push-off rather than total extension patterns.

Objective 1.3

In a supported sitting position, Kristy will consistently knock down a tower of blocks placed in various positions, with either hand, nine out of ten times.

Objective 1.4

Kristy will finger feed independently when food is placed close to her left hand.

Objective 1.5

Kristy will imitate either pat-a-cake or bye-bye eight out of ten times.

Part II. Score Sheet (Developmental Levels)

Section 1. Primarily Involuntary Arm-Hand Patterns (Positional-Reflexive)

Section 3: Pre-Writing Skills (Pencil Grasp and Drawings)

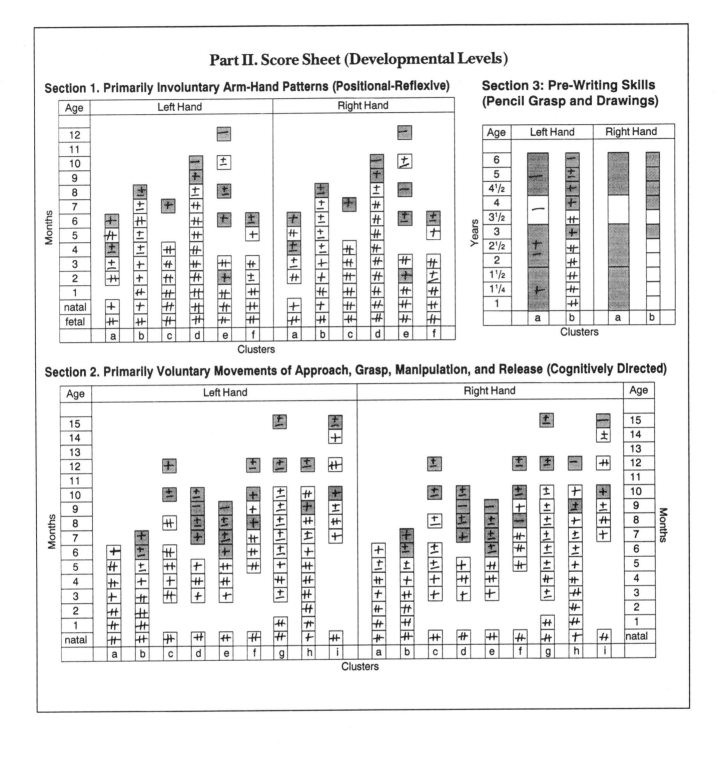

Section 2. Primarily Voluntary Movements of Approach, Grasp, Manipulation, and Release (Cognitively Directed)

Summary and Conclusions

Sensory Considerations

Kristy has a high threshold for tactile awareness, slow response time for sensory stimuli, and delayed fine motor skills due to central nervous system dysfunction related to cerebral palsy. Her visual and auditory systems bring her more interesting and usable information than her tactile system. Therefore, she has not been highly motivated to reach, touch, and explore objects, necessary to increase sensory as well as motor development. Types of sensory stimulation which can be carefully graded but can still reach Kristy's high threshold include proprioceptive (pressure, weight bearing), vestibular (movement such as swinging, spinning), and vibration (foam-enclosed vibrator). Tactile stimulation (textures and shapes) may be more effective when vision is occluded. Vision should of course be integrated into all functional skills; for example, use of the mirror for grooming.

Motor Considerations

Because of basic low muscle tone and difficulty grading movement, Kristy has increased tone proximally (spine, shoulders, and elbows) to achieve stability in antigravity positions, resulting in less mobility in those areas. She has more mobility and less stability in distal areas (wrists and fingers). Therefore, Kristy is able to manipulate only those objects that are within immediate reach of her arms and hands. Normalizing muscle tone, increasing range of motion, and improving midrange control can provide a balance of stability and mobility needed for skilled arm/hand function as well as assisted transitions.

Cognitive Considerations

While cognitive function is demonstrated by certain hand skills, fine motor development is also dependent on cognitive levels of functional awareness and the ability to generalize skills to similar but not identical situations. Kristy has demonstrated some awareness of functional cause and effect, such as spoon to mouth, switch operation, and pulling the towel off her head. As Kristy's motor skills continue to improve, some new cognitive abilities may emerge. She needs opportunities to participate in cognitively directed activities (imitation, means-end, scheme actions, spatial relations, causality) matched to her achievable fine motor abilities.

Recommendations

Occupational therapy and physical therapy with continued NDT emphasis is recommended to improve tactile awareness, postural control, and upper extremity use.

Sample IEP (Individual Education Plan) Occupational Therapy Components

Present Level of Function

Kristy is able to participate *independently* in the following activities: eye gaze to indicate choices of food or clothing, electronic keyboard.

With minimal to moderate assistance she also participates in spoon feeding, corralling cup to drink from straw, switch operation for television, music, drink, transitions from sit/stand/sit.

She needs maximum assistance and adaptations for dressing, bathing, and grooming.

Goals and Objectives

Goal #1
To independently use an augmentative system for communicating her needs/desires

Objective 1.1
Kristy will operate an adaptive switch to ask for a drink three times daily for two consecutive months. She will locate the switch with her eyes, reach with her arm, and grasp or press it.

Objective 1.2
Kristy will use an adaptive switch to turn on a music video on a VCR at least one time daily for one month.

Chapter Twelve
A Synthesis of Theory, Assessment, and Treatment

Treatment Planning

Use of the Taxonomy

Through formal and informal evaluations, as much information as possible has been collected about each child's muscle tone, reflex activity, and developmental levels. This Knowledge has been Comprehended, Applied, and Analyzed in each evaluation report. Synthesis, leading to solution of problems, depends on both the scientific and creative processes.

Designing the Program

Just as the architect has gathered large amounts of information about the client's functional and esthetic needs and is ready to blend all the structural components into an appropriate building, the therapist is faced with an almost overwhelming collection of data from which relevant facts must be selected. To be useful, the child's profile of strengths and weaknesses must be arranged in a hierarchy of steps toward a goal. As with building a structure, the end shapes the means. Since the basic premise in both professions is that good foundations serve as building blocks or prerequisites for higher levels, using what has been learned from past experiences to improve or replace missing components is crucial when formulating new plans (Smith et al. 1982).

In addition, just as the architect integrates components of the electrical, plumbing, and heating/cooling systems, the therapist similarly must consider cognitive, language, and social developmental levels, as well as motor, in designing an appropriate treatment program.

If this process is competently executed, the plan will be one that allows the structure or individual to interact more efficiently with the environment.

The practice of science demands two apparently paradoxical qualities in the professional who designs such complex systems: first, the capacity to doubt and question, and second, the confidence and desire to persist and dream (Connolly 1977).

Implementing the Program

When the architect's plan is completed, the process of implementation will involve contractors, plumbers, electricians, carpenters, bricklayers, and painters, essential members of the construction crew.

The therapy team may include occupational therapists, physical therapists, speech pathologists, teachers, nurses, and physicians, as well as parents and other family members, friends, students, aides, and most important, the child.

Because the treatment program encompasses the child's total environment, both home and school, every significant person in it is an essential team member. Therapeutic structuring of that environment is necessary to get the child's active participation and adaptation, which, with repetition, becomes automatic and internalized.

The child needs this team, not only for handling to be consistent, but equally vital, for sharing information, so the program can be constantly modified and improved. Each team member possesses special skills. For example, the parent knows the child better than anyone else. Therapists offer professional information based on training and experience with other children. Teachers are able to contribute knowledge from classroom observation of the child's response to educational tasks and interaction with peers. Aides have the advantage of frequent daily handling.

Most new skills taught to the child with a disability need to be modified and adapted. The key to valid task analysis lies in perfecting observational skills. The child usually indicates needs to the alert observer, most often by wanting to try something new. If tasks are presented at a level that gives the child a good chance for success, the child will continue to try and will not resort to persistent manipulative behavior, such as avoidance or aggression (Knickerbocker 1980).

Team members who are comfortable with their own roles are able to focus on the needs of the child. They respect the opinions of others as well as their own and are not threatened by differences of opinion. As information is shared and combined, even questioned and challenged, as different individuals react and discuss problems, awareness of each others' skills grows and communication deepens. The child's program ultimately becomes more and more relevant and comprehensive.

Basic Treatment Principles

Preparation

- Inhibit primitive reflexes.

- Normalize muscle tone, increasing or decreasing as necessary.

- Provide joint stability, especially proximally.

- Teach new skills in postures where child is most stable and tone is most normal.

- Provide no more postural support than necessary to allow child to use what is available.

- Position child as nearly symmetrically as possible.

- Break up total flexion or extension patterns.

Facilitation

- Strengthen present skill level to prepare for the next.

- Introduce next skill level concurrently.

- Try to fill all skill gaps in the young child.

- Focus only on necessary skill gaps in the older child.

- Carefully grade all stimulation (auditory, visual, tactile, and proprioceptive) to elicit movements that are as nearly automatic as possible and performed without excess effort.

- Direct the child's attention to what the child is doing rather than how the child is doing it.

- Require eye pointing before voluntary hand movements.

Adaptation

- Place child in correct position and ask the child to maintain it (placing and holding), gradually reducing external support.

- Experiment with movement, trying wider ranges, as long as child maintains normal patterns.

- Vary the speed of movement according to the child's needs.

- Grade the size of objects; for example, start with a small cube, increasing the size, but begin with a large pellet, decreasing as skill improves.

- If atypical patterns appear, return to lower skill levels, provide more postural support, or increase external control.

- Offer a variety of alternate activities for repetition, internalization, and generalization, and encourage the child to invent new ways of solving problems (Erhardt 1974; Erhardt, Beatty, and Hertsgaard 1981; Gilfoyle, Grady, and Moore 1981; Trombley and Scott 1977).

The Creative Process and Practice of the Art

Joanne: May 1, 1970 (CA: 19 months)

Supervision of the exercises by the pair of volunteers had just been completed. Joanne's mother, Gloria, asked an interesting question.

"Why can't Joanne reach out and hug me?"

"What do you mean?" I said.

"Well, you know how she puts her head against my cheek and says m-m-m. That's her way of saying that she loves me. We're doing all these exercises for her arms. Why can't she put her arms around me like her sister Valerie does?"

As Joanne sat in my lap I moved her shoulders and arms in all directions, realizing immediately that limitation of movement was present throughout the shoulder girdle and spine, due to spasticity. How many other therapists also focused so much attention on arm and leg (appendicular) exercises that important axial joints were ignored?

A quick task analysis, to determine which muscles were needed for reaching upward, outward, and forward, made me realize that an anatomy course taken 20 years before seemed hopelessly distant. It was necessary to go back to the text to find new solutions to these puzzling problems.

By the following day, I had developed a two-page list of additional exercises for Joanne, including neck flexion, extension, rotation, and lateral flexion; scapular elevation, depression, abduction, adduction, upward and downward rotation, and anterior-posterior movement; and spinal rotation and flexion, both laterally and anterior-posteriorly.

Within two months, the volunteers' work resulted in a new skill when Joanne began reaching for toys in the prone position, bringing both hands together to midline to hold those toys, and, several months later, hugging her mother around the neck, using both arms.

"I love you too, Joey," Gloria said as she hugged her back. Joanne grinned and giggled with delight. She seemed almost to be saying, "You do understand!"

Later we realized that Joanne, even at the age of 19 months, had been using problem-solving skills. She wanted so much to return her mother's hug that when she adapted by leaning forward with her trunk and head to give the same body contact and the same vocalization, she got her message across.

Joanne: July 16, 1970 (CA: 21 months)

To promote hand-to-mouth movements, Joanne's fingers were dipped into food and guided into her mouth. Messy exploration was encouraged to motivate manipulation of textures, begin sensorimotor feedback, and learn new movements through accommodation.

"Why don't we try a spoon?" Gloria suggested. She found one with a long handle and a small bowl, placed it in Joanne's left hand, and helped her scoop the food and bring it to her mouth. "Now it's your turn." Joanne promptly grasped the spoon and threw it on the floor.

Realizing that the stage of throwing or dropping things in order to make interesting sights last precedes that of using objects functionally, I suggested that Joanne may be telling us she's not ready. An adapted spoon seemed logical.

Joanne was intrigued by the elastic strap that kept her hand on the built-up handle of the adapted spoon. Because the task was slightly easier, she was willing to try. We watched her intense effort, which caused her shoulders to hike up, both arms to flex, and the opposite hand to fist. That was definitely not a normal pattern.

"Gloria, let's try this for a while and see how it goes."

A few weeks later I watched Joanne use the adapted spoon again. The same undesirable patterns were present. Gloria tried to remember when Valerie began using a spoon.

"Normal children usually start playing with one at about 12 months, but they don't really use it functionally until 16 or 18 months," I said.

"And what do you estimate Joanne's developmental level to be, in the fine motor area?" Gloria asked.

"About 6 months! Wow, we really are premature, aren't we? Even though she's almost 2 chronologically, her developmental level is nowhere near where she needs to be to use the spoon without excessive effort. Perhaps we'd better get back to finger feeding. The last thing we want is for her to practice the wrong movements so they become a permanent part of her feeding patterns."

Two years later, even though her fine motor development was still at less than a 1-year level, Joanne mastered the skill of feeding herself with a regular spoon. The importance of independent feeding to her social growth as an independent 4-year-old made acquisition of the skill vital, despite slight shoulder elevation and mild fisting of the opposite hand.

Joanne: January 19, 1971 (CA: 2 years)

Joanne was now crawling on her belly, but she could not push up on extended arms to prepare for crawling on hands and knees. When placed in a hands-and-knees position, she remained totally flexed. Various methods of achieving weight bearing on extended arms by working on the floor with Joanne were very difficult for her mother, because of a back problem.

"Come into the living room," Gloria greeted me. "I've got something to show you." She sat in a large rocking chair with Joanne facing her in her lap. With Joanne's elbows straight and her open hands flat against her mother's chest, she was rocked back and forth.

"Isn't this a good way to give Joanne the sensation of weight bearing on extended arms, like she'll need for crawling?"

"I think it's a terrific idea, because it's a natural way for you as a mother to relate to your child, making it a part of everyday play, rather than 'therapy.'"

Seven months later, Joanne began to crawl with a symmetrical pattern (bunny hop). By the time she was 3 years old, she had begun to crawl reciprocally up the stairs, originally motivated by the desire to reach her brother's guitar, placed strategically on the top step.

Joanne: September, 1973 (CA: 4¹/2 years)

Since state statutes at this time required the local school district to provide necessary services for handicapped children from age 4, Joanne was mainstreamed into a private nursery school. Her total program was planned and coordinated by a team that included the director of special services, a school social worker, the director of the nursery school, the school speech clinician, the school nurse, the occupational therapy consultant, an aide, and the parent.

For the next nine years, as various school systems in different communities provided Joanne with direct occupational therapy services, my involvement was minimal, more as a friend than as a professional.

Patrick: December 4, 1978 (CA: 3 years)

My evaluation of Patrick had been completed, and we were ready to begin setting up a home program. His mother, Sallie, was curious about the homemade table I had brought. I explained that a friendly volunteer carpenter built it, as well as many other things for our children. This table would help us in designing one specifically for Patrick.

As Patrick sat in a folding commercial corner sitter, I pulled the table close to him and set an inclined chalkboard on the surface.

"Why are those dowels sticking out on each side?" Sallie asked.

"That's for his right hand to grasp, to keep the shoulder forward, while he's drawing with his left."

Patrick had difficulty reaching and grasping the dowel. His mother helped, but as soon as she removed her hand, his fell away.

"The evaluation showed that he still has some remnants of the Avoiding Response, which is activated by light touch to the palmar surfaces of his fingers," I explained. "You need to keep your hand on his; in fact, you should probably push his forearm toward the dowel at the same time, so it is pressing firmly into the web space of his thumb."

"Hold tight, Patrick."

"We also need to have the dowel further away on the table to get more elbow extension. Otherwise he's into a total flexion pattern." I pulled out my pad and pencil and started taking notes.

Patrick's Progress Notes

December 4, 1978

To: Mr. and Mrs. John M.

Re: Occupational therapy for Patrick

- **Activity:** Posture at desk

  Response: When Patrick tried to draw with his left hand, his right arm retracted.

  Recommendations: Patrick's right hand should grasp a dowel on his desk while he performs skilled activities with his left. A table should be built with dowels placed to require full elbow extension. Adult should control his hand in grasping the dowel, reducing control when possible. His elbow can be extended by pressure on it at the same time his forearm is pushed toward the dowel, with the web space in firm contact.

Developmental Hand Dysfunction

Patrick: January 29, 1979

Sallie and I were having a cup of tea and discussing Patrick's feeding skills.

"You know, he's trying to feed himself with a spoon, but that darn 'flying hand' is still there when he tries anything new. I've tried to get him to hold the dish or even put his hand flat on the table, but it just flies up."

"Do you have a C-clamp, Sallie?"

"Whatever for?"

"You'll see."

Sallie found a small clamp. I tightened it on the table near Patrick's right hand. He understood exactly what it was for and grabbed it immediately. Because of the work he and his mother had been doing with sustained grasp on the desk dowel, he held on easily while bringing the spoon to his mouth with his left hand.

"Look how his head is in midline!" Sallie exclaimed. "Why can't we take that C-clamp wherever we go, to friends' homes, or restaurants?"

"Why not?"

Kristy: June 30, 1980 (CA: 2 years)

Kristy had been evaluated with the 1979 EDPA as part of a total evaluation for a home program. Her developmental level was estimated at 2 to 4 months. I asked Kristy's mother, Carmon, what her short-term goals were; that is, what did she most want Kristy to do soon. She replied that she wanted Kristy to be able to sit alone and showed me what happened when she tried. When Kristy was placed on the floor, she simply collapsed forward.

"Sit up, Kristy, come on, let me see you," Carmon tried. "Tracy, can you get Kristy to look at you?"

"Kristy, Kristy, peek-a-boo," her sister cajoled. With great effort Kristy lifted her head a few inches from her lap, resting it back on her shoulders. Her hips remained flexed and her arms limp. I explained that in order to sit alone, the baby needs head control, back extension, and weight bearing on extended arms.

I asked to see some of the activities that had been done in her previous therapy program. Tracy brought a padded wedge and helped her mother place Kristy on it in a prone position.

"We've never had much success with this," said Carmon, as she tried to get Kristy to push up with her arms and lift her head.

"That activity should help Kristy," I thought aloud, "because it incorporates many of the components needed in sitting."

Instead of pushing down on her arms, however, Kristy hyperextended her back and hips, asymmetrically, so she almost rolled off the wedge. When her hips were stabilized, I felt strong hip extension and abduction. By adducting her legs and pressing firmly down on her hips, I enabled Kristy to extend her head, although her arms remained somewhat flexed.

"Carmon, let's raise the wedge and see if we can get Kristy's arms straight. I'll try giving her some joint compression to her shoulders, elbows, and wrists first, to give her the feeling of weight bearing."

We also observed Kristy flat on the floor, watching her arms retract to her sides, joining her head, back, and hips in the same total extension pattern. Even her feet were plantar-flexed and toes clawed. When Kristy's arms were brought forward in extension in this position, she could not lift her head.

Kristy: October 20, 1980 (CA: 2½ years)

I was eager to share with Carmon the exciting new information gained at an NDT Refresher Weekend in Chicago. That information needed to be applied to children such as Kristy, to help work through the blocks that were interfering with their progress.

"Carmon, I have so much to tell you about the workshop that I don't know where to start. How about if we review the new information in my notes about the prone position during the first 5 months? Let's get down on the floor and try these postures." We duplicated as best we could the head, neck, shoulder, arm, elbow, wrist, hand, finger, and even thumb positions, as well as those of the trunk, pelvis, and lower extremities.

By the time we had finished, we both had realized that Kristy had never experienced physiological flexion that the newborn uses to provide stability when

Kristy's Progress Notes

June 30, 1980

To: Mr. and Mrs. Mike C.

Re: Occupational therapy for Kristy

- **Activity:** Weight bearing in prone on the wedge

  Response: Kristy hyperextended her back and hips and abducted her legs; her arms remained flexed, with hands fisted.

   Recommendations: Joint compression should be given first to shoulders, elbows, and wrists. Then a stimulus at eye level can help get head lifting while her hips are stabilized and legs adducted. To increase her strength, she can be moved forward on the wedge or be required to keep her head up longer.

- **Activity:** Prone on floor with arms extended forward

  Response: Kristy was not able to lift her head.

   Recommendations: Attempts should be made to motivate Kristy to raise her head in this position.

August 29, 1980

- **Activity:** Weight bearing in prone on the wedge (see 6-30-80)

Response: Kristy's right arm was extended, but the left was still slightly flexed.

 Recommendations: Prone on the wedge, Kristy should look slightly to the left to get more left elbow extension (utilizing remnants of the ATNR). Stimulus should gradually be moved toward midline as elbow extension maintains.

- **Activity:** Prone on floor with arms extended (6-30-80)

  Response: Kristy did not appear to be motivated to raise her head.

  Recommendations: Kristy can be placed in prone on adult's stomach (in supine), with arms forward.

September 25, 1980

- **Activity:** Prone on floor (see 8-29-80)

  Response: Kristy disliked prone positioning, crying until someone changed her position.

  Recommendations: Prone positioning should be continued. If Kristy cries, she can be talked to, rather than picked up. She should also be placed prone during speech therapy, as an alternate working position.

---

lifting the head against gravity. Expecting her to bear weight on extended arms was developmentally inappropriate. She needed to go through earlier stages, beginning with arms flexed and adducted under her body, gradually abducting, externally rotating, and coming forward as head control improved. Convinced that we were on the right track, I spent a great deal of time discussing this theory with Carmon, Tracy, and Mike, Kristy's father, so that the correct prone positioning could be carried out throughout Kristy's daily living activities.

Kristy: August 12, 1981 (CA: 3 years)

Kristy was re-evaluated with the EDPA as part of a total evaluation in preparation for development of an IEP for entrance into a preschool program. Her fine motor developmental level had increased from 2 to 4 months to a range of 3 to 6½ months. Team members present at the IEP staffing would include the preschool teachers, pre-K coordinator, psychologist, physical therapist, occupational therapist, NDT therapist consultant, OT/PT coordinator, speech pathologist, and parent.

Kristy: September 18, 1981

The team agreed that Kristy's needs included a half-day program in the pre-K handicapped classroom, direct services by a registered physical therapist, direct services by a therapy aide supervised by an NDT-certified occupational therapist, and consultation by a speech pathologist.

Kristy: September 23, 1981

Carmon and Mike asked me to come to their home to help them prepare for Kristy's first day at school. We needed to decide which essential handling and positioning techniques should be shared with the school staff. We also were planning to bring Kristy's adapted desk and chair, which her father had built, to the school for use in the classroom.

Entering their home, I noticed that Mike was reading a story to Tracy. His foot was propped against Kristy's right elbow while she looked into a mirror (figure 12.1).

"Mike," I asked, "Why do you have your foot behind Kristy's elbow?"

"Didn't you tell us not to let Kristy's elbows slide back when she lifts her head?"

"Yes, but I didn't realize that you were actually listening! That is very creative of you."

"That's me, creative Mike."

"Where is this table and chair I've been hearing about, the one you made out of cardboard, that Patrick's mother designed?"

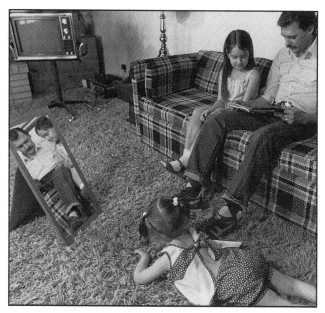

Figure 12.1. Kristy's father using his foot to keep her right elbow forward while reading to her sister (photo by Sheldon Green)

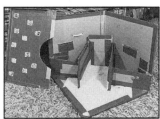

Figure 12.2. Construction of the two-piece cardboard desk system (photo by Sheldon Green)

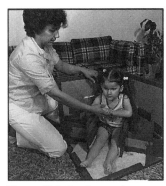

Figure 12.3. Seating system providing trunk support and preventing hip abduction (photo by Sheldon Green)

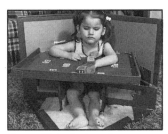

Figure 12.4. Desk surface providing arm support at appropriate height (photo by Sheldon Green)

Carmon pulled the heavy cardboard two-piece set into the middle of the room and placed Kristy in it (figures 12.2 to 12.4). I liked the way it prevented her legs from abducting and provided trunk support only to the middle of her back and sides. The desk appeared to be at the proper level for her arms to rest on without elevating her shoulders.

"It looks good. Is that duct tape holding it together?"

"You got it," said Mike. He closed the book he was reading to Tracy, put his arm around her, and leaned back to watch us work with Kristy, trying not to look too pleased with himself.

"What shall we do first?" I asked Carmon.

"Well, I'm very concerned that Kristy is lifted and carried correctly, because there will be so many times a day when she'll be handled by so many people."

"Yes, and the usual way we all pick up babies just reinforces the total extension pattern that we're trying to get rid of in Kristy. Why don't you pick her up the wrong way so we can demonstrate that to the staff first?"

Carmon reached for Kristy as she lay on her back on the floor. She put her hands underneath Kristy's arms and lifted (figures 12.5, 12.6). Kristy immediately stiffened and hyperextended her head (figures 12.6 to 12.8).

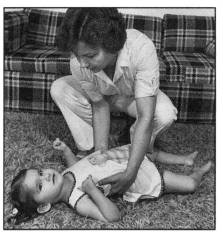

Figure 12.5. Demonstration by mother of inappropriate lifting from supine (photo by Sheldon Green)

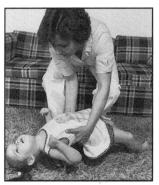

Figure 12.6. Stiffening and hyperextension due to inadequate support (photo by Sheldon Green)

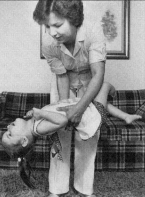

Figure 12.7. Increased hyperextension pattern during lifting in supine (photo by Sheldon Green)

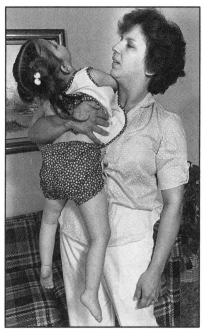

Figure 12.8. Neck hyperextension in supported upright position (photo by Sheldon Green)

Developmental Hand Dysfunction

"Gee, I can't believe I used to lift her this way. It feels so wrong!"

"Now try it the right way, rolling her to sidelying first."

There, that feels a lot better, doesn't it, Kristy?" (figures 12.9 to 12.13).

"Can you hold her the same way on the other side?"

"Sure. You're going to school, Kristy. What do you think of that?"

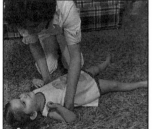

Figure 12.9. Mother's preparation for more appropriate lifting by passive rolling to sidelying (photo by Sheldon Green)

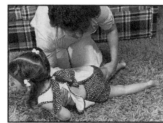

Figure 12.10. Providing support under chest and between legs (photo by Sheldon Green)

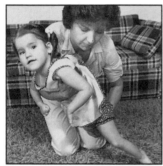

Figure 12.11. Transition from sidelying to upright position (photo by Sheldon Green)

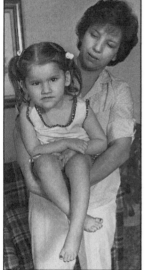

Figure 12.12. A position providing adequate support for Kristy without stress for mother (photo by Sheldon Green)

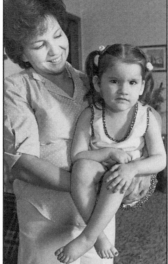

Figure 12.13. Alternative position on other side (photo by Sheldon Green)

Patrick: December 30, 1981 (CA: 6 years)

Re-evaluation with the Erhardt Developmental Prehension Assessment revealed that Patrick had regressed in fine motor skills compared with a previous test on April 20, 1981. Additional positional components (Arms in Supine and Prone) in the current version pinpointed developmental gaps in head control and shoulder stabilization, which had resulted in compensatory patterns such as shoulder elevation. Patrick's parents requested that the school hold a meeting to review his Individual Educational Plan. Team members present at that meeting would include the kindergarten teacher, principal, OT/PT coordinator, occupational therapist, physical therapist, parents, and Neuro-Developmental Treatment (NDT) consultant therapist.

Patrick: February 2, 1982

Patrick's teacher reported that during the last few months his sitting balance had significantly decreased. His aide needed to be nearby most of the time because of unexpected falls. Attention span and general alertness were noticeably reduced, and he had not retained many previously acquired academic skills. Absenteeism may have contributed to his regression.

The occupational therapist described the lack of progress in fine motor activities that were designed to meet the objectives in his IEP, such as pincer grasp, poking forefinger, and the use of scissors. The physical therapist stated that the quality and consistency of Patrick's gross motor skills had declined.

Because of Patrick's frequent absences from school, as well as the holiday season, the NDT therapist had not consulted with the team for three months. The evaluation performed in December, which had indicated regression in fine motor skills, had not yet been fully interpreted and was not ready for dissemination.

Patrick's parents explained the problems the family was having with medication regulation and seizure control, and that Patrick had been hospitalized seven times between September and January for status epilepticus (prolonged seizures). Their physician, who was working with them to adjust drug levels, had listed side effects of some of the drug combinations: poor balance and coordination, drowsiness, dizziness, irritability, severe emotional swings, and mental confusion. They expressed concern that Patrick had missed not only so much school but also his therapies. His mother suggested that until the medications were stabilized, transferring his therapy program to the home was an option she would like the team to consider. In fact, since the NDT philosophy integrated "therapy" into all daily living activities, including positioning, handling, and mobility, she had really always been Patrick's therapist and would be willing to resume that role.

The team agreed to a temporary change in Patrick's IEP, designating his mother as the direct service provider, with weekly consultation by the NDT therapist and monthly consultation by the school physical therapist.

Kristy: February 22, 1982 (CA: 3¹/₂ years)

Kristy's school team met to discuss the integration of the therapy program with educational activities. Seated around the large mat in the classroom used for therapy were Kristy, her mother, both classroom teachers, a classroom aide, the OT/PT coordinator, the NDT therapist consultant, and the therapy aide. The physical therapist joined the group and asked if they could talk that day about the problems Kristy was still having with total extension patterns, especially during rolling. The teachers noted an increased frequency of this new skill, Kristy's only way of moving around the room to be with the other children. They had positioned her in prone as much as possible, to help meet the objectives in Kristy's IEP, but felt that much of the action was above her eye level, since most of the children were ambulatory.

The physical therapist then showed the group how Kristy's extension increased when she worked on balance reactions in prone on the rocker board. The NDT therapist asked the therapy aide to demonstrate how she was able to break up the total extension-abduction pattern on the rocker board by keeping Kristy's arms flexed underneath and using a strap to keep her legs together while achieving head extension and weight shifting through eye contact.

The group decided that Kristy could be placed prone on a higher surface such as a table, with a teacher or aide assisting in keeping her arms flexed and legs together as she raised her head appropriately to watch activities at eye level. When prone on the floor, Kristy could be encouraged to roll to the right by placing her advantageously near a group of children.

The new classroom aide asked to see the special techniques for lifting and carrying Kristy, because she also found a great deal of stiffness and extension when handling her. Kristy's mother reviewed what she had found to be effective handling methods and helped several of the group try them out on Kristy. A date was set for another team meeting the following month.

Patrick: March 23, 1982 (CA: 6¹/₂ years)

Sallie, Patrick, and I sat down at the kitchen table.

"I want you to watch Patrick drink from a cup. Ever since we've had this drug problem, he has had such a hard time getting the cup to his mouth without spilling. It seems that all of the nice control he had gained is gone. First watch him using one hand," Sallie asked.

Patrick reached for the cup with his left hand, turned his head sharply to the left, and elevated his right shoulder as his entire right arm flexed.

"Do you see what's happening?" Sallie asked. "He's going into the ATNR again. Why?"

"Maybe to find stability," I ventured.

"Do we need to get the C-clamp back on the table again, to keep his right arm extended?"

"Maybe so, until his balance and coordination return. You could also give him a chair with more trunk support, so he doesn't need to 'fix' with his shoulders."

"He's never gone backward before. It's so depressing. Patrick, show us how you hold the cup with both hands."

Patrick tried, but as he drank, his shoulders again elevated, and his right hand began pulling downward, spilling the liquid and finally releasing the cup unintentionally. His mother shook her head and frowned.

"Patrick, try putting your elbows on the table after you grab the cup," I suggested, "and try to keep your head in the middle. Good. That works better, doesn't it?"

"I can't believe it. I've been trying to figure this out for days, and you think of an answer in 10 seconds. Why?"

"I don't know. Sometimes I can't solve a problem, either. That's why we all need to work together. I'll write this down in my progress notes and send you a copy. For the time being, give him more support and more stability, in every way possible, until his coordination returns after the medication settles down."

Patrick's Progress Notes

March 23, 1982

To: Mr. and Mrs. John M.

Re: Occupational therapy for Patrick

- **Activity:** Cup drinking using one hand

  Response: Patrick lifted the cup with his left hand, turned his head sharply to the left, and elevated his right shoulder as his entire right arm flexed.

  Recommendations: The right hand should grasp a C-clamp to reduce associated reactions and to keep head more in midline. Positioning in chair should be concerned with total trunk support to reduce need for compensatory fixing at shoulders or with total flexion patterns.

- **Activity:** Cup drinking using both hands

  Response: Patrick tried to lift the cup with both hands, but as he drank, his shoulders elevated, and his right hand began pulling downward, spilling the liquid and finally releasing the cup unintentionally.

  Recommendations: Patrick should be guided to rest his elbows on the table after he has grasped the cup with both hands. His weight should be centered, rather than on one side or the other. Head should be in midline. Positioning in chair should be concerned with proper level of table to enable elbows to rest comfortably on surface. If Patrick needs to empty the cup, he will probably have to lift his elbows from the table.

Patrick: April 1, 1982

Sallie had fixed up Patrick's bedroom as a therapy room. An extra mattress on the floor provided a safe place to practice falling with arms outstretched. A long rocker board faced a large wall mirror, and his custom-made table and chair were placed against a window.

As we began our therapy session, Sallie expressed her fear that Patrick's arm control seemed to be getting worse all the time. "His feeding is still bad," she said, "and look, his whole shoulder joint is so loose, especially the right. Take his arm and move it around. Do you see what I mean?"

Patrick's very unstable joint was no surprise. He had always lacked proximal stability and had compensated from infancy by retracting and elevating his shoulders. "His medication is finally stable, isn't it, Sallie?"

"Yes, it is, and his general balance and coordination are improving all the time. Even his behavior has been great. So why is he having so much trouble with his arms and hands? You know, I've been doing all that shoulder inhibition you showed me, to get his shoulders down. Maybe we shouldn't be doing it, or maybe I'm doing it wrong."

"Patrick, come on over here and lie down on your back. I want you and mother to show me the shake-shake game."

Patrick loved games. He crawled quickly to us. Sallie placed her hands on his shoulders, rapidly shaking and rotating them until she felt the tone decrease. She kept her hands pressing downward firmly between each shake, and I was pleased to see that when she removed her hands, the elevation had decreased. Suddenly I realized that Patrick's neck was longer than I had remembered!

"Sallie, you're doing it exactly right. I think you've accomplished a lot in a short time. His neck is definitely longer."

"Oh, yes," she agreed. "We've noticed that. Look how skinny it is, though."

"Of course, the muscles have been inactive because of the overcompensation of shoulder elevators. Wait a minute! I think I know what's happening to Patrick's arm control. Why didn't I think of it before? It makes so much sense! Yes. I'm sure of it."

"What? What? What?"

"Wait, I've got to make sure I explain it right. Let me think a minute. . . . Okay. I think what has happened is that you have done such a good job inhibiting those shoulders and getting rid of the artificial stabilization Patrick has used all these years to compensate for poor head control and joint stability, that he now has hardly any stabilization at all. What he needs to learn now is what normal joint stability feels like. We need to do lots of joint compression as well as the prone rocker board stuff. Patrick, we have a new game."

I showed Sallie how to keep Patrick's shoulder down while giving him intermittent compression from the elbow (figure 12.14). Then I did the same thing to her so she could feel it herself (figure 12.15).

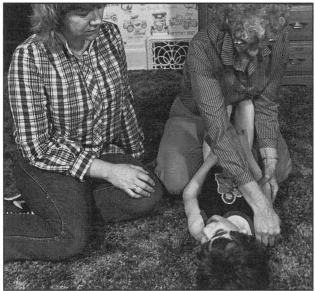

Figure 12.14. Demonstration of therapy technique on Patrick by therapist (photo by Sheldon Green)

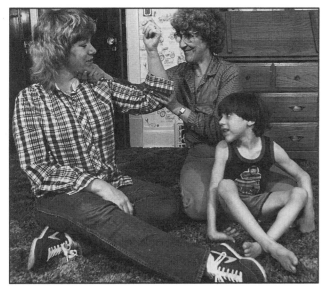

Figure 12.15. Technique performed on mother by therapist (photo by Sheldon Green)

"Hey, you're going to break my shoulder."

"Are you trying to tell me I'm pushing too hard? Look at me and see if I do it better this time."

I placed my hands on Sallie's as she tried it with Patrick, so she could tell how much pressure to use (figure 12.16). Finally, she did it herself as I watched (figure 12.17).

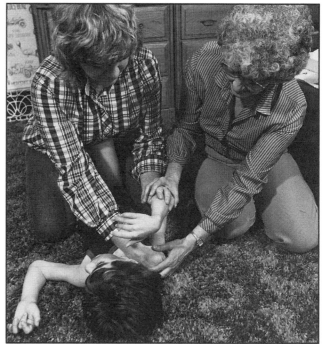

Figure 12.16. Therapist's hands on mother's hands to teach appropriate pressure (photo by Sheldon Green)

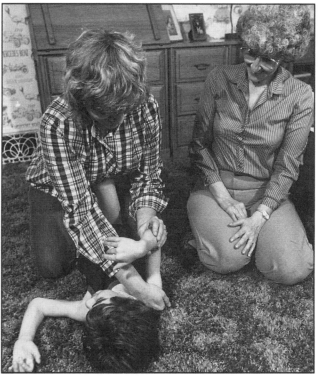

Figure 12.17. Observation by therapist of mother's technique (photo by Sheldon Green)

Developmental Hand Dysfunction

Patrick's Progress Notes

April 1, 1982

To: Mr. and Mrs. John M.

Re: Occupational therapy for Patrick

- **Activity:** Joint compression to shoulder joints

  Response: Patrick's shoulder joints were extremely mobile, right more than left.

  Recommendations: In supine, Patrick's arm should be compressed into his shoulder in three directions: upward, sideward, and forward. 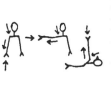 Adult's hand should stabilize the shoulder, keeping it down, while other hand controls at the elbow.

April 27, 1982

- **Activity:** Joint compression to shoulder joints (see 4-1-82)

  Response: Improvement was seen in shoulder stability.

 Recommendations: Compression with elbow straight can begin to prepare for active resistive pushing.

May 25, 1982

- **Activity:** Joint compression to shoulder joints (see 4-27-82)

  Response: Patrick was able to tolerate compression with elbow straight and keep his shoulder down with minimal adult assistance.

  Recommendations: Active pushing should be done with adult's hand on shoulder, gradually reducing pressure as he maintains shoulder depression.

Patrick: June 1, 1982

Patrick's IEP staffing included the following team members: OT/PT coordinator, preschool coordinator, physical therapist, speech pathologist, kindergarten teacher, extended pre-K teacher, principal, NDT consultant therapist, and both parents.

The NDT therapist interpreted the prehension evaluation administered in December, which revealed regression in fine motor skills, described the home program in effect for the past two months, and emphasized the focus on normalizing the shoulders to achieve higher fine motor skills.

Patrick's kindergarten teacher reported that both his academic skills and his behavior had improved since the last staffing.

The physical therapist stated that Patrick's posture and pelvic control showed much improvement, and he could now voluntarily lower his shoulders. Athetosis seemed decreased, and protective extension had improved.

Patrick's speech therapist had stressed articulation and conversational skills; during the past year, Patrick's proficiency had fluctuated with his drug levels.

Patrick's parents felt that his primary problem area was seizure control, since it affected his behavioral performance throughout his day. They had observed that he was particularly susceptible to seizures when emotionally excited because of special events and holidays, and when dehydrated, especially after increased physical activity.

The team agreed that Patrick's needs for the next school year included full day programming (half in kindergarten, half in pre-K, for more individual attention to conceptual skills), a classroom aide, occupational therapy, physical therapy, speech therapy, and NDT consultation. The present service delivery program would continue for 30 days at the beginning of the school year, after which a review would be held to write goals and objectives and revise the program, if necessary.

As the meeting was ending, Patrick's father said, "I think that in September you're going to see a totally different boy."

Patrick's mother smiled sweetly. "Yes," she said, "we're trading him in for another child."

Joanne: June 3, 1982 (CA: 13 years)

Communication with Joanne and her mother increased when the Erhardt Developmental Prehension Assessment had been administered, the evaluation report sent, and treatment recommendations made available to the current therapists.

The telephone rang. Gloria was calling long distance.

"Joanne is doing something different. I think it's important, because it seems to be filling a developmental gap that she missed."

"What is it?"

"She's started raising her arms over her head and saying 'so big.' She never was able to do that as a baby. Why is she doing it now?"

"I don't know. Is she imitating someone? I know that she's been playing basketball. That could be a factor."

"Yes, but you know how hard it has always been for her to push the ball up toward the basket, and she's been trying for a long time."

"What else is going on in her life that involves a new shoulder movement?"

"The only thing I can think of is bowling," Gloria said.

"Is it possible that she's beginning to get more separation between arm and scapula because of it? Do you remember after I did the evaluation that I told you of my concern about the muscle atrophy between the shoulder blades?" I wondered if 12 years ago, when we did all those shoulder mobilization exercises, we achieved plenty of separation between the spine and scapula but very little between the scapula and arm. It may be very important now to make sure that the muscles that adduct the scapula are strengthened to provide stabilization as her arm moves forward and upward.

"Will Joanne be having therapy this summer, Gloria?"

"Yes, she'll be going to the Easter Seal Center."

"Good. Would you ask her therapist to call me so we can discuss it?"

"Yes, I think we need more heads on this so we can figure out what Joanne is trying to tell us," Gloria said. "The questions never stop, do they?"

I agreed. "It isn't only that Joanne is constantly growing and changing. Better evaluations are being developed, and more qualified people are available to search for and share new information. It's been a long process, hasn't it? We've had our failures and successes with Joanne."

"Yes, but we've achieved far more than we ever dreamed 13 years ago."

Patrick: June 7, 1982 (CA: 6^1/$_2$ years)

The telephone again.

"Hi. Patrick has something to tell you. He wants to tell you himself."

"Rho . . . da?"

"Yes, Patrick?"

"I . . . went . . . potty . . . by . . . my . . . self."

"That's great, Patrick, really great."

Sallie took the phone. "He not only sat down and stood up all alone, but he managed all his clothing, except I cheated just a little bit and helped him pull his pants up in the back. And his shoulders stayed down most of the time."

"That's wonderful. May I talk to Patrick again?"

"Patrick, when I come to see you tomorrow, will you show me how you go potty by yourself?"

"May . . . be."

"Thanks, Patrick."

Kristy: June 11, 1982 (CA: 4 years)

Kristy's first year in school had ended. Her parents had asked to have an occupational therapy student work with her on a daily basis in the summer under

Developmental Hand Dysfunction

my weekly supervision. The day before the student was to start, Carmon and I planned which activities would be delegated to the student.

"I definitely want the student to work with Kristy in the prone position," Carmon said. "That still is a priority, isn't it?"

"Yes. Take a look at the score sheet of the last evaluation I did, especially Section 2, voluntary movements of approach, grasp, manipulation, and release. See how each cluster has well-established or emerging skills at each monthly level up to 6 or 8 months, except for approach in prone, which has all components missing at 1 and 2 months? If you look at the head-raising-in-prone cluster, you'll see some crucial components missing there, too, at the same levels. Those are important, as I have said before, because they prepare for pushing up to hands and knees and for sitting at 7 or 8 months."

Carmon frowned. "Does that mean I shouldn't be working on sitting? Let me show you something."

She sat cross-legged on the floor with Kristy on her lap, supporting her slightly at the hips. As she suddenly leaned sideward, Kristy reacted with beautiful righting reactions of head and trunk. I was impressed.

"That's not all," Carmon said. "Watch. Sit up, Kristy."

I watched as Kristy reached toward midline with her head and used appropriate trunk muscles to regain the upright position.

"Do it again, Carmon, and let her rest her forearm on your knee. Then offer her your finger to grasp with her other hand so she can pull up at the same time she pushes up from her forearm."

Carmon repeated the activity, but Kristy still used primarily head and trunk, despite the work we had done with tug-of-war activities and weight bearing on forearms.

"I think she needs all these to prepare for sitting, Carmon. What you are doing looks great, but we must continue building awareness of arm and forearm. The best way is through weight bearing, which provides a lot of proprioceptive input."

"I understand," Carmon sighed.

"It's been more than a month since I've seen Kristy. Let me see how she looks in prone." I placed her on the floor on her forearms, with arms somewhat internally rotated, elbows behind shoulders, and hands fisted. Her head control was excellent, her wrists were straight, not ulnar-deviated, and her hips showed more normal extension and abduction. When Kristy's elbows were placed under her shoulders, with arms in more external rotation, her head went into slight hyperextension, her wrists flexed and deviated, and her forearms lost contact with the surface.

Kristy's Progress Notes

June 11, 1982

To: Mr. and Mrs. Mike C.

Re: Occupational therapy for Kristy

- **Activity:** Sitting balance in adult's lap

  Response: When Kristy was pushed over, she caught herself on her elbow on adult's leg, then tried to sit up again, using head and abdominal muscles.

   Recommendations: Adult should offer a finger for Kristy to grasp, to pull up at the same time she pushes up with her other arm.

- **Activity:** Weight shifting in prone on rocker board

  Response: Kristy reacted with hyperextension of neck and back or shaking, if not provided enough support during weight shifting.

  Recommendations: Adult should straddle Kristy's legs behind her on the rocker board, while she looks at a mirror. Adult's hands should be on Kristy's elbows as much as necessary, but removed intermittently to allow her the opportunity to maintain the position. Tilting should be done slowly as well as quickly, stopping and holding, waiting for Kristy to right her head. Speed, range, and amount of control should be varied, as long as Kristy's movements and postures remain normal.

"Carmon," I said, "we are going to have to move Kristy's arms out and forward very, very gradually, so she maintains all these normal movements. Let's try her on the rocker board."

Lying prone facing Kristy, keeping her arms in position, I tried to rock the board back and forth. It wasn't easy. After watching me struggle for a few minutes, Carmon moved out of her chair. She had seen that Kristy was hyperextending.

"I've got an idea." She climbed on the rocker board and knelt behind Kristy. "Do you want to get me that mirror?"

I stood the mirror up in front of Kristy, so she would stop trying to turn around to look at her mother. Carmon controlled Kristy's elbows, taking her hands away as often as possible. She began tilting the board back and forth, sometimes slowly, sometimes quickly.

"You've got a good touch, Carmon. Try going to the side as far as possible and hold it. Wait for Kristy to right her head. You have three variables to play with: speed, range, and amount of control. May I try it, too?"

I crawled on the board, a little more cautiously than Carmon had, since I don't have the best balance in the world. When the board tilted to the side, I almost fell off. Carmon laughed merrily.

"Come on, Carmon. You know what low muscle tone I have. Good balance reactions depend on normal muscle tone."

Carmon was still smirking. "Don't feel bad. We all know that you were really a CP kid who has done very, very well."

"Thanks a lot, Carmon. Now will you help me off this board before I crash and take your kid with me?"

The Siblings' Perspective

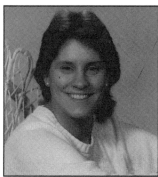

Valerie, Joanne's 24-year-old twin sister

May 19, 1993

Therapist: What activities have you and your sister done together in the past and recently?

Val: I don't remember very much when I was a child, mostly when we were teenagers. What I do remember when I was very little was thinking I was helping Joanne with her therapy, like playing on the carpeted barrel with her, but also thinking she got more attention than me. When we were 12, I went with her to day camp, but I was more like a junior counselor, helping all the kids with different activities.

Therapist: What kind of activities?

Val: The usual kind: swimming, crafts, games, everything. It was at a park. And all the time we were teenagers I actually took care of her every afternoon after school and all summer long when Mom was working.

(photo courtesy of Valerie Dosland)

We also had a regular weekly routine on Saturday mornings. I helped her get up and bathe and dress and everything, so that Mom could sleep in. Then Mom did all that on Sunday mornings and I had time to myself.

Therapist: What kinds of things could she do herself, and what things did she need help with?

Val: She could dress herself, but she needed help with cleaning, brushing her teeth, washing her hair, especially getting all the soap out.

Therapist: How much help did she need?

Val: She could do a lot if I was patient enough to wait and let her do stuff all by herself, but sometimes I would do it for her. That was my biggest problem. I was her protector, and it was hard to be patient and let her do things for herself.

Therapist: Could she dress herself independently, or were there things she really needed help with?

Val: She could do a lot, but she needed help for some things, like putting on her bra, and the hygiene things.

Therapist: Can you think of some other things that you did together, like recreation, in the community?

Val: Yes, we went bowling all the time, still do. We really like to do that.

Therapist: Have you seen her new adapted bowling ball, with the handle that retracts?

Val: Yes, she's had that a few years.

Therapist: So you still go bowling together?

Val: Yes, and we go to movies, too.

Therapist: What kind of movies does she like?

Val: Comedies, mostly. She likes to laugh. Another thing we did together when I was in college, and still do, is she used to visit me and stay overnight. She's coming for another visit soon. Being twins is interesting. Sometimes we seem to be feeling the same things, although we're so far apart. I'll call her and find out she's feeling low just like me that day, or we'll both be feeling good at the same time.

Therapist: What kinds of things will you do when she comes to visit?

Val: Probably go to the mall, walk around, see some monuments. We did that last time, and she liked it.

Therapist: How does cerebral palsy cause problems for Joanne in using her hands? What things can't she do because of it?

Val: I think hygiene is the biggest problem, and it's important.

Therapist: Is it because her hands aren't well coordinated, or is there more to it?

Val: Well, that's true, but also because her right hand isn't as strong as her left.

Therapist: When you were helping with those activities, did you ever think of things that would make it possible for her to do more for herself?

Val: Mostly trying not to help too much. Joanne will do what is expected of her, and if you don't expect much, she won't do much.

Therapist: So you're saying that the best thing to do is wait and let her do her own problem solving, because she will persist and keep trying. That's a real important point. Because she has difficulty, and because she's slower, there's a tendency for people to do things for her, and not let her tackle it.

Val: Yes, and I have that problem. My friends tell me that.

Therapist: When did you first realize that your sister had a handicap, that she had cerebral palsy and that she was different?

Val: I never really felt that. It always seemed natural that Joanne was the way she was. But sometimes I have wondered what it would be like to have a sister who was like a regular twin. I know we are identical but some people say we don't look alike so I doubted that for awhile. But I'm glad we're identical twins.

Therapist: Do you feel that your family had struggles as well as good times?

Val: Yes, that's true. I always thought she was the reason our parents had problems and broke up. And Joanne and I used to fight all the time when we were growing up, like other sisters.

Therapist: But you are also close, aren't you?

Val: Yes, we're very close, and we both felt really bad when I moved so far away to take a new job. I'm looking forward to this visit.

Therapist: I know you'll have fun, but will you irritate each other, too?

Val: Sure we will. She'll drive me crazy, and I'll probably bug her, too.

Therapist: How has Joanne's cerebral palsy affected you, in your life?

Val: Well, I always have to explain about her, first that I have a twin sister, and then about her handicap. And people always say they're sorry. They shouldn't be sorry.

Therapist: What do you think is the most important functional priority for Joanne's therapists to consider when planning intervention for better hand function? What is needed to prepare her for the future and allow her to do more and live more independently?

Val: I really think that hygiene, grooming, and things like that are the most important. Appearance matters in social situations, and Joanne loves being with people. She has a problem with drooling and eating behaviors, and it can turn people off. Also, Joanne used to do a lot of cooking at home when our mother was alive. She really enjoyed it, but she doesn't do much anymore.

Therapist: Yes, I understand that cooking isn't being encouraged, not only because of the drooling, but also because of safety factors. A feeding evaluation has been recommended, to see if oral-motor skills can be identified and improved, things like lip closure during chewing; sensory awareness inside the mouth for better control of tongue, lip, and cheek muscles; and manipulation of utensils, especially knife and fork.

Let's try a final question. What is your opinion about the therapy Joanne had early in her life, and what kind of difference did it make?

Val: It made a tremendous difference. She would have been in an institution without it.

Therapist: You realize that your mother was the one that made all that happen. She never stopped trying to get every kind of help for Joanne. She never gave up.

Val: And now our father is her guardian, and he's making sure her needs are getting met. Someday it will be up to me.

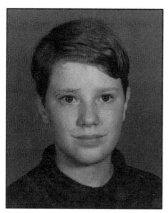

Ryan, Patrick's 11-year-old brother

April 24, 1993

(photo courtesy of Ryan Mooneyham)

Therapist: Ryan, let's talk about the things you and Patrick do together, and what you think his therapists should do to help him do things better in the future when he's all grown up. Let's start by talking about the kinds of things you and Patrick do now.

Ryan: Well, we play video games, we wrestle, we ride bikes in the neighborhood and down to my school.

Therapist: I saw a basketball backboard outside. Do you play basketball?

Ryan: Yeah, we shoot in the trash can sometimes, too.

Therapist: Is that because it's easier for Patrick? Whose idea was it?

Ryan: It was kind of his idea, because the first time he tried to shoot it up high, it hit the rim of the basket, and bounced down into the trash can.

Therapist: That's a great idea. You know, that's just like men in offices who crumple paper balls and throw them into the wastebasket. So, you are telling me that there is some problem solving going on, that you guys have adapted an activity to make it possible for you both to participate more nearly equally. Any more activities?

Ryan: Swimming.

Therapist: Where? In your pool?

Ryan: In all kinds of places. Neighbors' pools, too.

Therapist: What ages are the kids in the neighborhood?

Ryan: Mostly my age, but one across the street that goes to Patrick's school, his age, they're friends. Patrick also visits a lot with the mothers and fathers in the neighborhood, usually on his bike. Oh, another thing Patrick does independently. He goes out and gets the mail.

Therapist: Yes, I've seen him open the box, reach into it, take out the letters, and put them into his bike basket.

I have another question for you. What did you think, while you were growing up, about all his therapy? Did you ever watch it, did you participate in any of it? Do you remember?

Ryan: I remember a lot of it being fun. When Patrick would use his therapy ball, me and him would get on it, and the therapist would think of it as some kind of help for him. I would get on one side of the ball, and he would get on the other.

Therapist: So therapy was play for you? You were a helper, in a way? As you got older, did you see changes in Patrick, getting better, learning new things?

Ryan: Well, I do remember one thing. A long time ago, Mom had to feed him, and then one time he picked up the fork and fed himself.

Therapist: Yes, we all worked a lot on his hands. What do you think are other things he's learned to do with his hands? And also, what things are there that he still can't do, that you wish he could do, so you could do more things together?

Ryan: Well, a thing he couldn't do a long time ago was shake hands, but now he can real good.

Therapist: Yes, that's an important skill for social reasons and business. That's a very good observation, Ryan.

Ryan: And something he's getting better at, but still can't do very well, is catching a ball.

Therapist: What size ball?

Ryan: Basketball, mostly. When I pass it to him, he catches it against his stomach, and he always blinks when it comes at him.

Therapist: He uses both hands, but his right hand doesn't do as well as his left?

Ryan: Yeah.

Therapist: So for recreation activities with you and others, now and in the future, it would be nice if he could catch better. How is he at throwing?

Ryan: He throws pretty good.

Therapist: How does he do it?

Ryan: He starts holding it with both hands against his chest, and then straightens his arms out.

Therapist: You know, Ryan, we may be able to improve his catching by using balloons, which move more slowly and are so soft that Patrick may be able to control that defensive blink.

Ryan: Oh, I remember how one gym teacher used to let his class throw water balloons at the sidewalk. That's how Patrick got so good at throwing!

Therapist: Really? That makes sense. Well, after he gets good catching balloons, we could then use small beach balls, which move faster but are still soft.

Tell me, Ryan, do you and Patrick do things together more now, or less, or about the same?

Ryan: I think maybe more, because he's capable of doing more stuff than he was then.

Therapist: What other effects of cerebral palsy have you seen on his hands?

Ryan: He has trouble keeping them still. He'll put his hands on the table, and they'll move like this.

Therapist: Oh, yes, you know that's called athetosis, a form of cerebral palsy, involuntary movements; he can't help it. I think he's done some things to minimize that, don't you?

Ryan: Yeah, he used to go like, where he couldn't even keep his hands on the table, especially the right hand. But now he uses that hand to hold himself in place.

Therapist: Yes, that's a very important thing we've been working on, for Patrick to use the right hand to stabilize while he's using the left hand.

Here's another question. Do you remember a time, in the neighborhood or at school, when you started to realize that Patrick was different, that he had cerebral palsy?

Ryan: I think I was about 5. I was in kindergarten, and I saw that he was different from all my other friends.

Therapist: Did you notice how they reacted to him?

Ryan: They did look at him, and then it was like, who cares?

Therapist: People do look.

Ryan: Yeah. That's okay with me, as long as they don't, you know, stare.

Therapist: Yes. OK, here's another question. Do you think about your future? What kind of work you might want to do someday?

Ryan: I might want to be a teacher.

Therapist: Any particular kind?

Ryan: Well, maybe like a gym teacher, or a mathematician.

Therapist: Are you good at math?

Ryan: Yeah.

Therapist: Why do you think it would be fun to be a teacher? Why do you think you would be good at it, and be happy doing it?

Ryan: I like helping kids. I had a teacher, in my fourth-grade class, who taught me sixth-grade stuff.

Therapist: In the gifted program?

Ryan: Yes. And when other kids need help, my teacher now asks me to help them. I think it's also fun and satisfying when you teach a kid how to do new things.

Therapist: You're right. You know, your mom told me that even though you're in the gifted program, you also have certain learning styles that are different from other kids, and you have to learn certain ways, that you learn best through your ears, through listening. So as a teacher you would understand why each kid needs to learn in their own way. I think you'd probably be a very good teacher.

Let's talk now about Patrick's future. What kinds of things do you think he may be doing?

Ryan: Well, I think he'll be involved with computers, doing things like his own taxes.

Therapist: Yes, I agree. And the computer will also give him access to lots of jobs. Well, that means we must make sure that he has a computer that helps him do as much as possible. At this time, for his schoolwork, he uses a trackball and the keyboard with just his two index fingers. We might be able to improve his finger dexterity so his keyboard work would be faster.

I understand that your mom and dad have been thinking about buying a landscape/nursery business after retirement, and that Patrick could work in it, and eventually own it. He really likes gardening, and he could handle the business part of it with the computer. Do you think that might work for him?

Ryan: Yeah, I think so.

Therapist: Are you going to college? Do you want to go far away or stick around pretty close to home?

Ryan: I'd like to try a new place, see the sights, not have anyone hold me back, or for me to have anyone to worry about.

Therapist: A sense of freedom?

Ryan: Yeah. But after college I'd like to move back near my family.

Therapist: What do you think Patrick's life will be like? Do you think Patrick will live independently some day? That he won't need someone to take care of him? Do you think that's possible?

Ryan: Yes, I do. I think he'll have a lot of fun with computers, because he's always so interested in designing things and starting new programs. He was the first in our family to beat Oregon Trail, a computer game.

Therapist: So he's a problem solver?

Ryan: Yes, he had to make all kinds of choices in that game, like real life.

Therapist: Tell me, Ryan, do you think there's more we can do to help Patrick use his hands better?

Ryan: I heard something on the news about a new robotic chip that goes inside your body, for people who have uncontrollable movement, and the chip sends brain waves, to make you walk and stuff. I think that could help Patrick.

Therapist: Maybe. That would be great.

What about his independence in self-care? He can feed himself and dress himself and bathe himself, right?

Ryan: Almost. He needs a little bit of help washing his hair, especially on the right side.

Therapist: I guess the fingers on the right hand don't have the strength and control to dig in and scrub, especially up high like that. I wonder what other activities could improve that, first with his arms lower down. Maybe weeding in the garden. That's the same movement, and the dirt would give good resistance. He would be more stable, and could see his hand in that position.

Ryan, you've been a big help with your observations and your ideas, which help all of us think of other ideas. I hope you'll continue watching and thinking. We all have to be thinking now of what Patrick needs later. We can't just wait until he's all grown up, and then say, "Gee, we should have done this." We don't want to miss anything. We need everybody, not just parents and teachers and therapists, but people like you, who do things with him, to help us plan what he needs. Thanks a lot for your ideas.

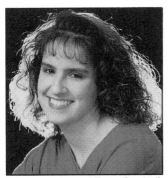

*Tracy, Kristy's
17-year-old sister,*

April 4, 1993

Therapist: What activities do you and your sister do together?

Tracy: Renting video movies on weekends, when her caregivers don't come in, so I'll stay home with her for the day.

Therapist: So you do some caregiving, as much as your schedule can allow? And you select the movies?

Tracy: Yes, usually something that's busy or colorful. Sometimes she'll get bored for a period of time, until something exciting starts to happen.

Therapist: So she likes sound and action. And you watch together?

Tracy: Yes, I'll sit at the corner of the couch and she can lean against me. She likes being close. When she gets bored, she'll try to purposely annoy me to get attention by putting her fingers in my ear or pulling my hair. She'll even reach for my face and start scratching. She loves grabbing at her caregiver's long blond hair.

Therapist: I didn't know that. She can touch you in different places? This is important hand function, and very appropriate at Kristy's developmental fine motor age level.

Tracy: I also take her shopping at the mall for an hour or so. She likes to see the people. Sometimes she gets crabby and cries, but I can talk to her and she'll calm down, sometimes even better for me than Mom and Dad.

Therapist: So there's a special relationship between you, and she feels that it's a real treat to be around her older sister, because you're pretty busy with school activities.

You're saying she's pretty good at aiming her hands and doing a variety of things with them. Anything else you do together? How much caregiving do you do?

Tracy: Every other weekend I relieve the caregiver, helping with feeding, dressing, bathing, toileting, things like that. Also other times, like last week because Mom and Dad were out of town for three nights, and there wasn't anyone to stay overnight. It's no problem for me to get up in the morning and dress her, fix her hair, and get her ready for school.

Therapist: Are there ways that you relate to her now that are different from when she was younger?

Tracy: Yes, the way I speak with her, and the way I handle her and play with her. The kinds of things we do. Another activity is looking at magazines, like *Seventeen*, instead of baby-type books. She likes looking at faces of kids her age. She'll grab at pages, too, and scratch at them.

Therapist: Do you think she wants to turn them or is pointing at them? Maybe there's a way we could facilitate that, since she's motivated, leading to new choices and decisions. Or does she do that simply to touch and feel things? Does she try to touch everything?

Tracy: No, not really, only certain things.

Therapist: Then it sounds to me like a purposeful action, rather than exploring, to communicate her desire to do something. That's a good idea for us to think about.

So you relate to each other as two teenagers now, rather than teen and child. Any other activities that are different now?

Tracy: Sometimes I'll read her stories, but not little kids' books anymore. I feel uncomfortable with those at her age.

Therapist: Well, you're right, those aren't age-appropriate anymore. She's 14. What stories do girls that age like? What library books are there about teenagers that have pictures, too? That would be hard to find. Some magazines have stories with pictures. How do we get her hands involved, besides turning pages? I wonder if we could have the caregivers use some of their time with Kristy to make looseleaf notebooks with pictures pasted in as well as textures for her to touch, like the *Pat the Bunny* book, but again, with an age-appropriate story. Kristy could even help if she had hand-over-hand assistance and verbal commentary.

How does her disability interfere with using her hands? What kinds of things do you wish she could do, and maybe could learn to do?

Tracy: Well, helping more in dressing, and in standing up, so it's not so much pressure on us.

Therapist: Using her hands to stabilize herself during transitions, to push up or pull up, because she doesn't have the muscle power. We do have that as a priority. I'm glad you feel the same way.

When did you first realize that your sister's cerebral palsy made her different?

Tracy: I don't know if I've ever really felt she was different, but I remember when I first realized that *other* people realized she was different. I was in fourth grade, and when Kristy had her reflux surgery, everyone in my class signed a card and sent a stuffed animal to the hospital. They would have done that for a classmate, but not usually for a classmate's sister. I was 3 years old when Kristy was born, so I never knew anything different. Friends of mine have said, "What's it like having a sister who is handicapped?" I find that my tolerance for certain children is lower, I get irritated at how demanding some of them are, because Kristy is so easy to be with, she never asks for anything. I like children, and I hope to work with them after I finish medical school, maybe.

Therapist: How has she affected your life?

Tracy: My mom always told me that since Kristy was born I've always responded well to different situations, like Kristy being in the hospital. I think I've matured a lot faster than other kids my age, understanding people's feelings, being more compassionate. Some people have a problem giving of themselves to help others, like the elderly, who need more help. I enjoy it, probably because I'm more used to it. I have the opportunity to see what it does for other people. It makes me realize different things about myself, and how I've grown.

Therapist: Many people don't understand this, do they? They think you're either a hero or they feel sorry for you when you have a child with a handicap in the family.

Tracy: Exactly.

Therapist: A person in your family, a real person whom you love, and who is who she is, so you don't sit around and think, "I wish she was different." You just don't do that.

Tracy: Yes. Sometimes people will ask me, "Do you have any brothers or sisters?" I'll say, "Yes, I have a younger sister." Then they ask what grade she's in, and I'll say, "She's not exactly in a grade. She attends junior high, but she has a handicap, cerebral palsy." Then I'll try to explain, and their usual response is "I'm sorry." That really bothers me. There's no need for them to be sorry. Maybe they just don't know how to respond.

Therapist: I think you're right, they don't know, and they get embarrassed. It's good that you try to explain cerebral palsy to them, but it's not easy to tell them how to respond, is it? I think it's getting better, because of the mainstreaming and exposure.

What do you think her future life will be like at home, in school, and out in the community? How do you think you will be involved?

Tracy: When I was younger I always thought, and still do, that our family will always be really close. I didn't think Kristy's needs would really change. I thought they would always be the same, and I always thought that Mom and Dad would be able to handle anything and everything. And now as we all grow older, I don't feel that way anymore. I now realize that it's a lot of work, and a lot of pressure, and that they'll need help as they get older. Even now they are looking for someone to care for her more. Most people who have children know that at some point their children will grow up and move on and become independent, and there would be time for themselves. That time hasn't come yet for my mom and dad. I know for sure my parents don't want Kristy to be put in a home, but they are thinking of all the possibilities. Their choice right now is to build a home with a separate section for Kristy, with a live-in caregiver.

Therapist: Yes, so they can have some freedom and privacy for themselves, still involved, but in a more normal living situation as Kristy becomes an adult. And Kristy could attend a day program, with structured activities.

Tracy: Yes, I can see that, with her out in the community. It's important for her, and it's important for other people to see her, and important for her to see normal people.

I see myself involved in the decision making, where Kristy will be, and who is going to care for her. I'm involved already, whenever new caregivers are hired. My mom really values my opinion, because I'm around the house, doing homework, cleaning, or in and out running errands, so I can see how they handle Kristy and how they handle new situations.

Therapist: I agree that you should share equally in the decision making with your parents. It is so important, especially as the years go by, and you may someday have to make decisions by yourself. Do you mind when I say that?

Tracy: No, it needs to be talked about. We can't act like it's never going to happen. And we need to be prepared in case of an accident or if something does happen.

Therapist: So I hear you telling me that as you and Kristy get older, as adults you would like to have the kind of relationship that other sisters have as adults: your own life, but a lot of interaction, and taking responsibility sometimes, but not the major responsibility of daily activities, and hopefully your parents won't need to, either. There are programs out there, trained caregivers and other services. And Kristy does like a variety of people, doesn't she?

Tracy: Yes, but I can tell if Kristy does or does not like a caregiver. She can tell if a person is there for her, or just for the job. She has one now that she absolutely loves, who takes her home every other weekend. She responds very differently to others.

Therapist: What do you hope for? How can she be more functional, doing, not just watching?

Tracy: Caring for her own needs. Like dressing in the morning, and eating on her own without any help, even though she does most of it now. Bathing is another thing. It's really hard when Kristy's wet, to get her out of the tub, so she needs to help more with transferring her weight. But the major thing I hope would happen is communicating, either by a communication board or a computer.

Therapist: Yes, we know she can activate a switch with her hand. She does that now, with the Help switch to get people to come. We also know that she is alert and very tuned in to what's going on. So what you're saying is that at this time your top priority is communication?

Tracy: Yes, I would love to know what she is thinking.

Comparisons of Normal and Atypical Prehension Development: Treatment Models in Childhood and during Transitions to Adulthood

The process of Analysis, the taxonomy level that follows Knowledge, Comprehension, and Application, was described previously as a way to compare normal and atypical development. The effects of three types of muscle tone on prehension development can also be compared by listing similarities and differences of each. Figure 12.18 presents an analysis of one EDPA cluster, The Arms at Rest and during Head Raising in Prone, illustrating these comparisons in development as well as in treatment models in childhood. Figure 12.19 compares normal and atypical prehension development and treatment models for function during transitions to adulthood, using the same EDPA cluster as an illustration.

Summary of a Theory of Prehension: Definitions

Developmentally appropriate patterns: normal movement and postural patterns appearing in sequence and at the normal developmental age.

Primary developmentally inappropriate patterns: normal movement and postural patterns appearing in sequence but delayed chronologically.

Secondary developmentally inappropriate patterns: combinations of several primary developmentally inappropriate patterns delayed and/or advanced (out of sequence), which result in atypical patterns.

Atypical patterns: patterns that are stereotyped (used for all movement, not adapted) and inefficient (leading to more compensations, substitutions, and eventually, deformities)

The Therapist: Architect of the Child's Treatment Program

The human body can be viewed as a unique architectural structure, with the ongoing capacity to change and grow, most rapidly before birth and during the first year of life. Movement, a response to stimuli, occurs as a part of the total, continuously adapting structure that houses the individual (Coley 1978). As the architect of the child's treatment program, the therapist prepares the child's internal and external environment, facilitates normal posture and movements, and helps the child adapt to participate actively in a happy, useful life.

References

Coley, I. L. 1978. *Pediatric assessment in self-care activities.* St. Louis, MO: C.V. Mosby.

Connolly, K. J. 1977. *The developmental origins of behavior.* Omaha, NE: Mayer Children's Rehabilitation Institute.

Erhardt, R. P. 1974. Sequential levels in development of prehension. *American Journal of Occupational Therapy* 28:592-96.

Erhardt, R. P., P. A. Beatty, and D. M. Hertsgaard. 1981. A developmental prehension assessment for handicapped children. *American Journal of Occupational Therapy* 35:237-42.

Gilfoyle, E. M., A. P. Grady, and J. C. Moore. 1981. *Children adapt.* Thorofare, NJ: Charles B. Slack.

Knickerbocker, B. M. 1980. *A holistic approach to the treatment of learning disorders.* Thorofare, NJ: Charles B. Slack.

Smith, M. A. M., B. Connelly, S. McFadden, C. R. Nicrosi, L. J. Nuckolls, M. N. Russell, and W. M. Wilson. 1982. *Feeding management of a child with a handicap: A guide for professionals.* Memphis, TN: University of Tennessee.

Trombley, C. A., and A. D. Scott. 1977. *Occupational therapy for physical dysfunction.* Baltimore, MD: Williams and Wilkins.

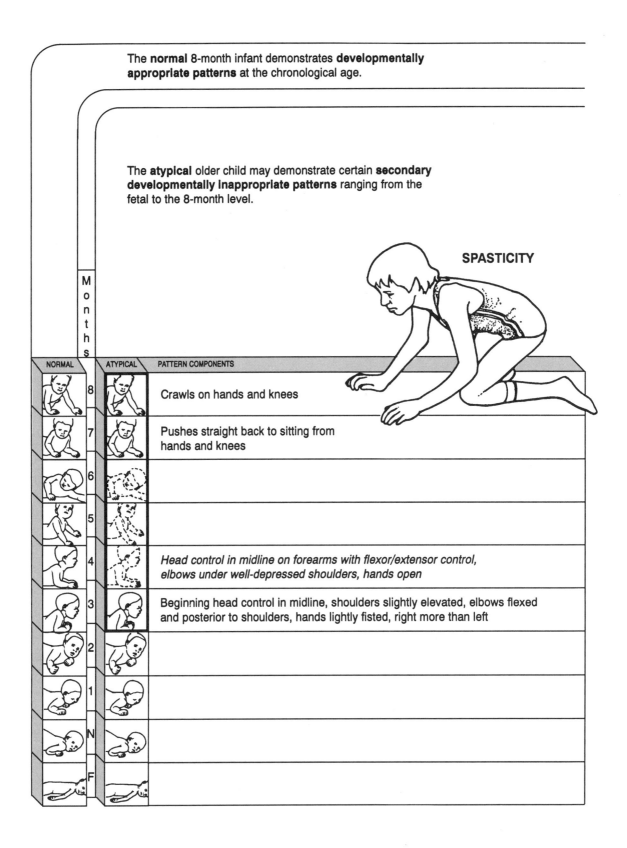

The **normal** 8-month infant demonstrates **developmentally appropriate patterns** at the chronological age.

The **atypical** older child may demonstrate certain **secondary developmentally inappropriate patterns** ranging from the fetal to the 8-month level.

SPASTICITY

NORMAL	Months	ATYPICAL	PATTERN COMPONENTS
	8		Crawls on hands and knees
	7		Pushes straight back to sitting from hands and knees
	6		
	5		
	4		*Head control in midline on forearms with flexor/extensor control, elbows under well-depressed shoulders, hands open*
	3		Beginning head control in midline, shoulders slightly elevated, elbows flexed and posterior to shoulders, hands lightly fisted, right more than left
	2		
	1		
	N		
	F		

Figure 12.18. A comparison of normal and atypical prehension development and treatment models for spasticity, athetosis, and flaccidity in childhood

Developmental Hand Dysfunction

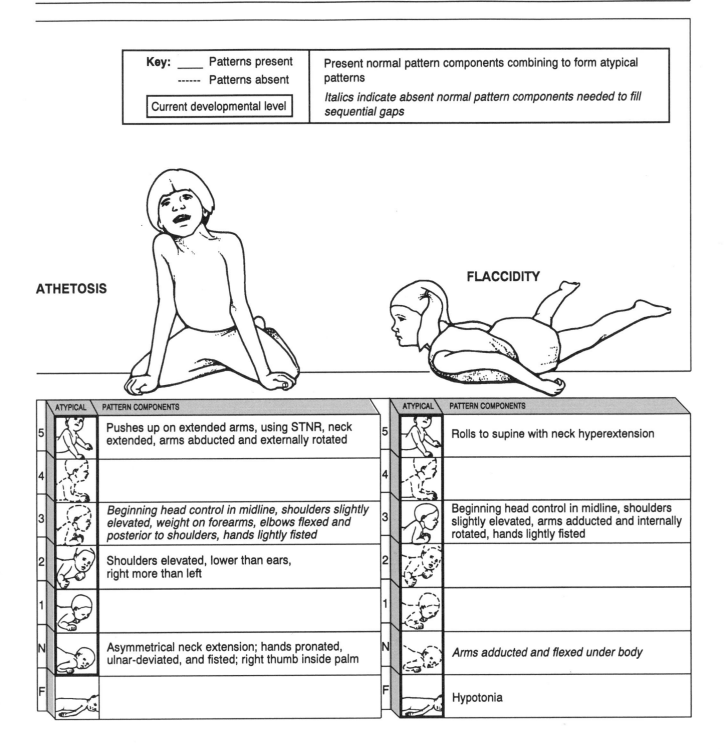

Key: _____ Patterns present
------ Patterns absent

Current developmental level

Present normal pattern components combining to form atypical patterns

Italics indicate absent normal pattern components needed to fill sequential gaps

ATHETOSIS

FLACCIDITY

ATYPICAL		PATTERN COMPONENTS
5		Pushes up on extended arms, using STNR, neck extended, arms abducted and externally rotated
4		
3		*Beginning head control in midline, shoulders slightly elevated, weight on forearms, elbows flexed and posterior to shoulders, hands lightly fisted*
2		Shoulders elevated, lower than ears, right more than left
1		
N		Asymmetrical neck extension; hands pronated, ulnar-deviated, and fisted; right thumb inside palm
F		

ATYPICAL		PATTERN COMPONENTS
5		Rolls to supine with neck hyperextension
4		
3		Beginning head control in midline, shoulders slightly elevated, arms adducted and internally rotated, hands lightly fisted
2		
1		
N		*Arms adducted and flexed under body*
F		Hypotonia

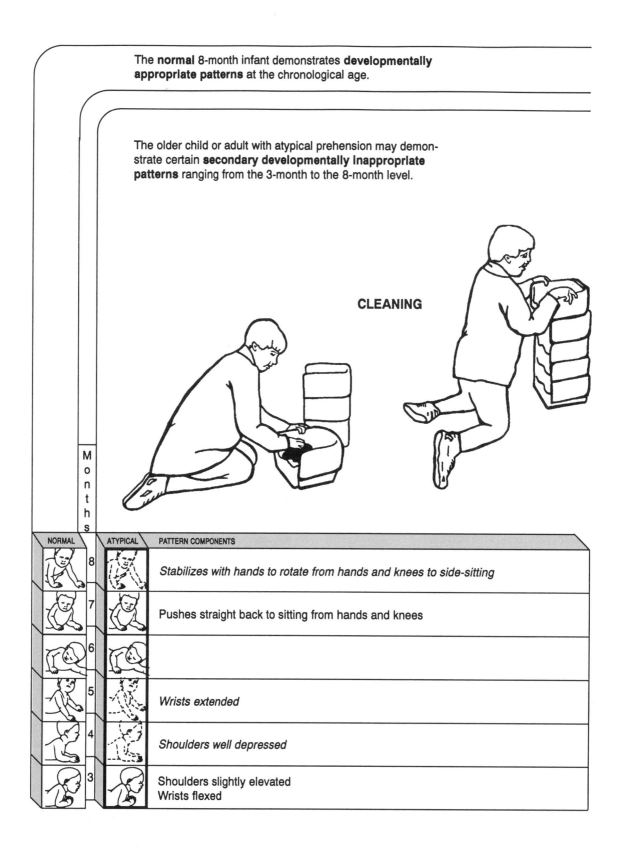

The **normal** 8-month infant demonstrates **developmentally appropriate patterns** at the chronological age.

The older child or adult with atypical prehension may demonstrate certain **secondary developmentally inappropriate patterns** ranging from the 3-month to the 8-month level.

CLEANING

NORMAL		ATYPICAL	PATTERN COMPONENTS
	8		*Stabilizes with hands to rotate from hands and knees to side-sitting*
	7		Pushes straight back to sitting from hands and knees
	6		
	5		*Wrists extended*
	4		*Shoulders well depressed*
	3		Shoulders slightly elevated Wrists flexed

Figure 12.19. A comparison of normal and atypical prehension development and treatment models for function during transitions to adulthood

Developmental Hand Dysfunction

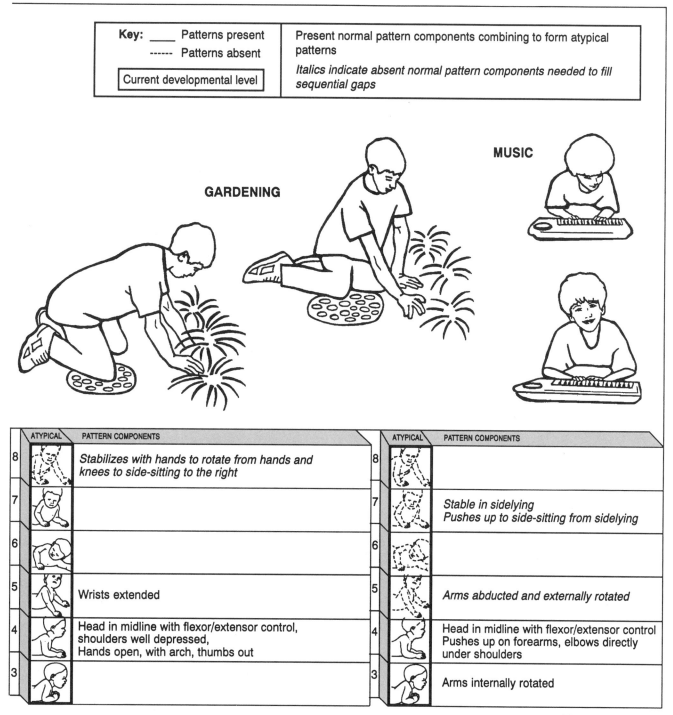

Key: ____ Patterns present
       ------ Patterns absent

Current developmental level

Present normal pattern components combining to form atypical patterns

Italics indicate absent normal pattern components needed to fill sequential gaps

GARDENING

MUSIC

	ATYPICAL	PATTERN COMPONENTS
8		*Stabilizes with hands to rotate from hands and knees to side-sitting to the right*
7		
6		
5		Wrists extended
4		Head in midline with flexor/extensor control, shoulders well depressed, Hands open, with arch, thumbs out
3		

	ATYPICAL	PATTERN COMPONENTS
8		
7		*Stable in sidelying* *Pushes up to side-sitting from sidelying*
6		
5		*Arms abducted and externally rotated*
4		Head in midline with flexor/extensor control Pushes up on forearms, elbows directly under shoulders
3		Arms internally rotated

(illustrations by author)

Subject Index

Note: numbers in italics indicate an illustration.

plans

    IEP (Individual Education Plan) xi, 100, 134, 170, 199, 200, 208, 211, 212, 215

    ISP (Individual Service Plan) xi, 100, 136

    ITP (Individual Transition Plan) xi, 100, 172

play (*see* functional activities)

position, positioning 4, 26, 29, 35, *36*, 37, 55, 59, 60, 61, 72, 121, 129, 153, 175, 176, 204, 209, 212, 213

    hands and knees 1, *22*, 25, *30*, 108, 109, *109*, 116, 142, 143, *143*, 144, 150, 177, *177*, 205, 217, *226*

    kneeling 26, 109, 146

    prone 8, *9*, 10, 14, 16, *22*, 25, 29, *30*, 32, 33, *33*, 35, 55, 58, 59, 60, 105, 108, 116, 117, *117*, 122, 139, 140, 142, 150, *151*, 154, 156, 158, 164, 173, 174, 175, 176, *176*, *177*, 184, *185*, 188, 190, 191, 196, 205, 207, 208, 212, 217

    sidelying 16, *30*, 55, 106, 109, *109*, 140, 142, *143*, *183*, 211, *211*

    side-sitting 60, 142, *143*, *176*, *177*, 185

    sitting 8, *9*, 10, *10*, 14, 16, *22*, 25, 26, 29, *30*, 32, *32*, 33, 36, 37, 55, 59, 105, 107, *107*, 108, 112, 118, 122, 126, 139, 146, 152, 153, 154, 156, 158, 164, 166, 173, *175*, 177, 180, 186, *186*, 188, 190, 191, 196, 198, 199, 207, 211, 217, *226*

    standing 16, 17, *22*, 36, 38, 55, 59, 107, *108*, *109*, 112, *112*, 146, 147, *151*, 223

    supine 8, *9*, 10, 14, 16, *22*, 23, 24, *25*, 29, *30*, 32, *32*, 33, 55, 59, 105, 106, 107, 114, 117, 139, 140, 149, 154, 156, 164, 173, 174, 175, *175*, 176, *176*, 182, *182*, 183, 188, 190, 196, *210*

    W-sitting *25*, 108

posture, postural 2, 3, *9*, *9*, 10, 14, 16, 18, 21, 22, 23, 24, 26, 29, 31, *32*, 36, 37, 38, 55, 58, 59, 60, 61, 107, 109, 117, *117*, 136, *152*, *153*, 177, 200, 204, 225

practice 11, 16, 17, 56, 57, 61

    blocked 57

    constant 57

    distributed 57

    massed 57

    part 57

    random 57

    variable 57

    whole 57

praxis 53

prehension *12*

    development of 9, 23, 24, 35-38, 43, 44, 46, *48*, *49*, *50*, 68, 70, 173, 225

    levels *9*, 10, 14

    schema *12*, 32, 124, 125, 160, 161, 192, 193

    theories of 4, 9, 13, 33, 43-51, *47*, 53, 68

prematurity, prematurely 1, *24*, 31

pronation *13*, 14, 23, *30*, 40, 50, 61, 118, 152, 164, 167, 186, *227*

prone (*see* position)

proprioception, proprioceptors 16, 17, 23, 31, 53, 54, 59, 200, 217

qualitative (*see* tests)

quantitative (*see* tests)

reciprocal

    assimilation *12*, 12, 124, 192, 194

    innervation 21, 23, 24, *24*, 26

reflexes 11, 17, 31, *32*, 61, 68

    asymmetrical tonic neck reflex (ATNR) 2, 23, *24*, 25, 26, *26*, *30*, 31, 35, *36*, 110, 144, *144*, 178, 208, 212

    avoiding responses 16, 23, 24, *24*, 25, 35, 113, 148, 181, 206

    flexor withdrawal 13

    grasp *12*, 23, 24, *24*, 25, 111, 113, 145, 148, 179, 181

    instinctive grasp reactions 23, 24, 35, 111, 145, 179

    Moro 29, *30*, 32

    protective extensor thrust, protective extension, protective placing 16, 23, 26, 112, *112*, 146, *147*, 180

    symmetrical tonic neck reflex (STNR) 17, 23, *24*, 25, *25*, 108, 142, *227*

    tonic labyrinthine reflex (TLR) 23, *24*, 24

release 9, 10, *15*, *22*, 35, 44, 46, 67, *128*, 129, *129*, *130*, *165*, *166*, 179, *196*, *197*, 217

    assistive *9*, 128, 129, *129*, 164, *165*, *196*, 197

    clumsy, crude *9*, 130, 164, 166

    controlled 166

    involuntary *9*, 10, *196*, 197

    precise *9*, 111, 128, 130, 136, 145, 159, 164, 166

    transfer 2, *9*, 23, 128, *129*, 130, *130*, 164, 166, 196

schema, schemata 10, 11, *12*, 12, 124, 125, 126, 160, 161, 162, 192, 193

seizures 26, 31, 55, 56, 139, 211, 215

sensation 11, 14, 15-16, 49, 53, 54, 55, 70, 175

    awareness 2, 124, 127, *127*, 194, *195*, 200, 220

    perception 7, 17, 59

    tactile 125, 134, 148, 161, 184, 194, *195*, 199, 200

sensory integration (*see* theory)

sidelying (*see* position)

social (*see* development)

spastic, spasticity (*see* cerebral palsy)

stability *4*, 14, 25, 26, 29, 31, 32, 33, 35, 47, 54, 55, 59, 60, 72, 107, 109, 117, *117*, 133, 150, *153*, 167, 175, 176, *197*, 199, 200, 204, 207, 212

standing (*see* position)

static tripod grasp (*see* grasp)

supination 14, 23, *50*, 61, 118, *119*, 121, *126*, 129, 152, *152*, 165, 193

supine (*see* position)

swiping (*see* approach)

tactile system (*see* sensation)

T'ai Chi (*see* functional activities)